3D Echocardiography of Structural Heart Disease

Hakimeh Sadeghian
Zahra Savand-Roomi

3D Echocardiography of Structural Heart Disease

An Imaging Atlas

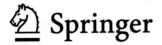

Hakimeh Sadeghian
Department of Echocardiography
Associate Professor of Cardiology and
  Echocardiography
Tehran University of Medical Science
Tehran
Iran

Zahra Savand-Roomi
Department of Echocardiography
Cardiologist and Echocardiographist
Kowsar Hospital
Shiraz
Iran

Additional material to this book can be downloaded from http://extras.springer.com

ISBN 978-3-319-54038-2   ISBN 978-3-319-54039-9   (eBook)
DOI 10.1007/978-3-319-54039-9

Library of Congress Control Number: 2017946311

Printed on acid-free paper

This Springer imprint is published by Springer Nature
The registered company is Springer International Publishing AG
The registered company address is: Gewerbestrasse 11, 6330 Cham, Switzerland

Dedicated to all my family and friends

Hakimeh Sadeghian

This book is dedicated to
my parents who taught me how to love other people,
my honorable husband,
my little daughter, Avina, who encouraged me to move on.
It is also dedicated to all my mentors, without whom none of this
would have been possible.

Zahra Savand-Roomi

Contents

List of Videos

Chapter 1 Degenerative Mitral Valve Disease

Case 1   Fibroelastic Deficiency, Prolapse of A2, Moderate Mitral Regurgitation (MR)
Case 2   Fibroelastic Deficiency+ (FED+), Severe Mitral Regurgitation, Prolapse and Rupture of Chorda of A2
Case 3   Fibroelastic Deficiency+ (FED+), Rupture of Chorda of A2, Severe MR
Case 4   Forme Fruste, Rupture of Chorda of P2, Severe MR
Case 5   Rupture of Chorda of P2, Severe MR, Barlow Disease
Case 6   Barlow Disease, Rupture of Chorda of P2, Severe MR
Case 7   Barlow Disease, Severe Mitral Regurgitation, Elongation of Chorda of P2
Case 8   Barlow Disease, Rupture of Chorda of Lateral Side of P2 (Between P1 and P2), Prolapse P1, P2, P3, and A2
Case 9   Barlow Disease, P2 Rupture, Severe MR
Case 10 Barlow Disease, Severe Mitral Regurgitation, and Rupture of Chorda of A2 and A3
Case 11 Severe Functional and Organic MR Due to Prolapse of A2 in a Post CABG Patient (Candidate for Mitraclip)

Chapter 2 Rheumatic Mitral Stenosis

Case 1   Severe Mitral Stenosis, Mild MR, Mild AS, Moderate AI, No LA, and LAA Clot Suitable for PTMC
Case 2   Severe MS, No MR, Mild AS, Mild to Moderate AI, and LAA Clot
Case 3   Severe MS, Mild MR, Mild AI, No LAA, and LAA Clot Suitable for PTMC
Case 4   Severe MS, Severe Spontaneous Contrast in LA, and LAA Clot
Case 5   Severe MS, Severe MR, Severe TR, and Severe Spontaneous Contrast in LA
Case 6   Severe MS, Moderate MR, and a Mobile Mass on Ventricular Side of Aortic Valve
Case 7   Severe MS, Mild MR, No LA, and LAA Clot
Case 8   Severe MS, Mild MR, Moderate AS, Moderate AI, No LA, and LAA Clot
Case 9   Severe MS, Mild MR, Moderate AI, No LA, and LAA Clot
Case 10 Mild Mitral Stenosis due to Severe Mitral Annulus Calcification and Senile Degenerative Changes of Mitral Valve
Case 11 Severe Mitral Stenosis, Severe Mitral Regurgitation, Severe Tricuspid Regurgitation, No LA, and LAA Clot
Case 12 Severe Mitral Stenosis, Mild Mitral Regurgitation, Severe Tricuspid Regurgitation, and Severe Spontaneous Contrast Impending to Fresh Clot Formation in LAA

Chapter 3 Aortic Valve Disease

Case 1   Severe Aortic Regurgitation
Case 2   Critical AS, Severe AI
Case 3   Moderate Valvular AS, Bicuspid Aortic Valve, and Interrupted Aortic Arch
Case 4   Bicuspid Aortic Valve with Moderate Valvular Aortic Stenosis
Case 5   Bicuspid Aortic Valve, Mild AS, Mild AI
Case 6   Low Flow, Low Gradient Severe AS

Chapter 4 Tricuspid Valve Disease

Chapter 5 Pulmonary Valve Disease

Chapter 6 Malfunction and Other Complications After Heart Valve Surgery

Chapter 7 Paravalvular Leak of Prosthetic Valves

Chapter 8 Infective Endocarditis (IE)

Chapter 9 ASDs and PFO

Chapter 10 VSD, PDA, Coarctation of Aorta, Subvalvular AS

Chapter 11 Cardiac Mass

Chapter 12 Intervention in Structural Heart Disease

Degenerative Mitral Valve Disease

Videos can be found in the electronic supplementary material in the online version of the chapter.
On http://springerlink.com enter the DOI number given on the bottom of the chapter opening page.
Scroll down to the Supplementary material tab and click on the respective videos link.

© Springer International Publishing AG 2017
H. Sadeghian, Z. Savand-Roomi, *3D Echocardiography of Structural Heart Disease*,
DOI 10.1007/978-3-319-54039-9_1

1.1   Introduction

There is a spectrum of degenerative mitral valve disease from fibroelastic deficiency to Barlow disease [1].

In fibroelastic deficiency, one segment is involved and has deficiency of collagen, mitral annulus is normal or mildly dilated and the chorda of affected segment is involved, thin, and/or ruptured.

With long-standing prolapse, secondary mitral valve change may occur resulting thick and excess tissue in affected segment (FED+).

In forme fruste, thick and excess tissue affects more than one segment but not all segments and not in large valve size.

In Barlow disease, multiple segments of mitral valve are involved, thick, and redundant, mitral annulus is more dilated, and chorda are involved, thick, elongated, and often ruptured [1] (◘ Fig. 1.1).

Patients with Barlow disease are younger and have significantly higher values of billowing height and volume. There is infiltration of mucopolysaccharidosis material in valve tissue and disorganization of elastin and collagen leading to excess tissue in valves and a vulnerability to annular calcification [2].

In a recent study by 3D echocardiography, mitral annular area and intercommissural diameter were smaller in FED compared to Barlow disease and in Barlow disease these indices increased during systole. Anteroposterior diameter was smaller in FED compared to Barlow disease and height was similar between the two groups. Saddle shape of mitral valve progressively increases from diastole to systole in FED, but is stable in Barlow disease. FED and Barlow disease have different mitral annular geometry and dynamics with larger annular dimensions and loss of saddle-shape deepening in Barlow disease [3]. This may affect surgical restoration of mitral annular shape and durability of repair in Barlow disease and the use of saddle-shaped ring annuloplasty in Barlow disease [3].

In a study by Chandra et al., billowing height >10 mm can discriminate degenerative mitral valve disease from normal and billowing volume >1.15 can differentiate between FED and Barlow disease [4].

In a study by Kovalva et al. mitral annular height >6.55 mm can discriminate between FED and Barlow disease [5]. This index is higher for Barlow disease. Barlow disease is characterized by dilation and vertical deformation of the mitral annulus (annulus height and height index increase), height index is measured by the ratio of mitral annular height/perimeter of annulus*100 [6].

In up to 20% of patients, exact detection between two groups is not possible.

In Barlow disease, there is billowing of body of leaflets and prolapse of margin of leaflets, mitral regurgitation is the result of prolapse of margin of leaflets, not billowing of the body of leaflets. If there is chordal elongation, mitral regurgitation will be mid or late systolic while if there is chordal rupture, mitral regurgitation will be holosystolic [2]. As excess tissue is a characteristic hallmark of Barlow disease, resection of excess tissue is a crucial point strategy for surgery and correction of marginal prolapse for correction of regurgitation is not adequate. Besides, all segments which are fed by an elongated chorda should be corrected [2]. Use of large annuloplasty ring will prevent systolic anterior motion [2].

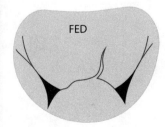
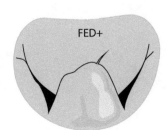
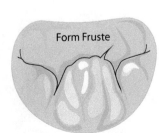
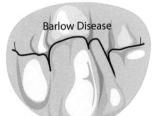

◘ **Fig. 1.1**   Spectrum of degenerative mitral valve disease from fibroelastic deficiency to Barlow disease

In fibroelastic deficiency, the average ring size is about 32 mm.

The ratio of commissural diameter to anteroposterior annular diameter is 4:3 in normal population and FED and is near one in BD in favor of more circular rather than oval-shaped mitral annulus.

In Chandra et al.'s study, there was no significant gender difference between BD and FED [4].

Detection of BD and FED is essential before surgery, in multisegment involvement and larger AMVL surface area a more complex repair is required, in addition restoration of saddle shape of mitral annulus in BD needs saddle-shaped ring annuloplasty, ring size is always between 36 and 40 mm. Barlow disease may require use of partial ring instead of rigid or flexible complete rings [4].

In classic prolapse, mitral leaflets are thick (>5 mm), and in nonclassic prolapse the mitral leaflets are not thick and show only billowing beyond annular plane of 2 mm.

Mitral annulus has a saddle shape appearance and in anteroposterior direction is concave upward and in medial to lateral direction is concave downward.

Based on the classic Carpentier classification, the mitral scallops are classified as P1, P2, and P3 and A1, A2, and A3 based on their indentation and from lateral (LAA) to medial (septum), A2 and P2 are laid near aorta and P1 is best visualized in apical four-chamber view [7]. Duran has classified mitral scallops based on chordal attachments, so anterior mitral leaflet has two scallops (A1 and A2) and posterior mitral leaflet has 4 scallops (P1, P2, PM1, and PM2). A1, P1, and PM1 have chordal attachment to anterolateral papillary muscle and A2, P2, and PM2 have chordal attachment to posteromedial papillary muscle [8]. Modified Carpentier classification is a combination of two nomenclatures which proposed by Pravin Shah, according to this classification, anterior mitral leaflet is classified into three scallops, A1, A2 lateral and A2 medial and A3, posterior mitral leaflet is also classified into three scallops, P1, P2 lateral and P2 medial and P3 [9] (◻ Fig. 1.2). In a study by Mayo Clinic, progression of MR occurred in 51% of patients (8 cm³ in a 1.5 year follow-up), and new flail segment and increase in annular diameter were two independent factors for prediction of MR progression [7]. Thickness of mitral leaflets more than 5 mm was a predictor of sudden cardiac death and endocarditis and progression of MR in some studies [10], but another study could not prove it [11]. In a large study including 833 patients over a period of 9 years, natural history of asymptomatic mitral valve prolapse was evaluated, the most frequent primary risk factors for cardiovascular mortality were mitral regurgitation from moderate to severe and, less frequently, ejection fraction <50%. Predictive of cardiovascular morbidity were slight mitral regurgitation, left atrium >40 mm, flail leaflet, atrial fibrillation, and age ≥50 years [12].

It is of notice that the presence of mitral flail has been associated with a widely varying prognosis and management decisions for patients with flail leaflet are like chronic severe MR and based largely on the presence or absence of clinical symptoms, the functional state of the left ventricle, and the feasibility of successful MV repair. The definition of flail is based on failure of coaptation of mitral leaflets and rapid systolic movement of flail tip into left atrium [13]. Tricuspid valve prolapse concomitant with mitral valve prolapse has a frequency of 40–50% [7], isolated tricuspid valve prolapse is rare [7].

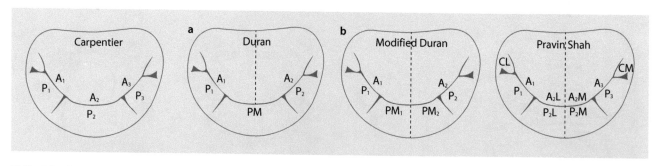

◻ **Fig. 1.2** Carpentier classification, Duran **a** and modified Duran **b** classification and Pravinshah classification

In conclusion, confronting mitral valve prolapse, the presence of mitral leaflets billowing and billowing of coaptation point into left atrium should be mentioned. The thickening of mitral valve leaflets if present and the severity and timing of mitral regurgitation, left atrial and ventricular dimensions and left ventricular systolic function, the presence of atrial fibrillation and pulmonary arterial systolic and diastolic pressure are cornerstones of diagnosis and treatment. Besides, differentiation between Barlow disease and fibroelastic deficiency, rupture or elongation of chorda, the involved scallops and mitral annulus dimensions should be mentioned. The decision about surgery is like other causes of severe chronic or acute mitral regurgitation and the type of repair is completely dependent on echocardiographic criteria.

One of the reasons for residual leaflet leak is separation of a leaflet cleft or indentation, uncorrected prolapse, or systolic anterior motion (SAM). SAM is due to undersized ring annuloplasty or excess valve tissue especially posterior leaflet. At the time of repair, a leaflet coaptation line about 5–8 mm should be restored [1]. Congenital cleft is not a characterizing feature of Barlow disease, but should be repaired for an adequate repair [2].

1.2   Case 1: Fibroelastic Deficiency, Prolapse of A2, Moderate Mitral Regurgitation (MR)

A 56-year-old woman presented with dyspnea on exertion functional class III of recent exacerbation.

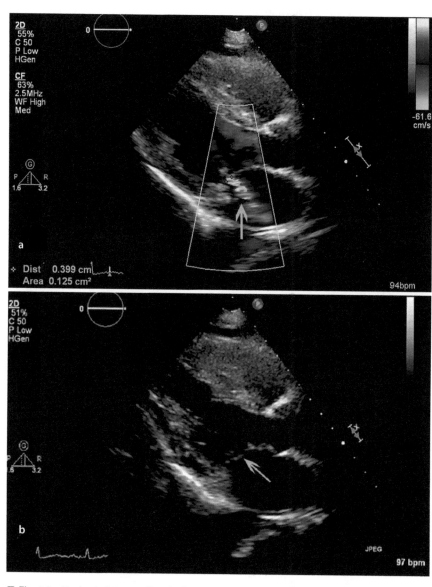

☐ **Fig. 1.3**   Moderate late systolic mitral regurgitation (*arrow*) (MR) is seen in parasternal long-axis view **a**, MR vena contracta measures 3.9 mm **a**, prolapse of A2 is also evident in this view (*arrow*) **b**, MR is eccentric toward lateral wall **a**

1.2 · Case 1: Fibroelastic Deficiency, Prolapse of A2, Moderate Mitral Regurgitation (MR)

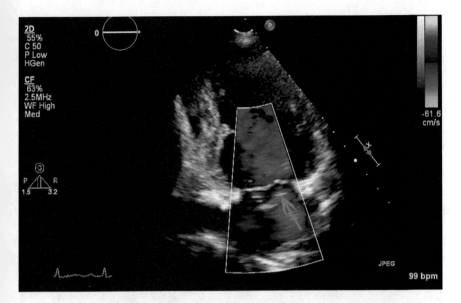

■ **Fig. 1.4** Eccentric moderate MR (*arrow*) is also visualized in apical two-chamber view

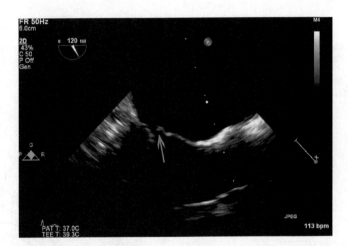

■ **Fig. 1.5** TEE long-axis view shows prolapse of A2 without thickness (*arrow*), other scallops are not prolaptic and thick

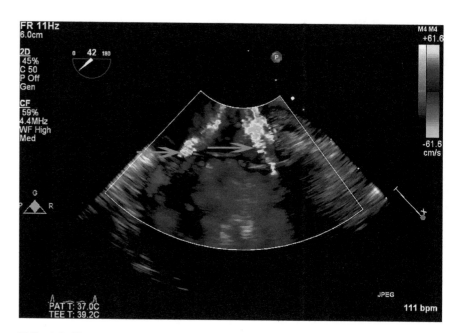

Fig. 1.6 There are two jets of MR from both commissures in TEE 42° view (*arrows*)

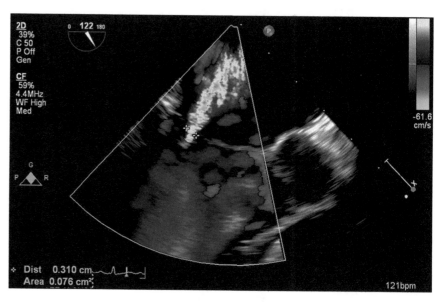

Fig. 1.7 MR vena contracta measures 3.1 mm in TEE long-axis view. It is of notice that MR vena contracta should be measured in orthogonal views like TEE long-axis or parasternal long-axis views

1.2 · Case 1: Fibroelastic Deficiency, Prolapse of A2, Moderate Mitral Regurgitation (MR)

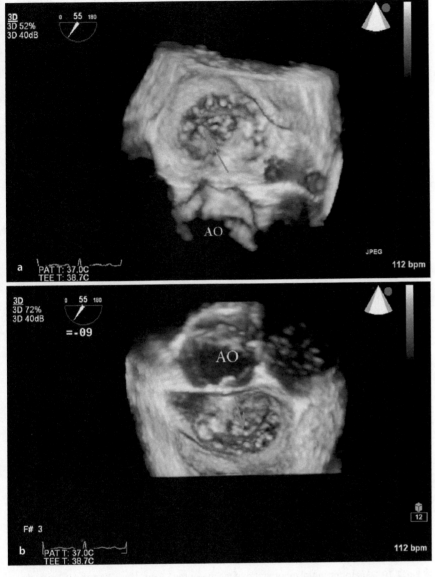

◼ **Fig. 1.8**   3D zoom shows prolapse of A2 from LA side (*arrows*) before Z rotation **a** and after Z rotation **b**

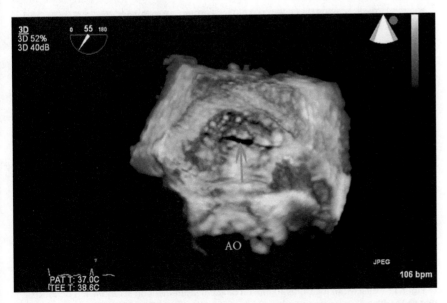

◼ **Fig. 1.9**   Failure of coaptation of MV leaflets in systole (*arrow*) is evident by 3D zoom from LA side

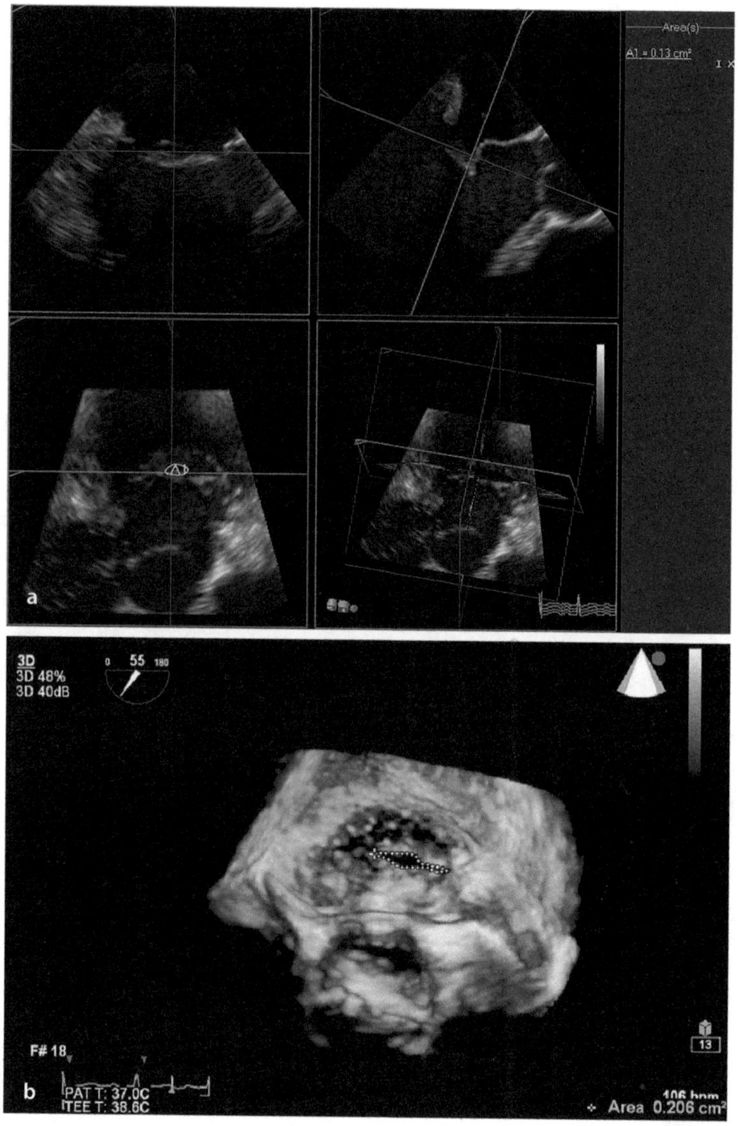

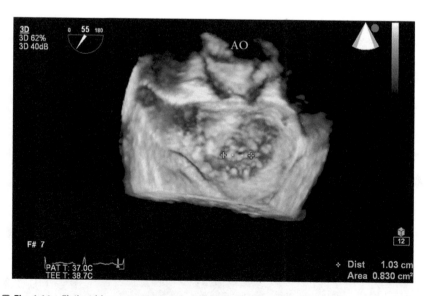

Fig. 1.10 Anatomic mitral regurgitation area measures 1.3 mm^2 by 3DQ **a** and 0.2 mm^2 by direct planimetry by 3D zoom **b**

Fig. 1.11 Flail width measures 10 mm on direct measurement on 3D zoom. It is of notice that flail width ≥15 mm was an exclusion criteria for Mitraclip in EVERST II study [14]

1.2 · Case 1: Fibroelastic Deficiency, Prolapse of A2, Moderate Mitral Regurgitation (MR)

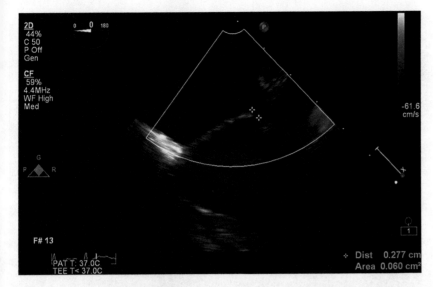

◘ **Fig. 1.12** Flail gap measures 2.7 mm by TEE 0° view. It is of notice that flail gap ≥10 mm is an exclusion criteria for Mitraclip according to EVEREST II study [14]

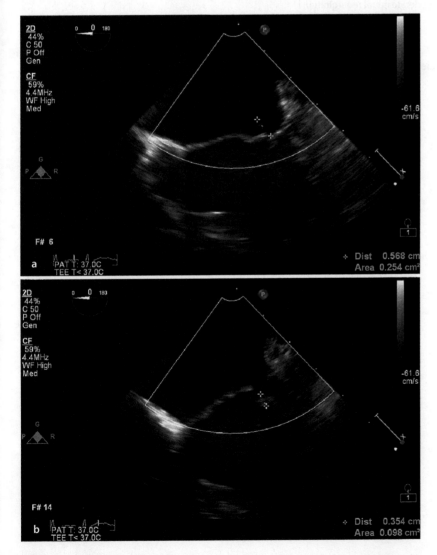

◘ **Fig. 1.13** Coaptation depth measures 6 mm and zona coapta (vertical coaptation length) measures 3.5 mm in TEE 0° view **a, b**. If leaflet tethering is present, coaptation depth >11 mm and zona coapta <2 mm were exclusion criteria for Mitraclip according to EVERST II study [14]

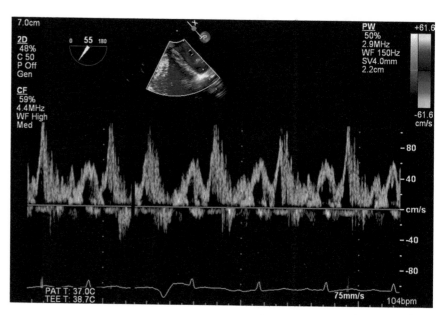

◘ Fig. 1.14 In left upper pulmonary vein, systolic flow is less than diastolic flow in favor of moderate mitral regurgitation

Diagnosis   Moderate MR due to prolapse of A2, A2 is not thick, fibroelastic deficiency (other scallops are not thick and prolaptic)

Comment   Follow up.

Lesson
1. This case is a typical form of fibroelastic deficiency, only one scallop of mitral valve is involved and prolaptic and not thick, other mitral valve scallops are not thick and prolaptic, there is no rupture of chorda.
2. For measurements with 3D echocardiography, 3DQ is a recognized and recommended method, direct measurement by 3D should be evaluated in future studies.
3. Exclusion criteria for Mitraclip according to EVEREST II trial were:
   a   Evidence of calcification in A2 and P2 scallops (grasping area),
   b   Presence of significant cleft in A2 or P2,
   c   Bileaflet flail or severe bileaflet prolapse,
   d   Lack of primary or secondary chordal support,
   e   Prior mitral valve surgery or valvotomy or any current mechanical device,
   f   Intracardiac mass or thrombosis or vegetation,
   g   History of active endocarditis or rheumatic heart disease,
   h   History of ASD or PFO with symptoms,
   i   MI in recent 12 weeks,
   j   Any endovascular therapeutic interventional procedure performed within 30 days prior
   k   EF <25% or LVESD >55 mm,
   l   Orifice area <0.4 cm^2,
   m   Severe mitral annular calcification,
   n   If leaflet prolapse presents: Flail gap ≥10 mm, Flail width ≥15 mm,
   o   If leaflet tethering present: Zona coapta <2 m, Coaptation depth >11 mm [14].

1.3   Case 2: Fibroelastic Deficiency+ (FED+), Severe Mitral Regurgitation, Prolapse and Rupture of Chorda of A2

A 70-year-old man presented with dyspnea on exertion of one month duration.

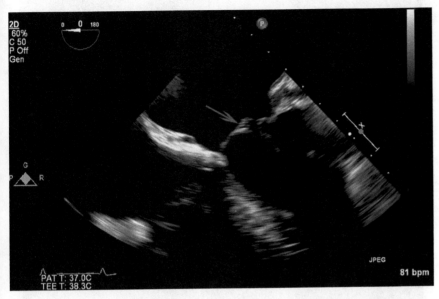

🔲 **Fig. 1.15** Prolapse of A2 is evident in this TEE 0° view (*arrow*), other MV scallops seem thin and non-prolaptic in this view, chorda are not thick, and mitral annulus is not dilated

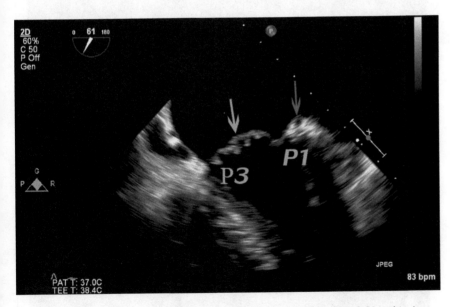

🔲 **Fig. 1.16** TEE 61° view shows prolapse and rupture of chorda of A2 (*arrow*), P3 in this view seems prolaptic but thin, P1 is not prolaptic, mitral annulus is not dilated, and LCX is seen in AV groove near LAA (*pink arrow*), when LAA is open the middle MV scallop is A2

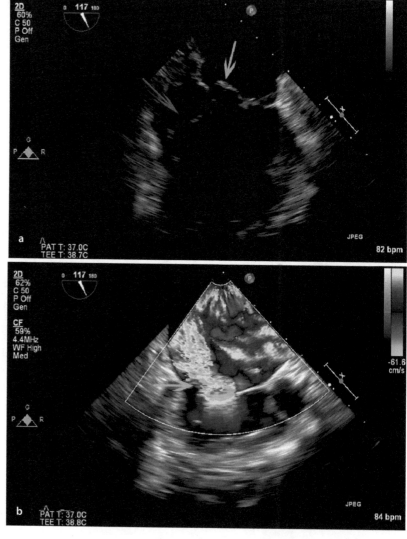

◘ Fig. 1.17 Severe eccentric MR is evident in TEE 61° view (*arrow*)

◘ Fig. 1.18 Prolapse of A2 (*arrow*) is evident in this TEE 117° view, other MV scallops are not prolaptic **a**, mitral valve chorda are not thick (*pink arrow*), severe eccentric MR toward lateral wall is relevant in this view by color Doppler study (*arrow*) **b** in favor of that main mechanism of MR is prolapse of A2

1.3 · Case 2: Fibroelastic Deficiency+ (FED+), Severe Mitral Regurgitation, Prolapse and Rupture of Chorda of A2

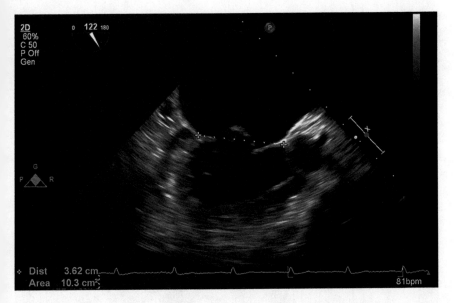

◘ **Fig. 1.19** MV annulus measures 36 mm in this TEE long-axis view (mildly dilated)

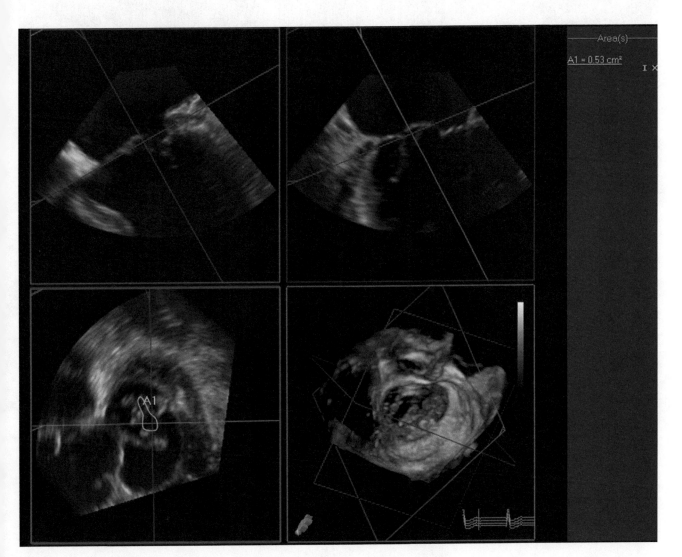

◘ **Fig. 1.20** Anatomic mitral regurgitation area measures 0.53 cm² by 3DQ method by 3D zoom

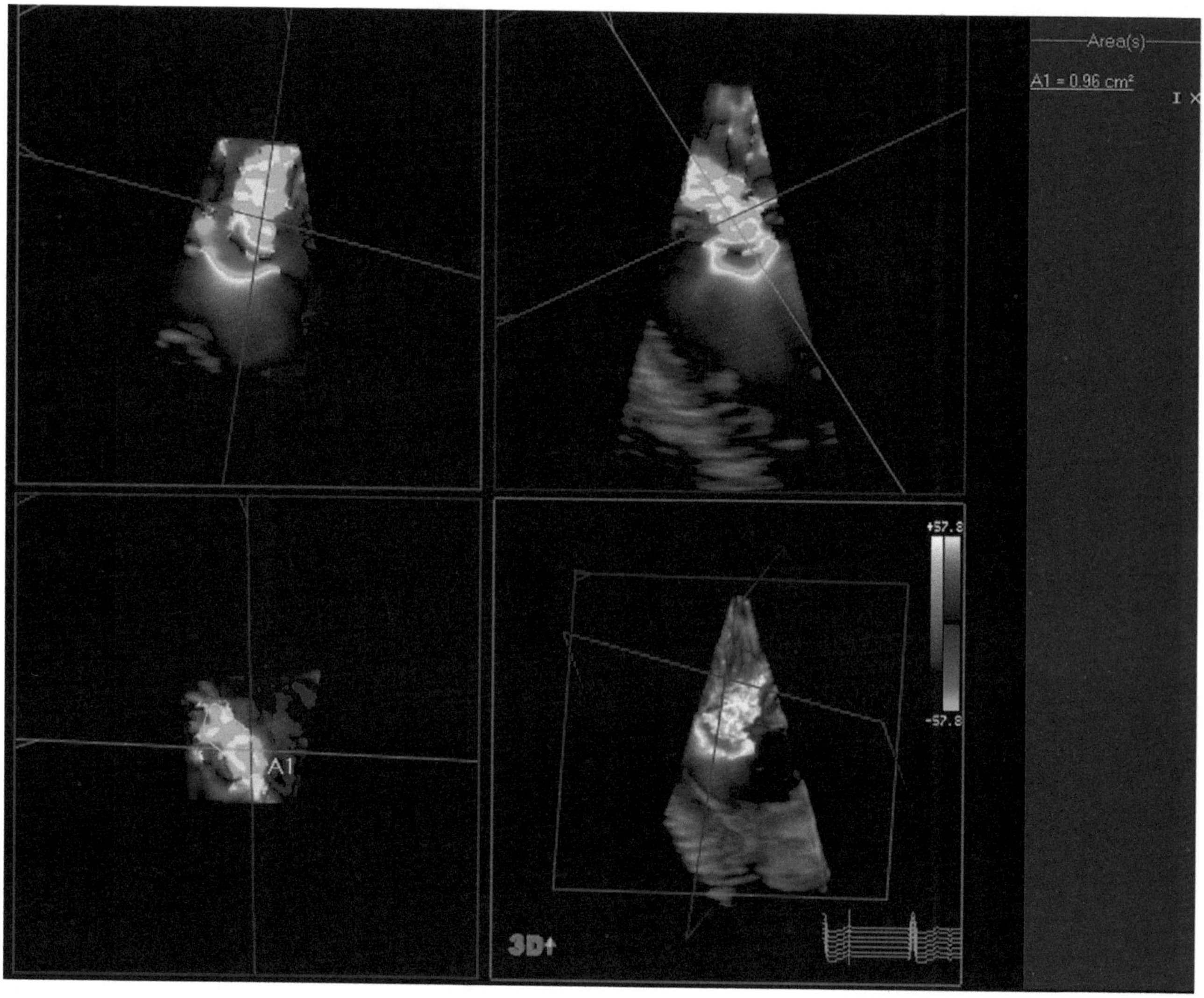

Fig. 1.21 Vena contracta area measures 0.96 cm² by color Doppler full volume 3DQ in favor of severe MR

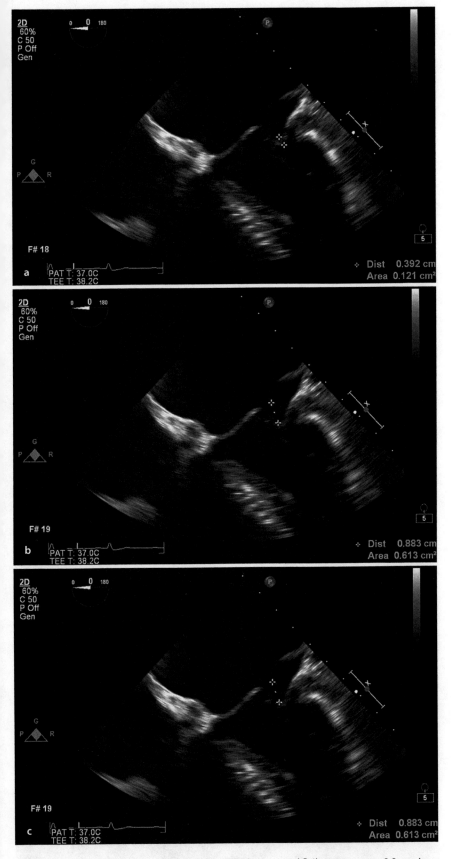

■ **Fig. 1.22** Zona coapta measures 3.9 mm in TEE 0° view **a** and flail gap measures 8.8 mm in this view **b** and coaptation height measures 7.6 mm in this view **c**

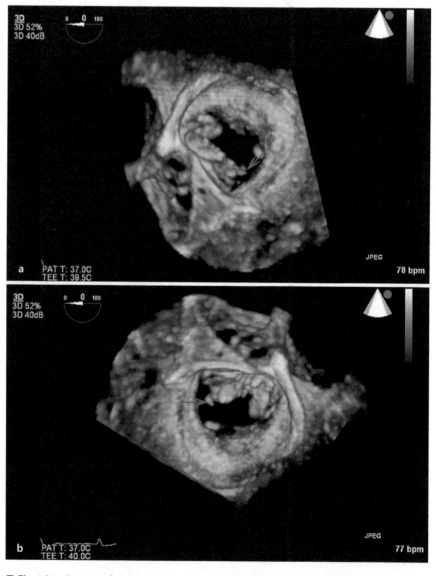

▢ Fig. 1.23 Flail width measures 15 mm by 3D zoom from LA side by direct measurement. *AO* aortic valve

▢ Fig. 1.24 Rupture of chorda of A2 (*green arrows*) is evident by 3D zoom from LA side **a**, **b**, (**a**, before Z rotation and **b**, after Z rotation), in addition stitch effect is seen (*pink arrow*) **b**)

Diagnosis   Severe MR due to FED, prolapse and rupture of chorda of A2, MV scallops are thin, only A2 and somehow P3 are prolaptic.

Comment   MV surgery.

Lesson
1. In FED, MV annulus is less dilated compared to BD, one or two segments are affected and MV scallops are not thick [1], repair is feasible, the only concern about repair in this patient is that A2 is affected and repair of A2 is difficult.
2. For Mitraclip, flail width should be less than 15 mm and flail gap should be less than 10 mm [14]. In this patient, flail width is 15 mm and so is not suitable for Mitraclip.

1.4   Case 3: Fibroelastic Deficiency+ (FED+), Rupture of Chorda of A2, Severe MR

A 74-year-old man who underwent AVR with bioprosthetic valve one year ago referred due to dyspnea on exertion functional class III.

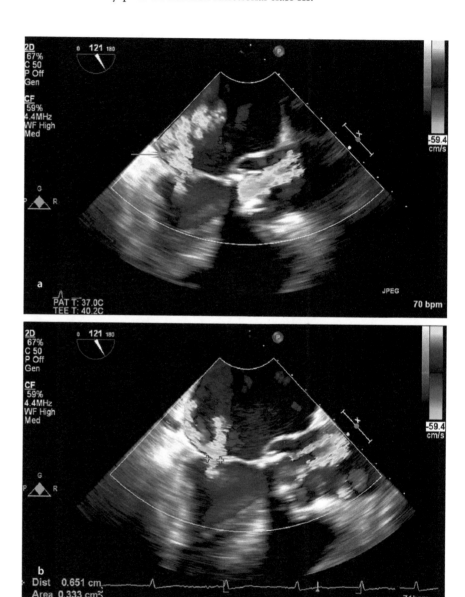

☐ **Fig. 1.25**   Severe eccentric mitral regurgitation is seen in TEE long-axis view (*arrow*) **a**, MR vena contracta measures 6.5 mm in this view **b**

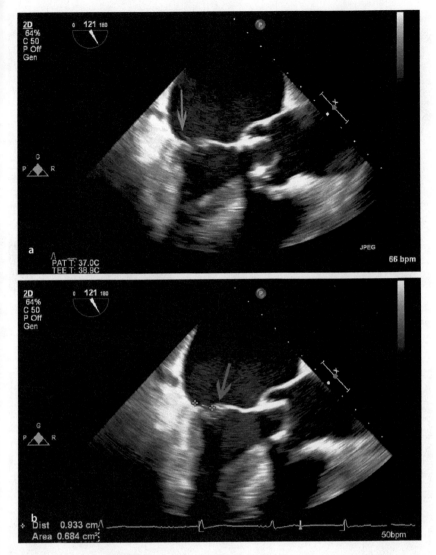

Fig. 1.26 A mobile mass is seen on atrial side of A2 in favor of rupture of chorda of A2 in TEE long-axis view (*arrow*) **a**, this mass measures 9 mm in size **b**, A2 is also thick in this view (*arrow*) **b**

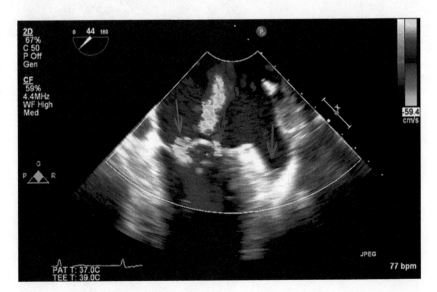

Fig. 1.27 Two jets of MR are evident by TEE short-axis view (*arrows*), LAA is not ligated in previous surgery (*pink arrow*)

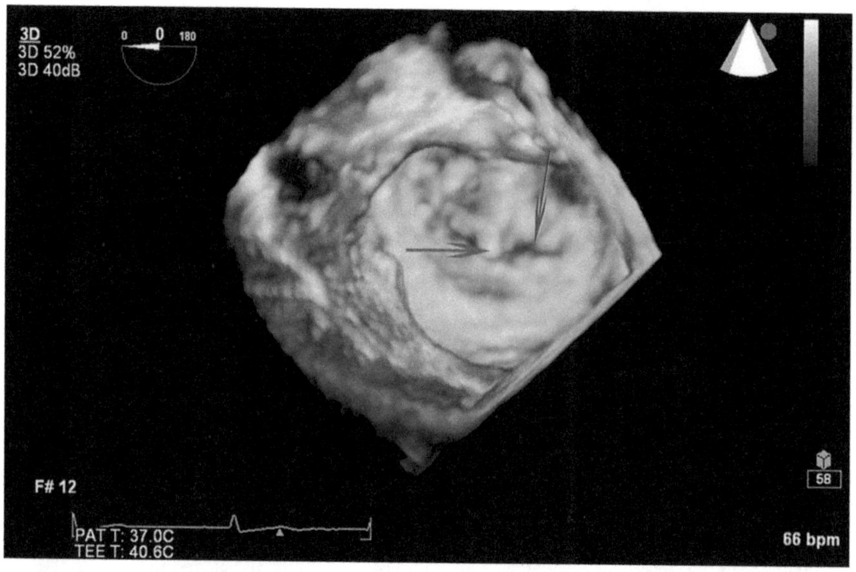

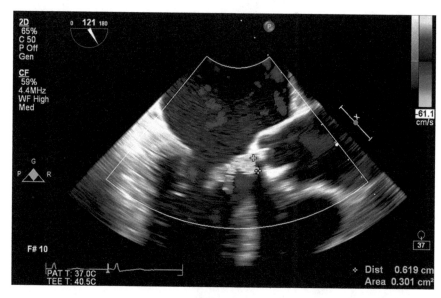

■ **Fig. 1.28**   Prolapse of A2 and rupture of chorda of A2 are evident by 3D zoom from LA side (*arrow*), besides failure of coaptation of mitral valve leaflets is evident in this view (*pink arrow*)

■ **Fig. 1.29**   Moderately severe aortic regurgitation is shown in TEE long-axis view, aortic regurgitation vena contracta measures 6 mm in this view

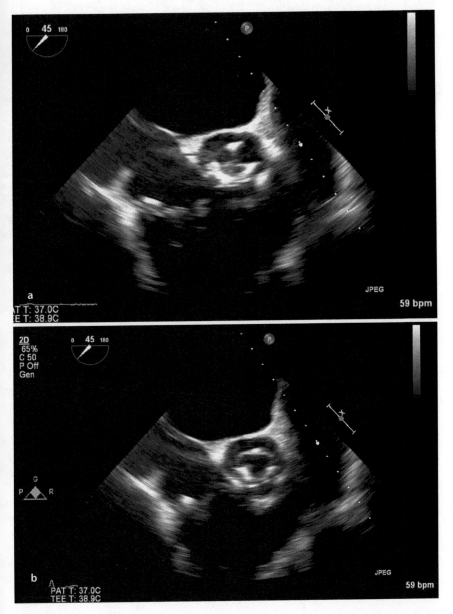

☐ **Fig. 1.30** Three leaflets of bioprosthetic aortic valve are evident by TEE short-axis view in diastole and systole **a, b**, failure of coaptation of aortic leaflets in diastole is evident (*arrow*) **a**

◻ Fig. 1.31   Moderately severe aortic regurgitation is also evident in TEE short-axis view (*arrow*), there is also a small patent foramen ovale (PFO) flow (*pink arrow*)

Diagnosis   Prolapse of A2 and rupture of chorda of AMVL (A2) and severe MR due to fibroelastic deficiency, moderately severe aortic regurgitation on bioprosthetic aortic valve. It is of notice that other scallops are not involved, so it is in FED category, with respect to thick A2 scallop, it will be categorized in FED+.

Comment   If the patient is symptomatic on medical treatment, mitral valve repair and AVR is recommended.

1.5 Case 4: Forme Fruste, Rupture of Chorda of P2, Severe MR

A 57-year-old woman presented with dyspnea on exertion functional class III of one month duration.

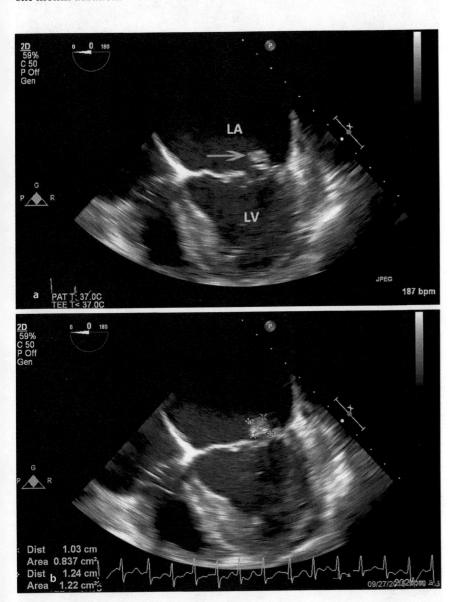

Fig. 1.32 A mobile mass is seen on PMVL in TEE 0° view (*arrow*) **a**, this mass measures 12*10 mm **b** in this view. *LA* left atrium, *LV* left ventricle

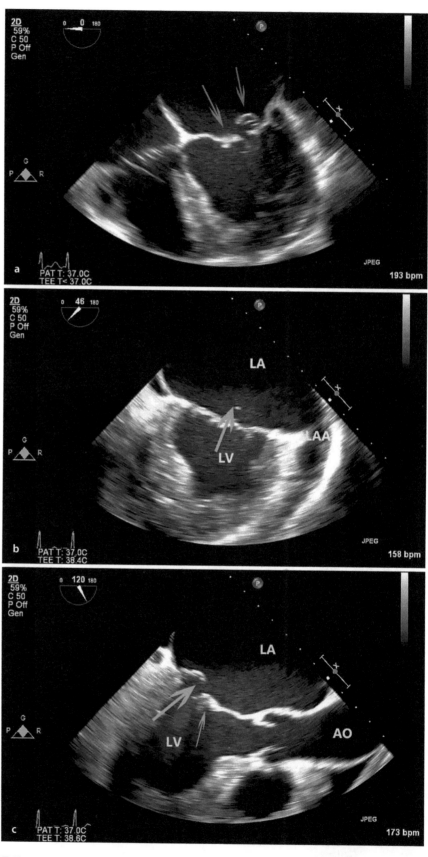

Fig. 1.33 The head of posterior mitral leaflet is turned toward left atrium in systole (*arrows*) in favor of complete flail of posterior mitral leaflet by TEE 0° view **a**, TEE short-axis view **b** and TEE long-axis view **c**, A2 is also thick and prolaptic in these views (*pink arrows*). Involvement of other segments in addition to main flail segment is in favor of forme fruste

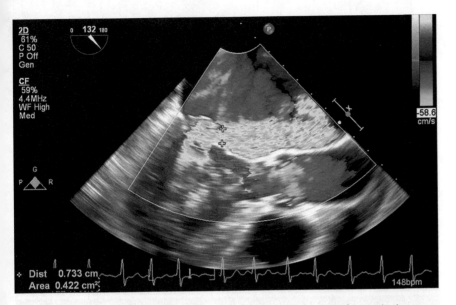

Fig. 1.34 Severe mitral regurgitation is seen in TEE long-axis view, mitral regurgitation vena contracta measures 7.3 mm in this view

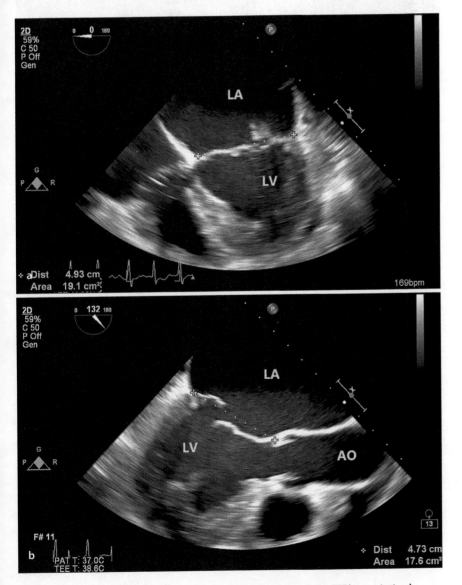

Fig. 1.35 Aortic annulus measures 49 mm in TEE 0° view **a** and 47 mm in TEE long-axis view **b**, severe annulus dilation is in favor of a form of degenerative mitral valve disease more complex than FED

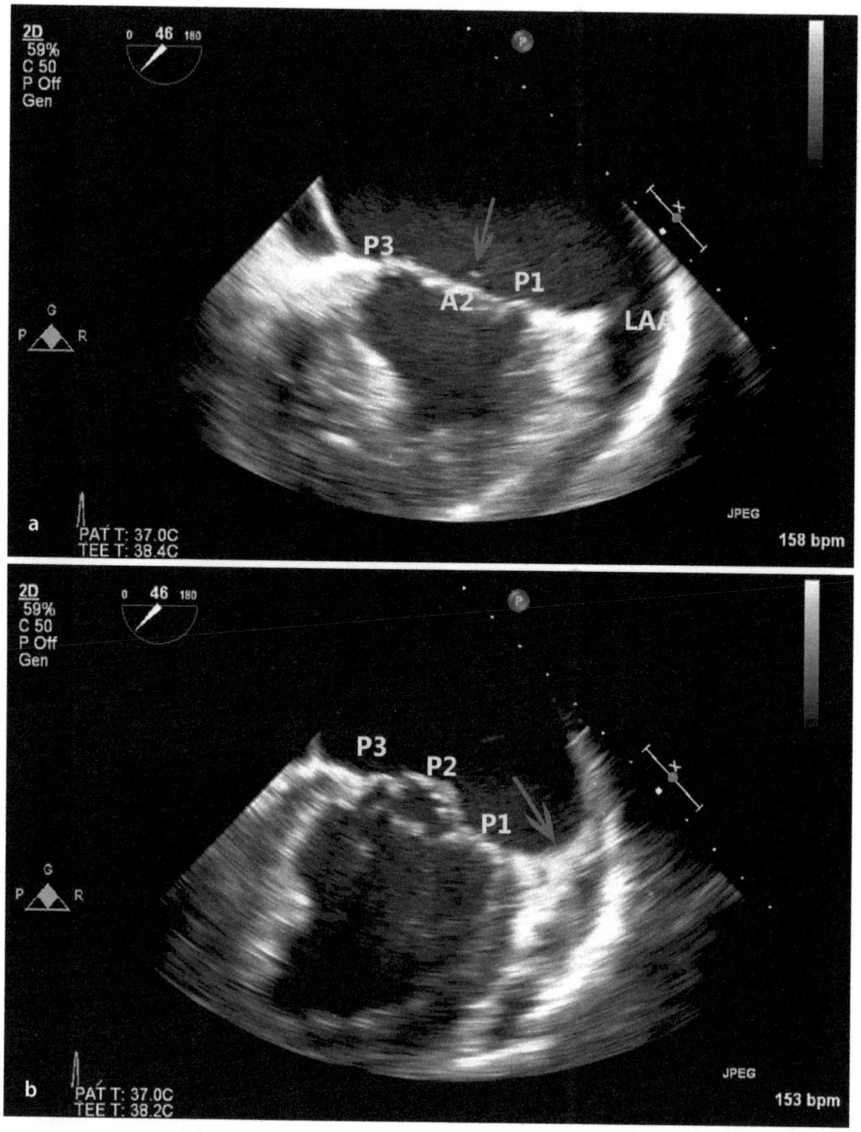

Fig. 1.36 P1, A2, and P3 are relevant by TEE short-axis view when LAA is apparent, head of ruptured P2 is also evident in this view (*arrow*) **a**, P1, P2, and 3 are evident in TEE short-axis view when LAA is not visualized (*arrow*) **b**, P2 is prolaptic and flail, P3 is also prolaptic **b**

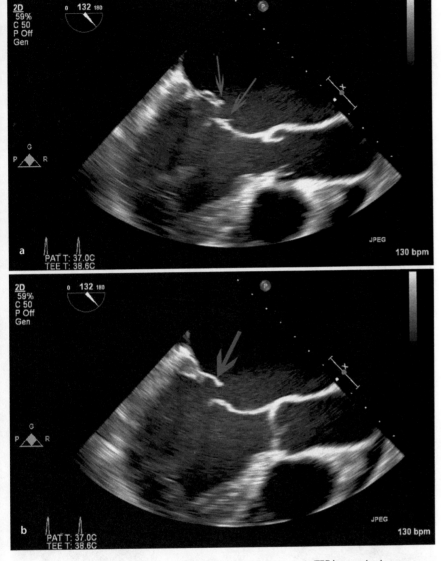

■ Fig. 1.37   Multiple masses and complete flail of PMVL are seen in TEE long-axis views (*arrows*) **a**, **b**, prolapse of A2 is also evident in this view (*pink arrow*)

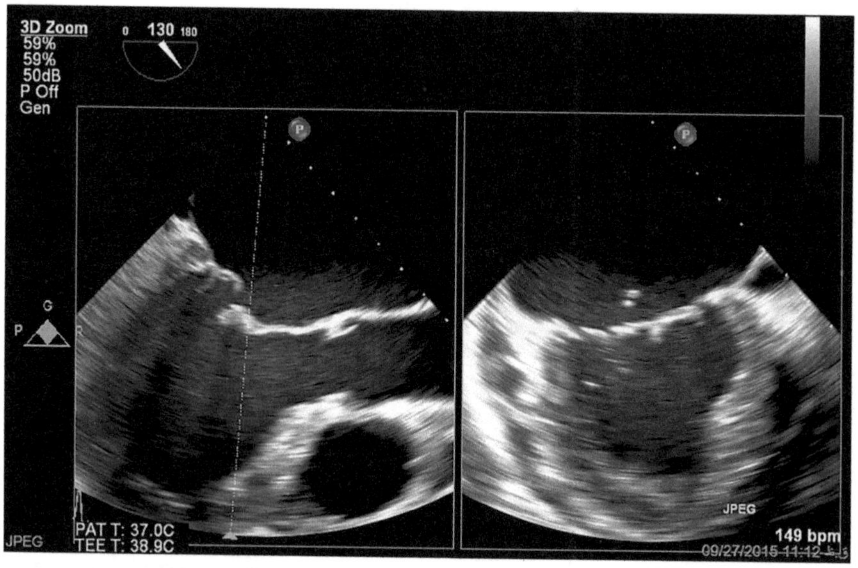

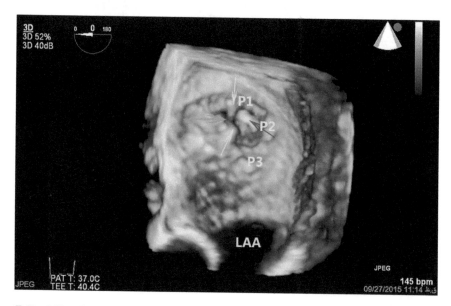

Fig. 1.38 Biplane view of 3D zoom shows mitral valve in two orthogonal views, complete flail of PMVL (*left figure*), and rupture of chorda of P2 (*right figure*)

Fig. 1.39 3D zoom of mitral valve from LA side shows failure of coaptation of MV leaflets (*green arrow*) and rupture of chorda of P2 (*pink arrow*), prolapse of A2 and P3 is also evident (*yellow arrow*), this view is without Z or on plane rotation, LAA in 6 o'clock

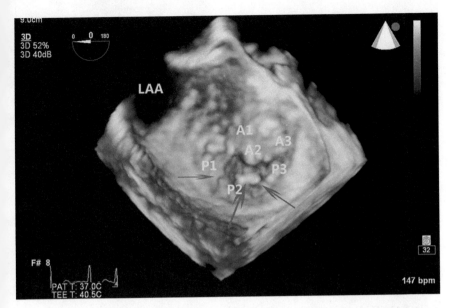

Fig. 1.40 All mitral scallops are marked in this figure and rupture of P2 is evident in this view (*pink arrow*) after Z rotation, LAA in 10 o'clock, indentation between P1 and P2 and P3 is evident in this view (*green arrows*), prolapse of A2 and P3 is also evident

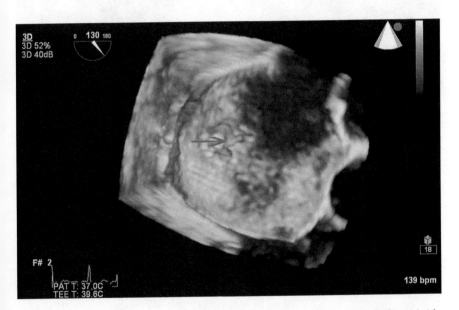

Fig. 1.41 Rupture of P2 (*pink arrow*) is evident by TEE long-axis view by 3D zoom from LA side

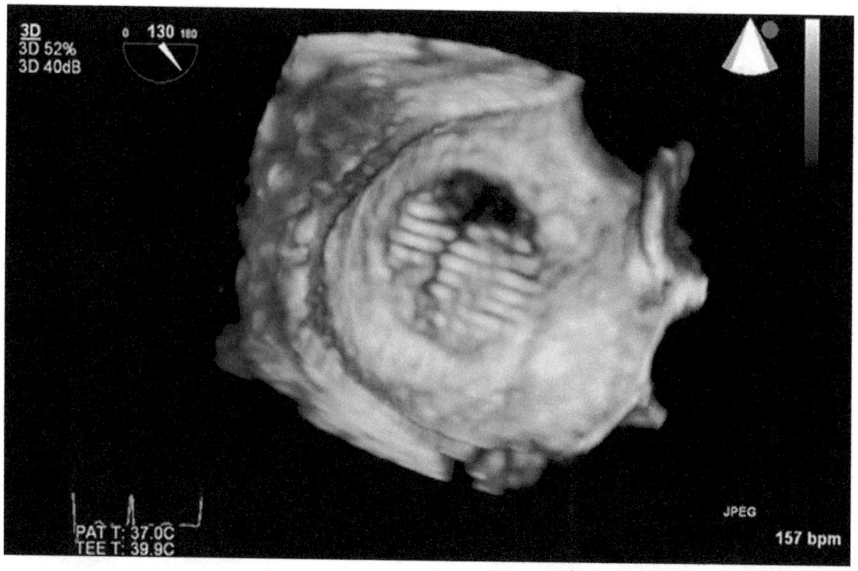

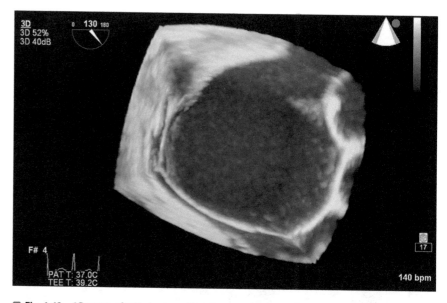

■ **Fig. 1.42**   TEE long-axis view by 3D zoom from LA side with stitch effect (*arrows*)

■ **Fig. 1.43**   3D zoom of mitral valve with gain more than 60% nearly shows nothing

1.5 · Case 4: Forme Fruste, Rupture of Chorda of P2, Severe MR

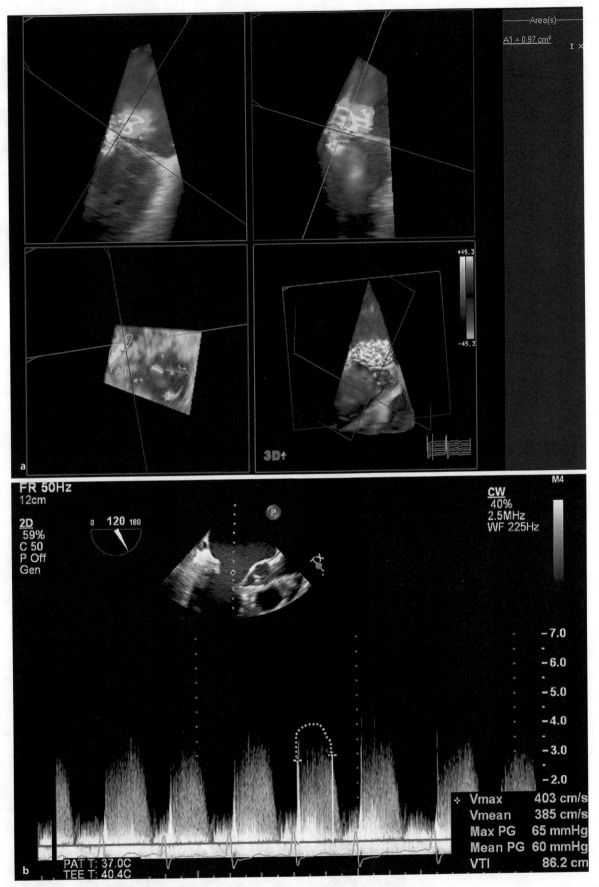

◻ Fig. 1.44　MR VC area measures 0.97 cm² by full volume **a**, VTI of MR is equal to 86 cm **b**, so MR volume measures as follows: MRVC area*MR VTI = 0.97*86 = 83 cm³. Vena contracta area more than 0.4 cm² and MR volume more than 60 cm³ are in favor of severe MR

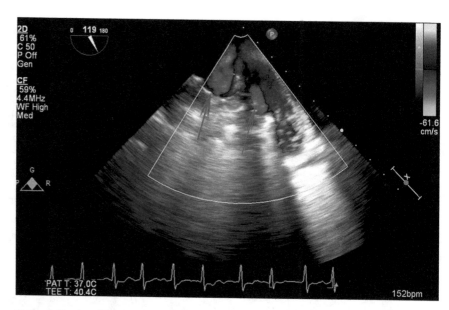

Fig. 1.45 Systolic reversal flow is seen in TEE long-axis view (*arrows*)

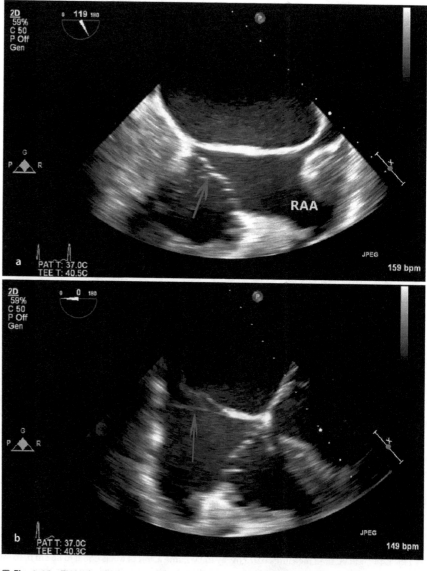

Fig. 1.46 TV is also prolaptic in TEE long-axis (*arrow*) and TEE 0° views **a**, **b**. Eustachian valve is also evident in this view (*arrow*) **b**, RAA is evident in TEE long-axis view **a**

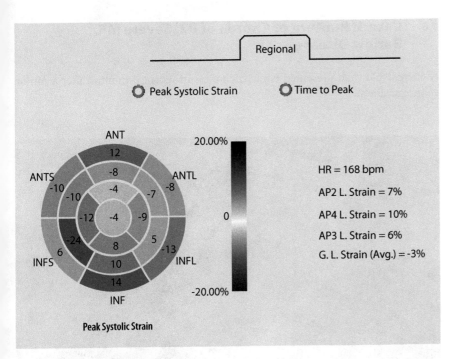

Fig. 1.47 Global longitudinal strain measures −3%

Diagnosis Severe eccentric MR due to degenerative mitral valve disease and rupture of chorda of P2. A2 and P3 tricuspid valve are also prolaptic. In this patient, more than one segment is affected so it is a more complex disease compared to FED, but still it does not fulfill criteria for Barlow disease and not all MV scallops are affected. Mitral valve annulus is dilated.

Comment The patient referred for surgery (MV repair).

Lesson Although LVEF is within normal limits, global longitudinal strain is reduced in favor of subclinical LV systolic dysfunction.

1.6   Case 5: Rupture of Chorda of P2, Severe MR, Barlow Disease

A 50-year-old man presented with palpitation in recent 2 months after a motor vehicle accident.

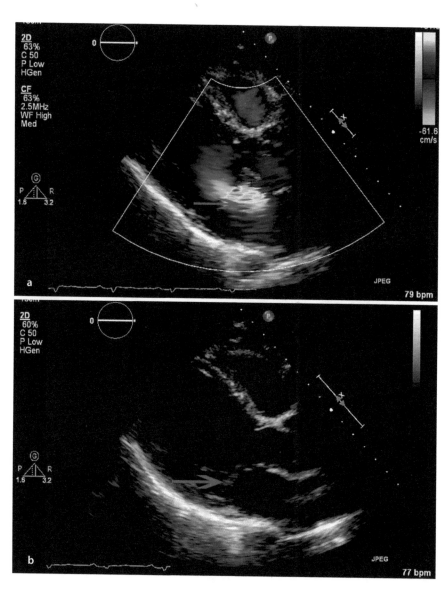

◘ Fig. 1.48 Parasternal long-axis view shows severe eccentric MR toward IAS (*arrow*) **a**, prolapse of both mitral leaflets especially P2 is evident in this view (*arrow*) **b**

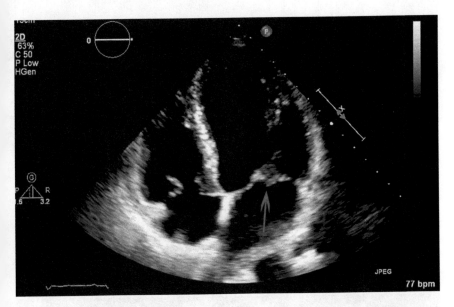

■ **Fig. 1.49** Apical four-chamber view reveals a mobile mass (*arrow*) on atrial side of PMVL (P2) in favor of rupture of chorda of PMVL (P2)

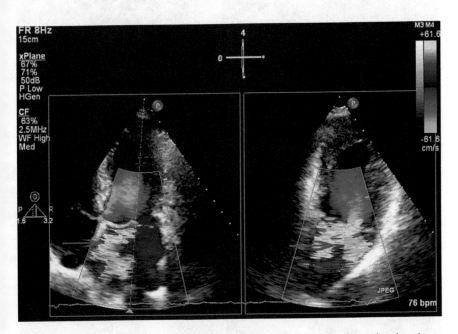

■ **Fig. 1.50** Severe MR (*arrows*) is also evident in apical four-chamber and two-chamber views by 3D zoom biplane view (before 3D reconstruction)

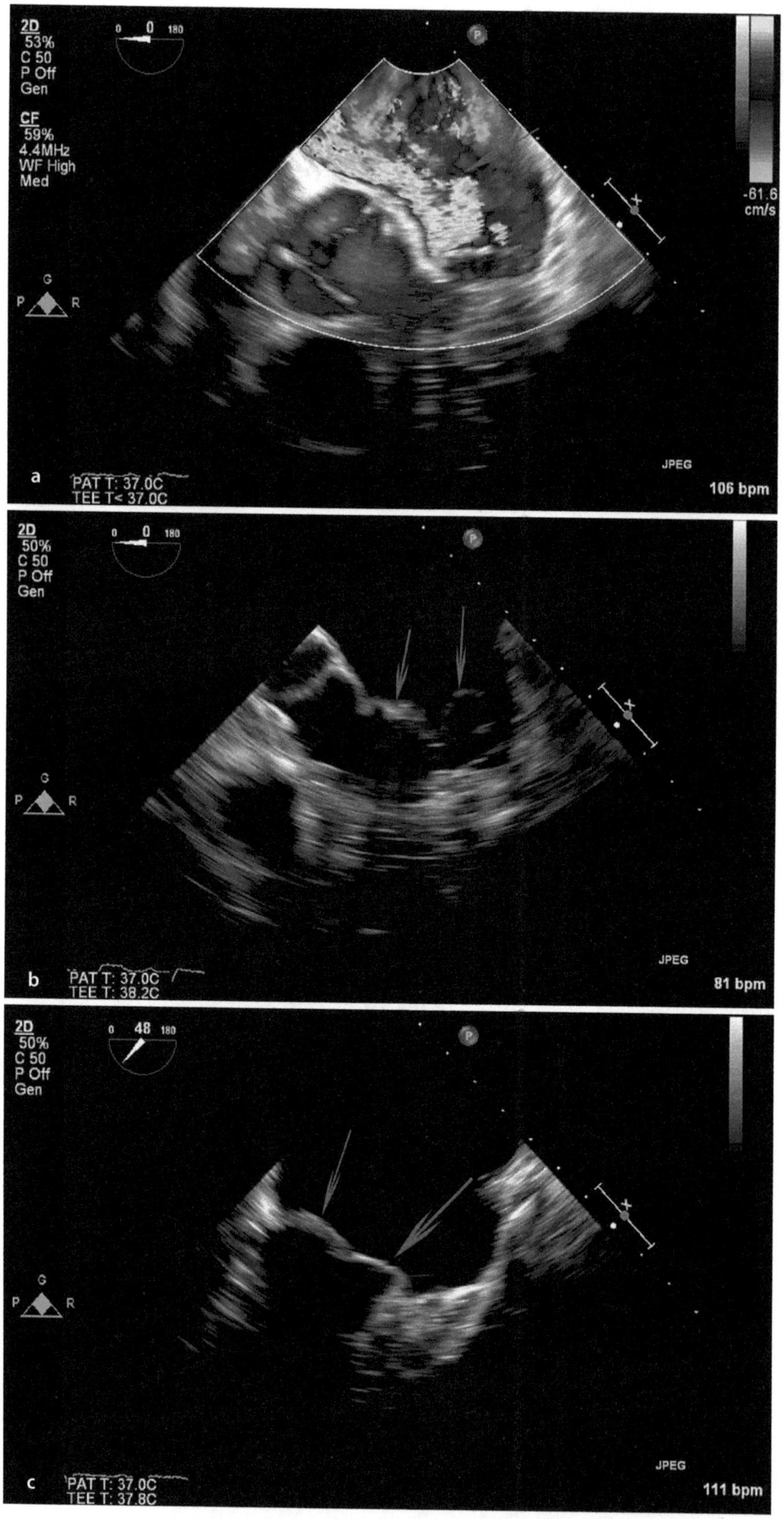

■ **Fig. 1.51**   Severe eccentric MR toward IAS (*arrow*) **a** is evident in TEE 0° view, thickening and prolapse of both mitral leaflets (nearly all scallops) are evident in TEE 0° **b** and TEE short-axis views **c**

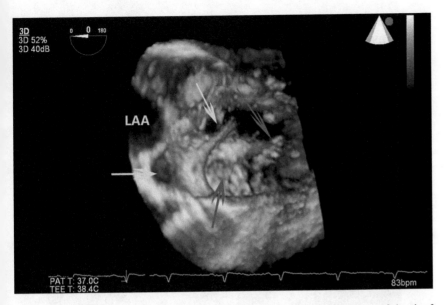

☐ **Fig. 1.52** TEE 3D zoom of mitral valve from LA side reveals prolapse and rupture of chorda of P2 segment (*arrow*), this is a surgical view and LAA is in 9 o'clock, P1 is also prolaptic (*pink arrow*), left pulmonary veins are obvious in this view (*yellow arrows*)

Diagnosis   Severe eccentric MR due to prolapse of both mitral leaflets (A2 and P2) and rupture of chorda of P2 by 3D echocardiography.

Comment   The patient referred for surgery of MV repair with saddle-shaped ring annuloplasty.

Lesson   This patient was a case of Barlow disease but after a trauma, rupture of chorda of P2 occurred, so the symptoms of patient developed during recent 2 months.

1.7   Case 6: Barlow Disease, Rupture of Chorda of P2, Severe MR

A 60-year-old man presented with dyspnea on exertion functional class III of recent duration.

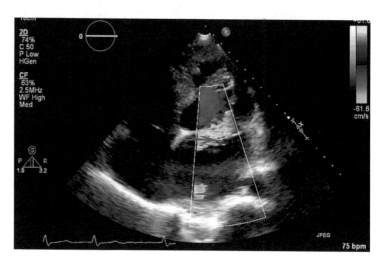

◘ Fig. 1.53   Severe eccentric MR toward inter-atrial septum is seen in apical four-chamber view (*arrow*)

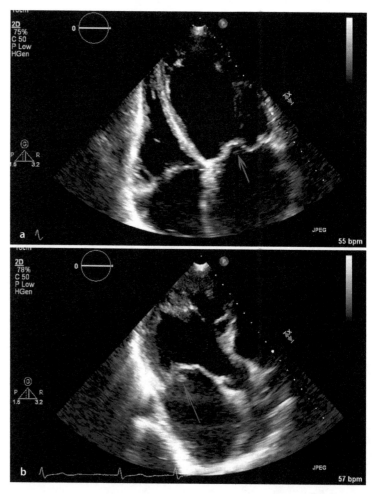

◘ Fig. 1.54   Rupture of chorda of PMVL (P2) and prolapse of P2 are evident by apical four-chamber **a** and apical three-chamber views **b** (*arrows*)

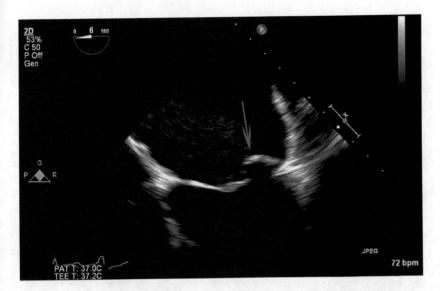

◘ Fig. 1.55 TEE 0° view shows that the head of PMVL turns toward LA in systole in favor of rupture of chorda of PMVL (P2) (*arrow*)

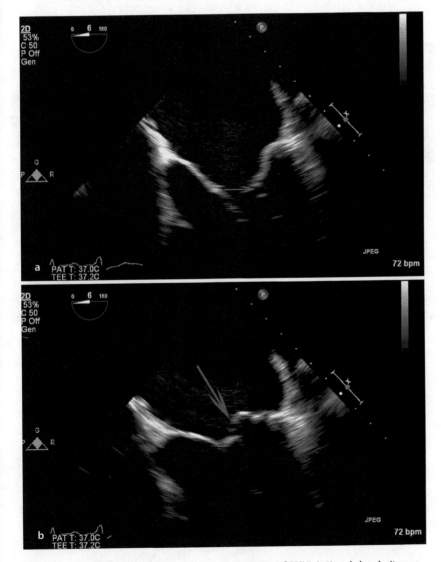

◘ Fig. 1.56 The site of rupture of chorda is in the junction of PMVL (p2) and chorda, it goes into LV in diastole **a** and it returns into LA in systole (b) (*arrows*)

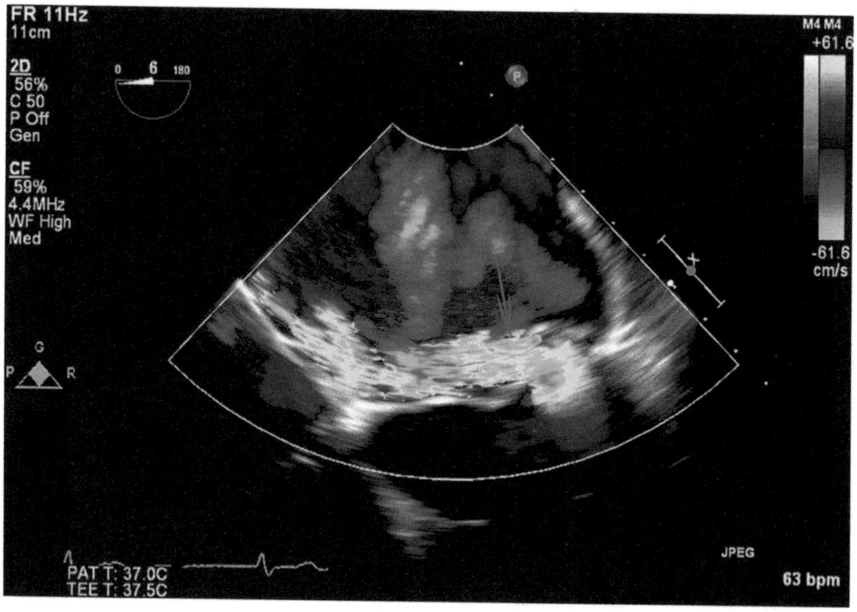

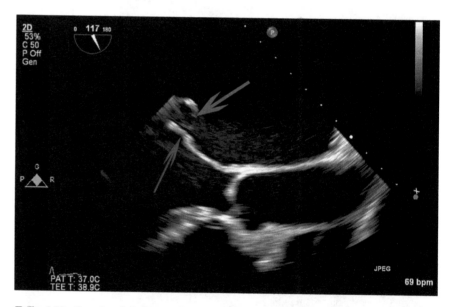

◘ Fig. 1.57 TEE 0° view shows severe eccentric MR toward inter-atrial septum (*arrow*)

◘ Fig. 1.58 Complete flail of P2 is relevant in TEE long-axis view (*arrow*), A2 is also prolaptic (*pink arrow*)

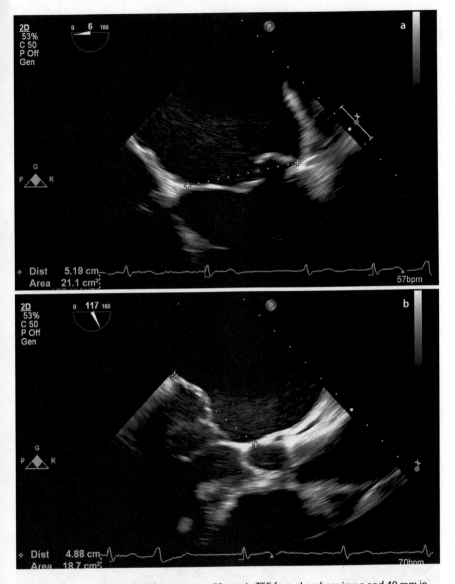

Fig. 1.59 Mitral valve annulus measures 52 mm in TEE four-chamber view **a** and 49 mm in TEE long-axis view **b**, and is severely dilated

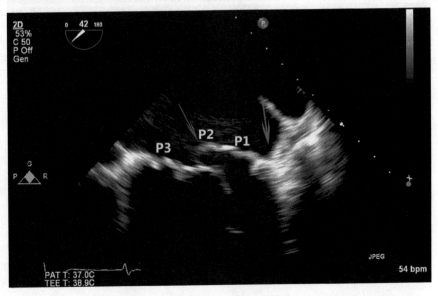

Fig. 1.60 TEE short-axis view when LAA is closed (*green arrow*) reveals P1, P2, and P3, rupture of P2 is evident in this view (*pink arrow*)

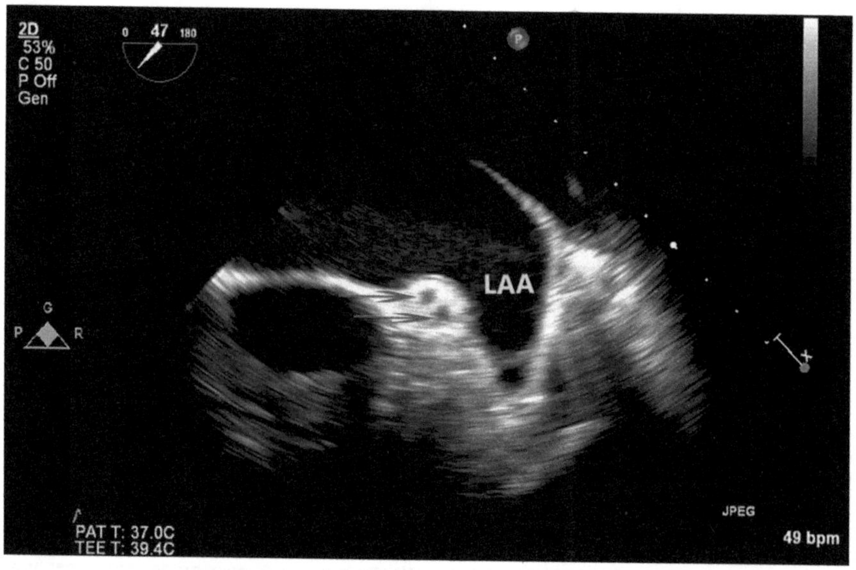

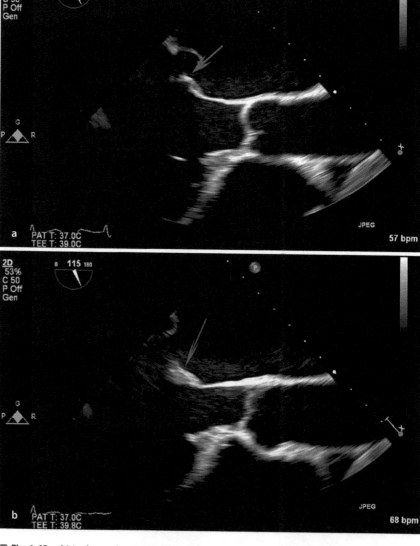

Fig. 1.61 TEE short-axis view reveals LAA and LCX (*green arrow*) and great cardiac vein (*pink arrow*)

Fig. 1.62 A2 is also prolaptic (*arrow*) **a** and thick (*arrow*) **b** in TEE long-axis view

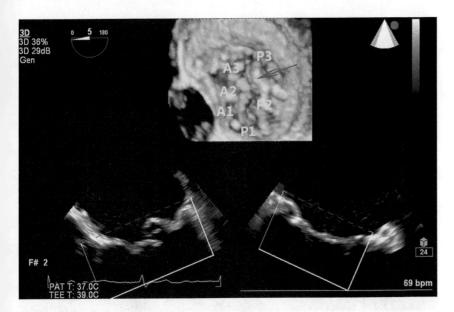

☐ **Fig. 1.63** Rupture of chorda of P2 (*arrow*) and prolapse of P2 are evident by 3D zoom with i-crop, P2 is thick, P3, A2, and A3 are also prolaptic

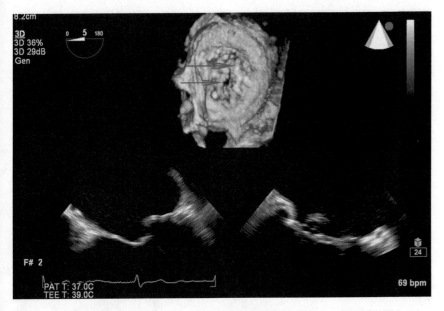

☐ **Fig. 1.64** Rupture of chorda of P2 (*green arrow*) is evident by 3D zoom, mitral valve is open in systole (*pink arrow*)

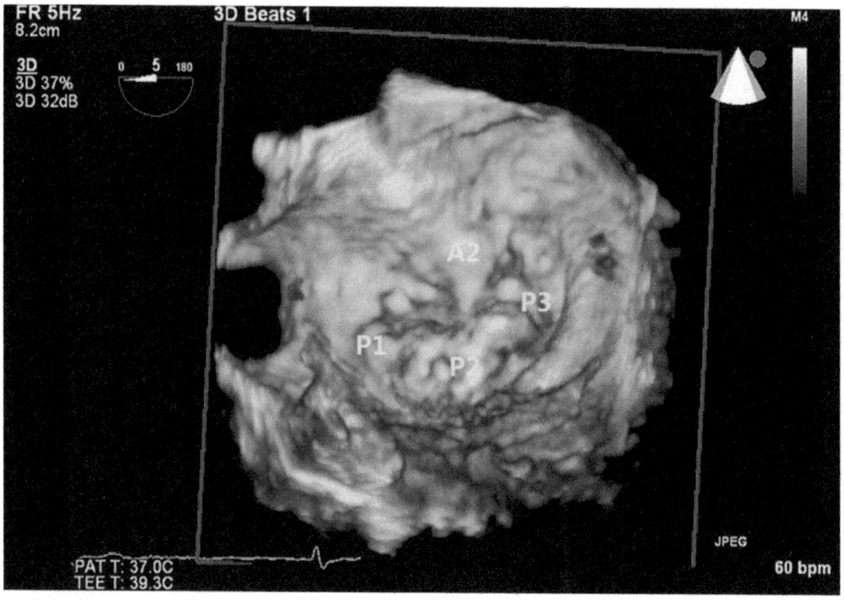

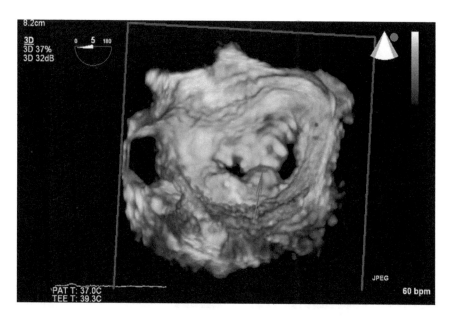

■ **Fig. 1.65**   Prolapse of P2 extends toward P1 and P3, A2 is also prolaptic

■ **Fig. 1.66**   P2 remains prolaptic even in diastole (*arrow*) by 3D zoom from LA

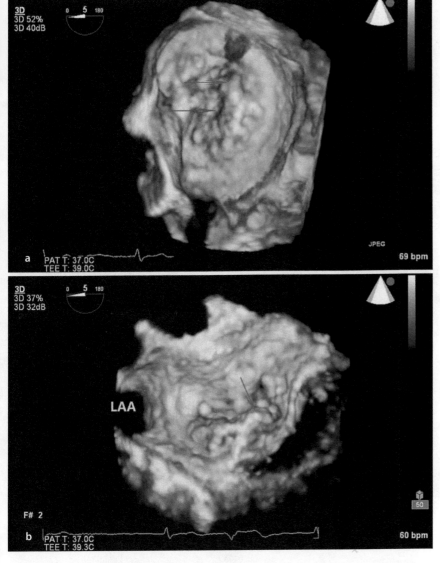

Fig. 1.67 Complete flail of P2 is evident by 3D zoom from LA side (*arrow*), besides, failure of coaptation of mitral leaflets in systole is evident in this view (*pink arrow*) **a**, head of ruptured chorda is fully evident by this view (*green arrow*) **a. a** Before Z rotation, all mitral valve scallops are prolaptic but P2 is flail (*green arrow*), **b**, 3D zoom of mitral valve from LA side after Z rotation, LAA is in 9 o'clock

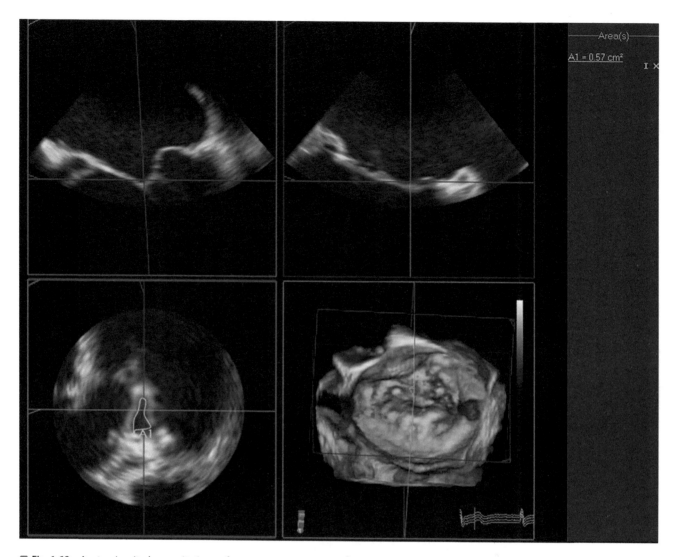

☐ Fig. 1.68   Anatomic mitral regurgitation surface area measures 0.57 cm² and has a relatively circular shape

Diagnosis   Severe MR due to rupture of chorda of P2 and Barlow disease.

Comment   MV repair with saddle-shaped ring annuloplasty.

Significant asymmetry of vena contracta area in functional MR occurs compared with organic MR [15].

Anatomic mitral regurgitation surface area more than 25 mm² can differentiate moderately severe MR and ≥40 mm² suggestive for severe MR, LA views provide more accuracy for measurement compared to LV views [16].

1.8   Case 7: Barlow Disease, Severe Mitral Regurgitation, Elongation of Chorda of P2

A 34-year-old man presented with dyspnea on exertion functional class II of recent 1 year.

Transthoracic echocardiography shows moderate left ventricular dilation, LVEDD = 64 mm, LVEDV = 190 cm^3, LVEDS = 42 mm LVESV = 77 cm^3, LVEF = 56% by 4D, moderate TR with PAPs = 40 mmHg, upper limit of normal RV size and normal systolic function.

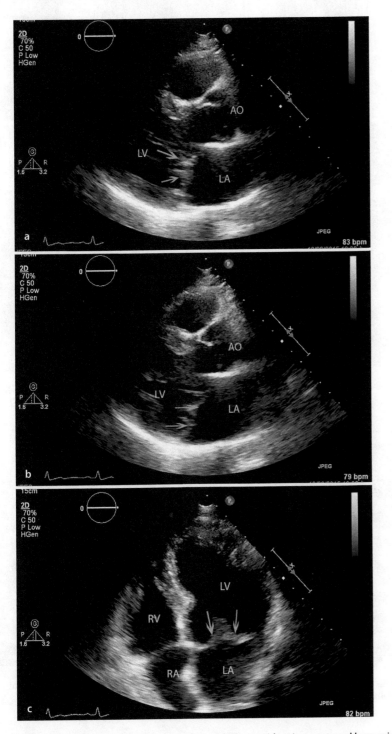

◘ Fig. 1.69 Prolapse and severe thickening of A2 and P2 are evident in parasternal long-axis view (*arrows*) **a**, **b** and apical 4C view **c**

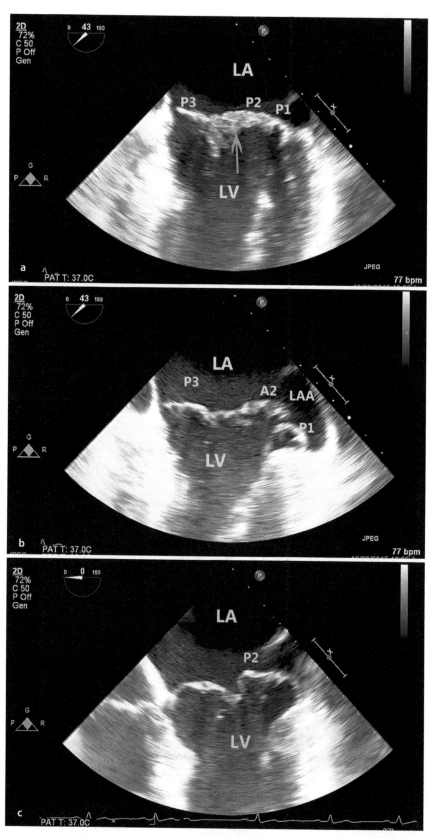

■ Fig. 1.70   Prolapse of P1 and P2 and A2 is evident in TEE short-axis view (*arrow*) **a**, **b**, but prolapse of P2 is more evident (TEE 0° view) **c**

Lesson   When LAA is not open in TEE short-axis view, the mitral scallops are P1, P2, and P3 but when the LAA is open in TEE short-axis view, the mitral scallops are P1, A2, and P3 due to anterior position of A2 and posterior position of P2.

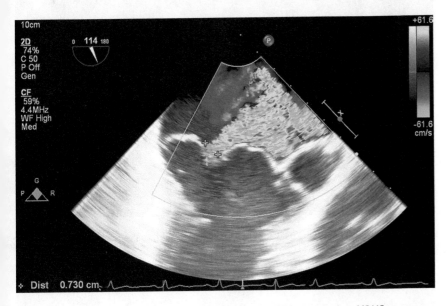

◘ **Fig. 1.71**   Severe eccentric MR toward IAS is evident by TEE long-axis view, MR VC measures 7.3 mm

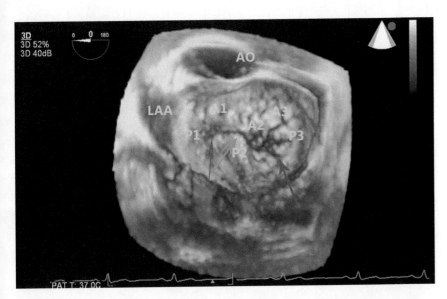

◘ **Fig. 1.72**   The main mechanism of MR is prolapse of P2 (*green arrow*), indentation between P2 and P3 (*red arrow*) is evident by 3D zoom from LA side (gain about 57%), indentation between P1 and P2 is shown by *pink arrow*

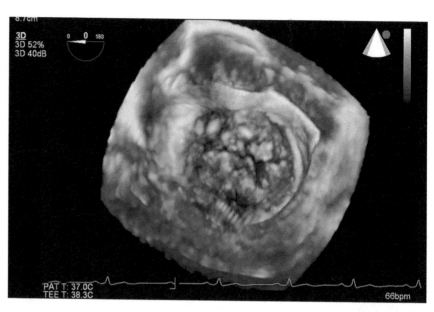

▫ Fig. 1.73   With lowering the gain about 50, the image of mitral valve is not interpretable

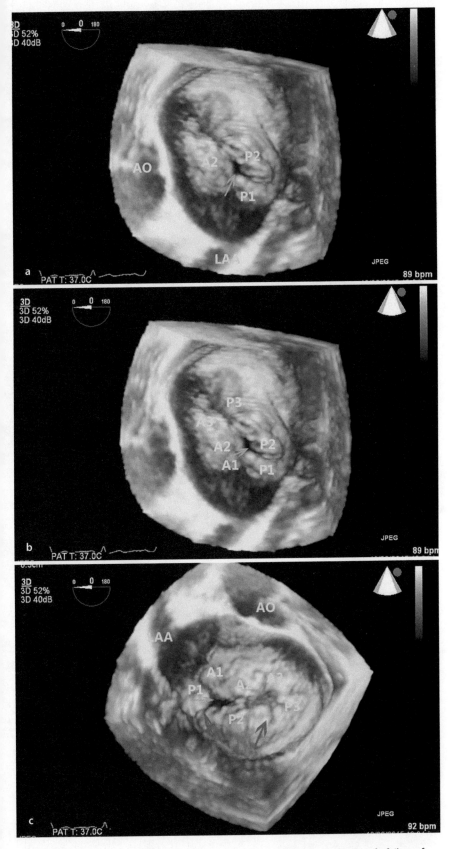

☐ **Fig. 1.74** P2 is more prolaptic by 3D zoom but A2 and P1 are also prolaptic **a**, **b**, failure of coaptation of MV leaflets in systole is also evident (*green arrows*) **a**, **b**, *red and pink arrows* **c** refers to the indentation between P1 and P2 and P2 and P3

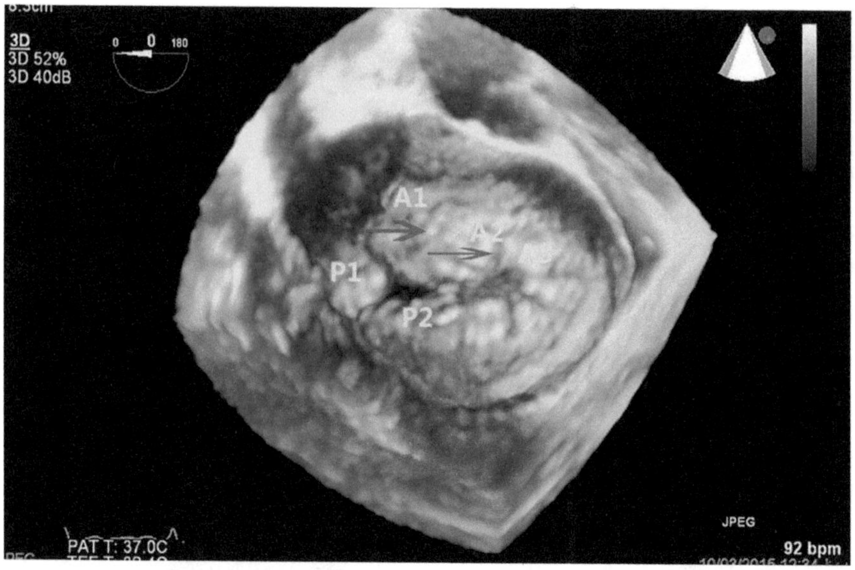

■ **Fig. 1.75**   The indentation between A1 and A2 and A3 is evident by *pink arrows*, failure of coaptation of mitral valve leaflets also lies between P1 and P2 and anterior mitral leaflet

1.8 · Case 7: Barlow Disease, Severe Mitral Regurgitation, Elongation of Chorda of P2

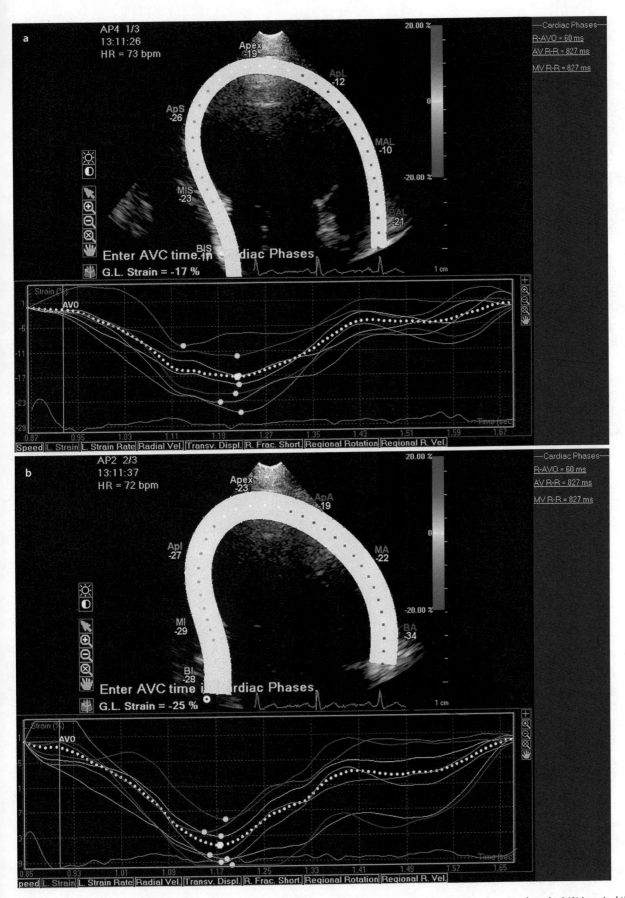

Fig. 1.76 Longitudinal strain is equal to −17% in apical four-chamber view **a**, −25% in apical two-chamber view **b** and −24% in apical three-chamber view **c**. Global longitudinal strain measures −21% **d**

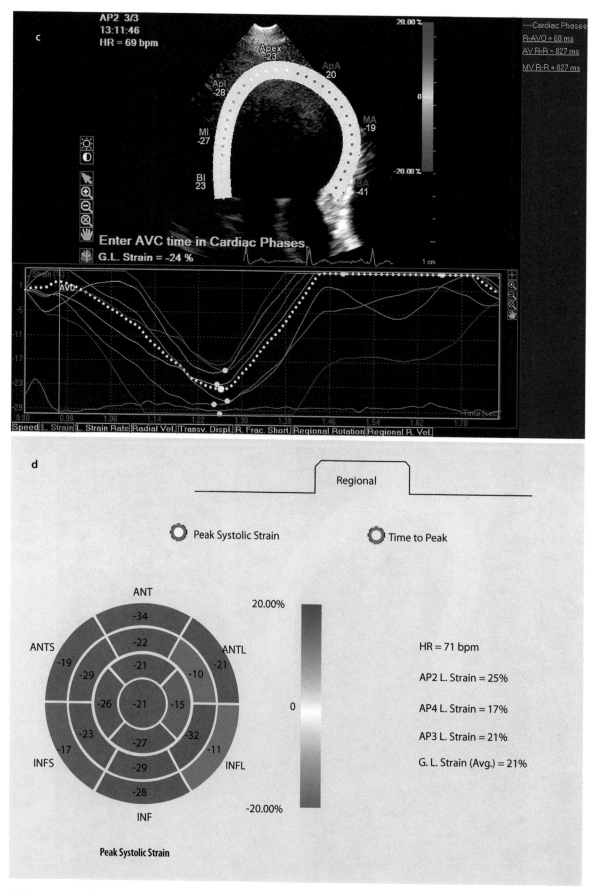

■ **Fig. 1.76**   (continued)

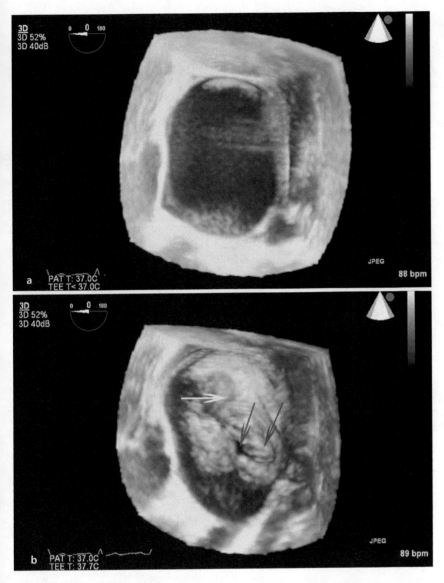

□ **Fig. 1.77** 3D zoom of mitral valve before lowering the gain **a** and after lowering the gain **b**, prolapse of P2 (*green arrow*) and failure of coaptation of MV leaflets (*red arrow*) and some stitch effect (*yellow arrow*) are evident in this view

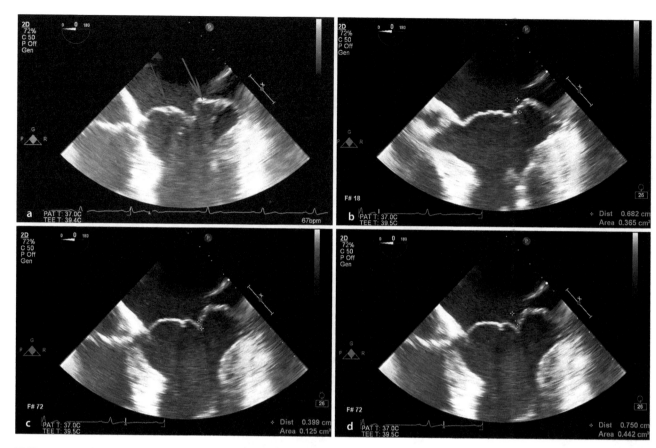

☐ **Fig. 1.78** Prolapse of A2 and P2 is evident by TEE 0° view **a**, flail gap measures 6.8 mm **b**, zona coapta measures 4 mm **c** and coaptation depth measures 7.5 mm in this view **d**

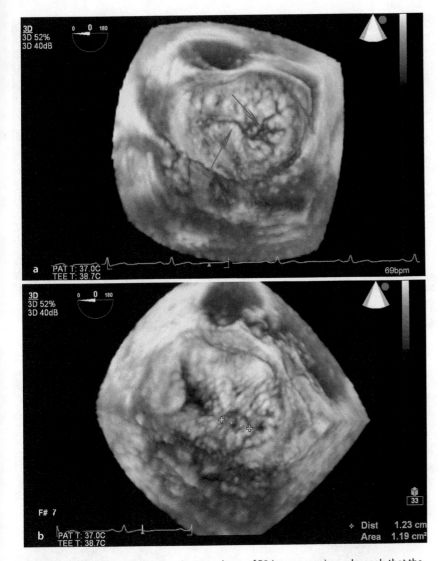

Fig. 1.79 3D zoom of mitral valve shows prolapse of P2 (*green arrow*) **a** and reveals that the most coaptation failure is between P3 and AMVL (*pink arrow*) **a**, coaptation width measures 12.3 mm in this view **b**

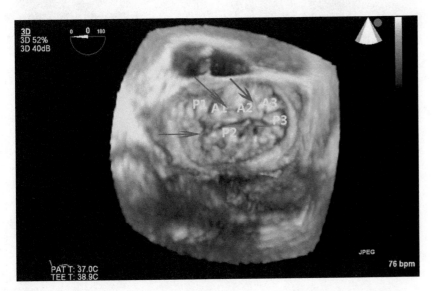

Fig. 1.80 Mitral valve scallops with indentations (*arrows*) between them are visualized in this 3D zoom view

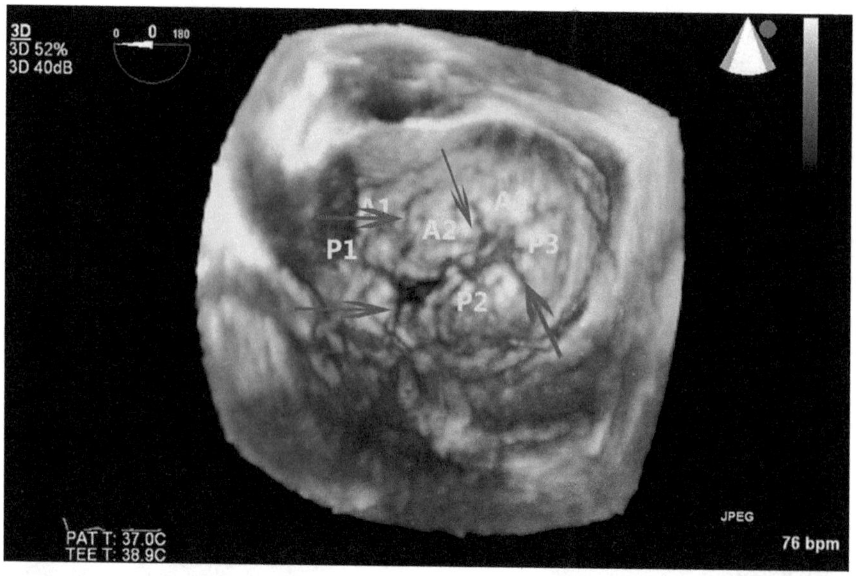

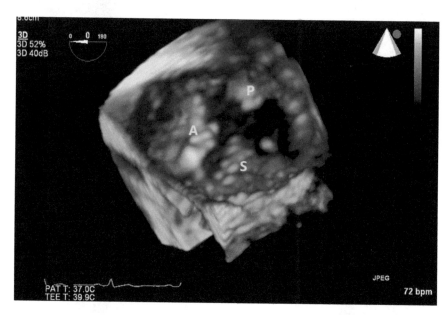

Fig. 1.81 The indentations between anterior mitral scallops are shown by *pink arrows* and the indentation between posterior mitral leaflets is marked by *green arrows*

Fig. 1.82 The anterior **a**, septal (S) and posterior (P) tricuspid leaflets are shown from RA side by 3D zoom of tricuspid valve

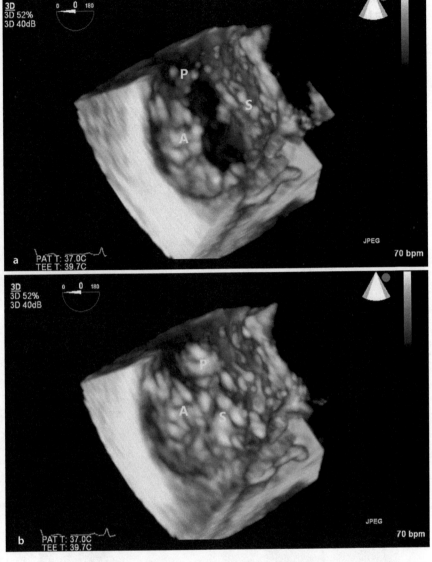

◘ Fig. 1.83 The anterior tricuspid leaflet is a large leaflet and has a major role in systolic coaptation of tricuspid valve **a** and **b**, 3D zoom of tricuspid valve from right atrial side by TEE, **a**, early systole, **b**, midsystole A, anterior; S, septal and P, posterior tricuspid leaflets

Diagnosis Severe eccentric MR due to Barlow disease, main mechanism is prolapse of P2 and elongation of chorda of P2.

Comment The patient referred for surgery (MV repair).

Lessons
1. Mitraclip is class IIb for this patient.
2. Barlow disease affects more commonly young persons with involvement of more scallops.
3. Global longitudinal strain is within normal limits in this patient, although global LVEF is 56% and mildly impaired.
4. In Barlow disease, use of saddle-shaped ring annuloplasty or partial rings instead of complete or more flexible rings is recommended [4].

1.9   Case 8: Barlow Disease, Rupture of Chorda of Lateral Side of P2 (Between P1 and P2), Prolapse P1, P2, P3, and A2

A 56-year-old man presented with dyspnea on exertion functional class III of two months duration.

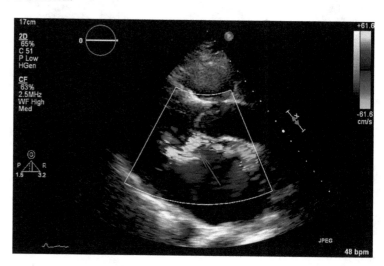

Fig. 1.84 Severe eccentric mitral regurgitation toward inter-atrial septum is evident in parasternal long-axis view (*arrow*)

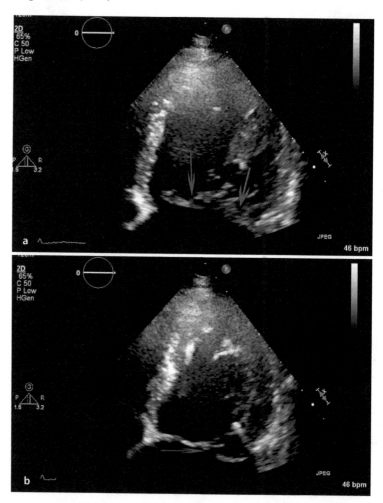

Fig. 1.85 Both mitral leaflets are thick and prolaptic in apical four-chamber view (*arrows*) **a**, Rupture of chorda of PMVL is evident by apical four-chamber view (*arrow*) **b**

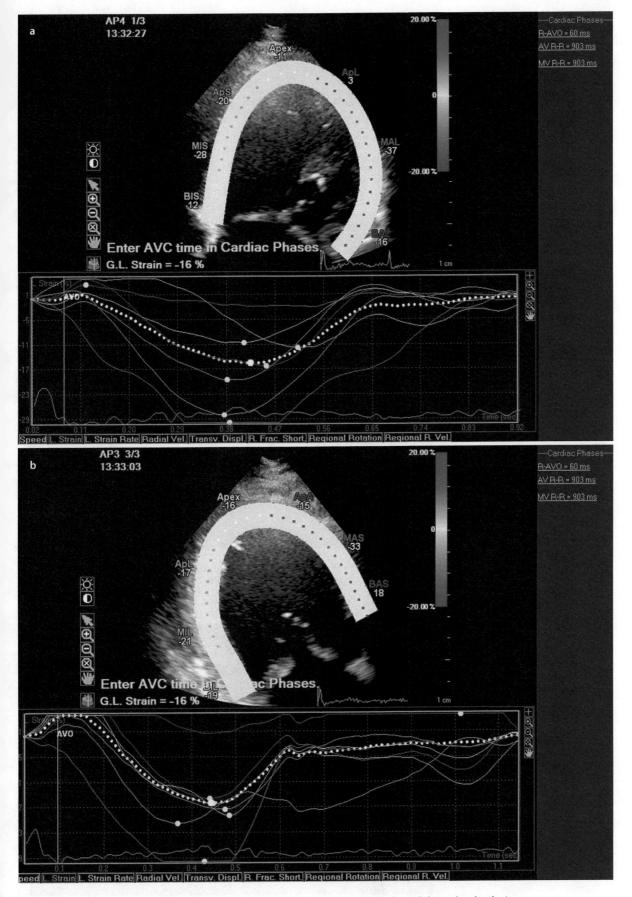

■ **Fig. 1.86** Global longitudinal strain measures −16% in apical four-chamber **a** and apical three-chamber **b** views

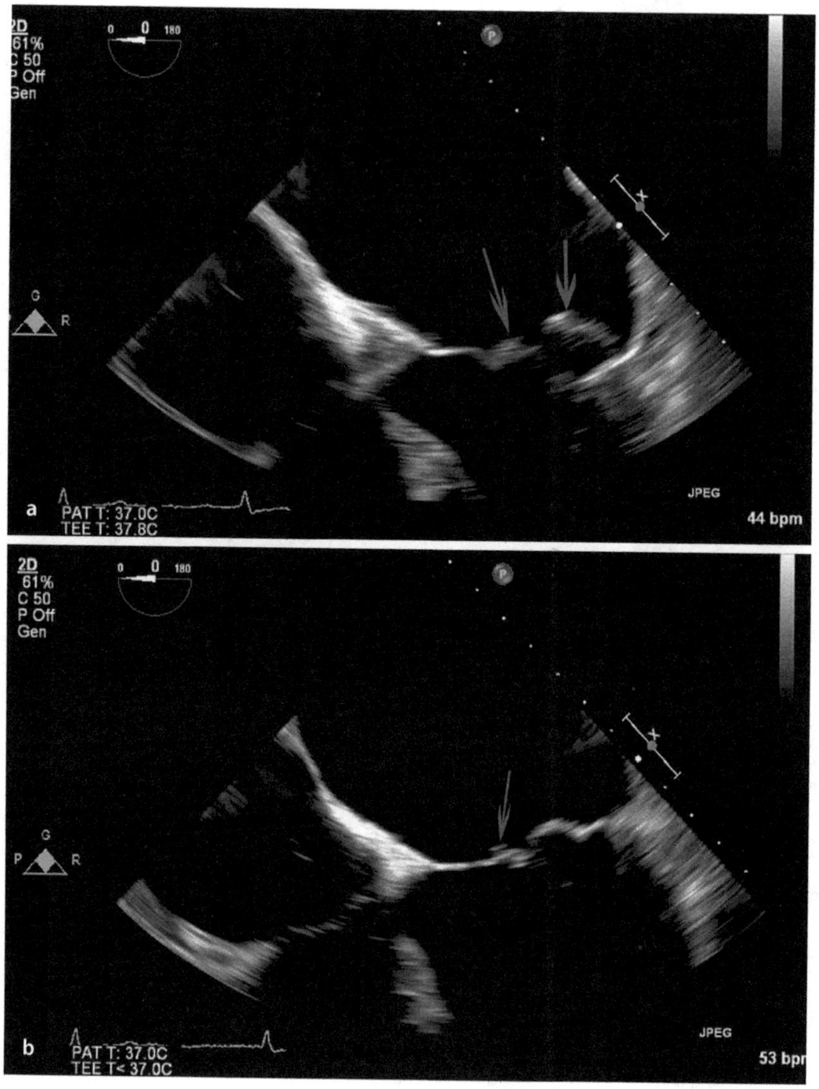

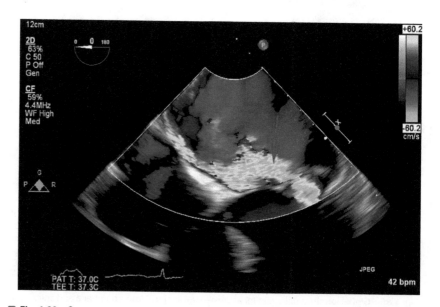

Fig. 1.87   Prolapse of A2 and P2 is evident by this TEE 0° view (*arrows*) **a**, rupture of chorda of PMVL is evident by TEE 0° (*arrow*) **b**

Fig. 1.88   Severe eccentric MR toward inter-atrial septum is evident by TEE 0° view (*arrow*)

1.9 · Case 8: Barlow Disease, Rupture of Chorda of Lateral Side of P2 (Between P1 and P2), Prolapse P1, P2, P3, and A2

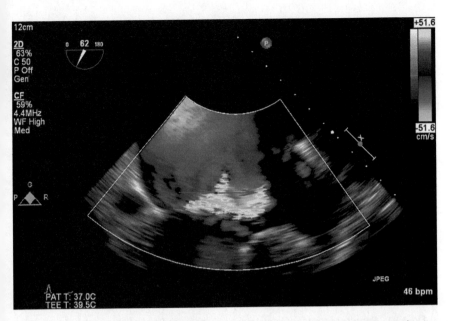

🔲 **Fig. 1.89** Severe MR is evident by TEE short-axis view, there are two jets of MR (*arrows*)

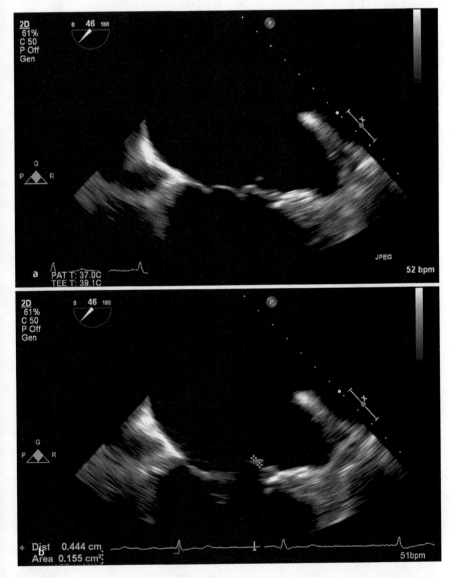

🔲 **Fig. 1.90** TEE short-axis view reveals head of chordal rupture (*arrow*) **a**, this mass measures 4.4 mm in this view **b**

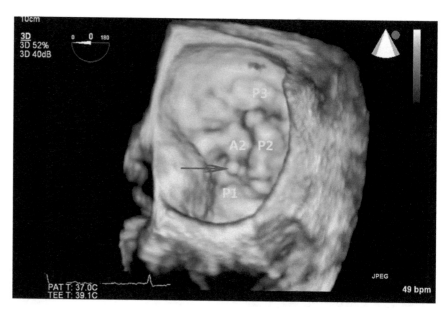

■ **Fig. 1.91**   Rupture of chorda of lateral side of P2 (between P1 and P2) (*arrow*) and prolapse of all posterior mitral leaflet scallops and A2 are evident by 3D zoom from LA side

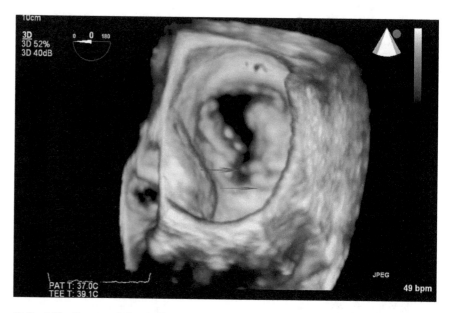

■ **Fig. 1.92**   Rupture of chorda of P2 (*green arrow*) (near P1) is evident by 3D zoom from LA side, indentation between P1 and P2 is shown by *pink arrow*

1.9 · Case 8: Barlow Disease, Rupture of Chorda of Lateral Side of P2 (Between P1 and P2), Prolapse P1, P2, P3, and A2

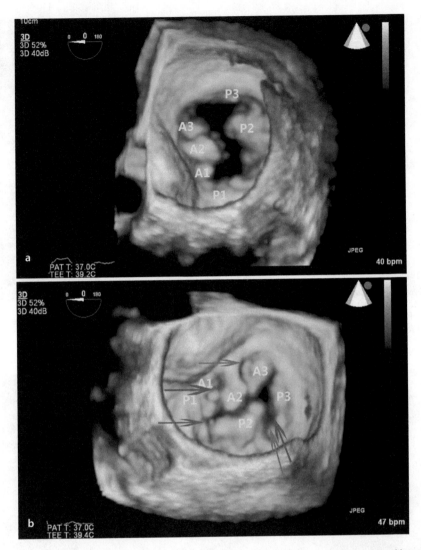

☐ **Fig. 1.93** The three scallops of anterior and posterior mitral leaflets are fully visualized by 3D zoom of mitral valve in diastole **a**, indentation between anterior mitral leaflet scallops is shown by *pink arrow* and between posterior mitral leaflets is shown by *green arrow*, indentation between P2 and P3 (*double green arrow*) is like a cleft (pseudocleft) **b**

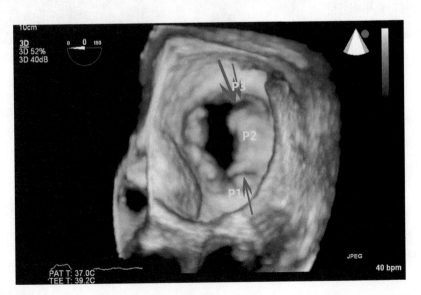

☐ **Fig. 1.94** The indentation between P1 and P2 is marked by a *green arrow* and between P2 and P3 by *double green arrow* and is like a cleft (pseudocleft)

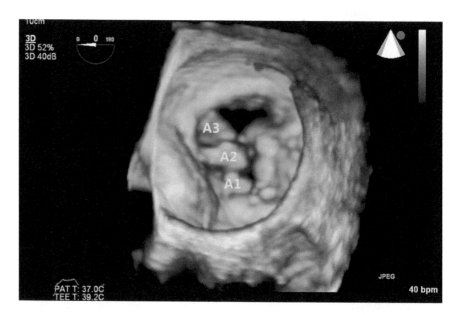

Fig. 1.95 Three anterior mitral leaflet scallops are fully visualized by 3D zoom from LA side before Z rotation

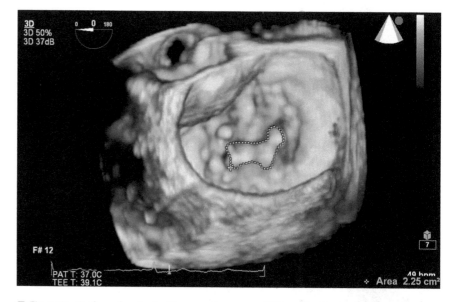

Fig. 1.96 Surface of prolaptic P2 segment measures 2.25 cm² by direct planimetry

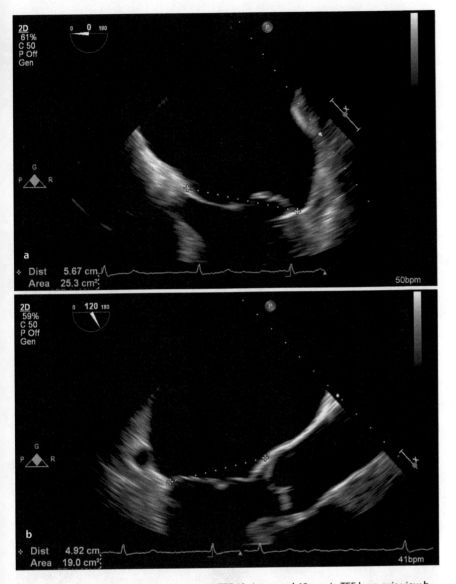

■ Fig. 1.97   MV annulus measures 57 mm in TEE 0° view **a** and 49 mm in TEE long-axis view **b**

Diagnosis   Barlow disease, prolapse of A2 and all posterior mitral leaflet scallops and rupture of chorda of P2.

Comment   Surgery, MV repair.

1.10   Case 9: Barlow Disease, P2 Rupture, Severe MR

A 34-year-old woman presented with dyspnea on exertion functional class III of recent duration.

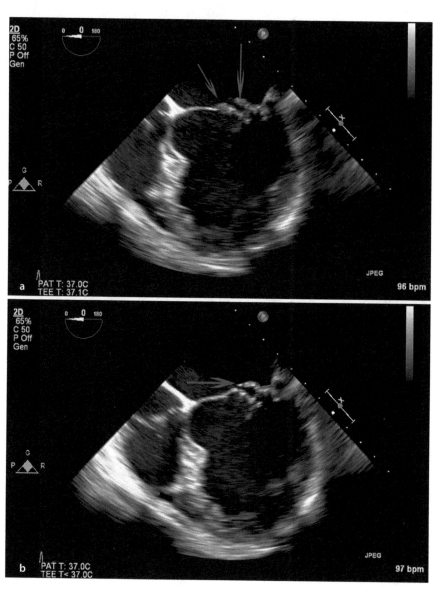

☐ **Fig. 1.98**   Prolapse of A2 and P2 and rupture of chorda of P2 are evident by TEE 0° views (*arrows*) **a, b**

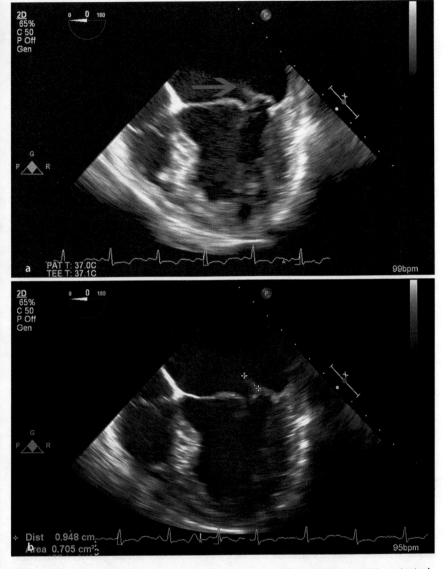

Fig. 1.99 There is a mobile mass on atrial side of P2 (*arrow*) **a**, this mass measures 9.5 mm in size **b**

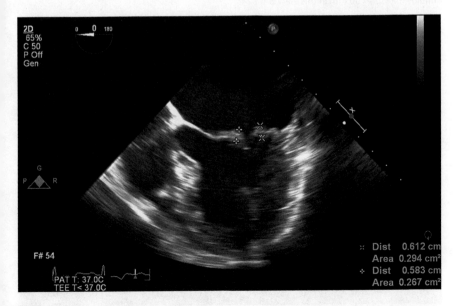

Fig. 1.100 Both mitral leaflets are thick, anterior and posterior mitral leaflets thickness measure 6 and 6 mm in TEE 0° view, respectively

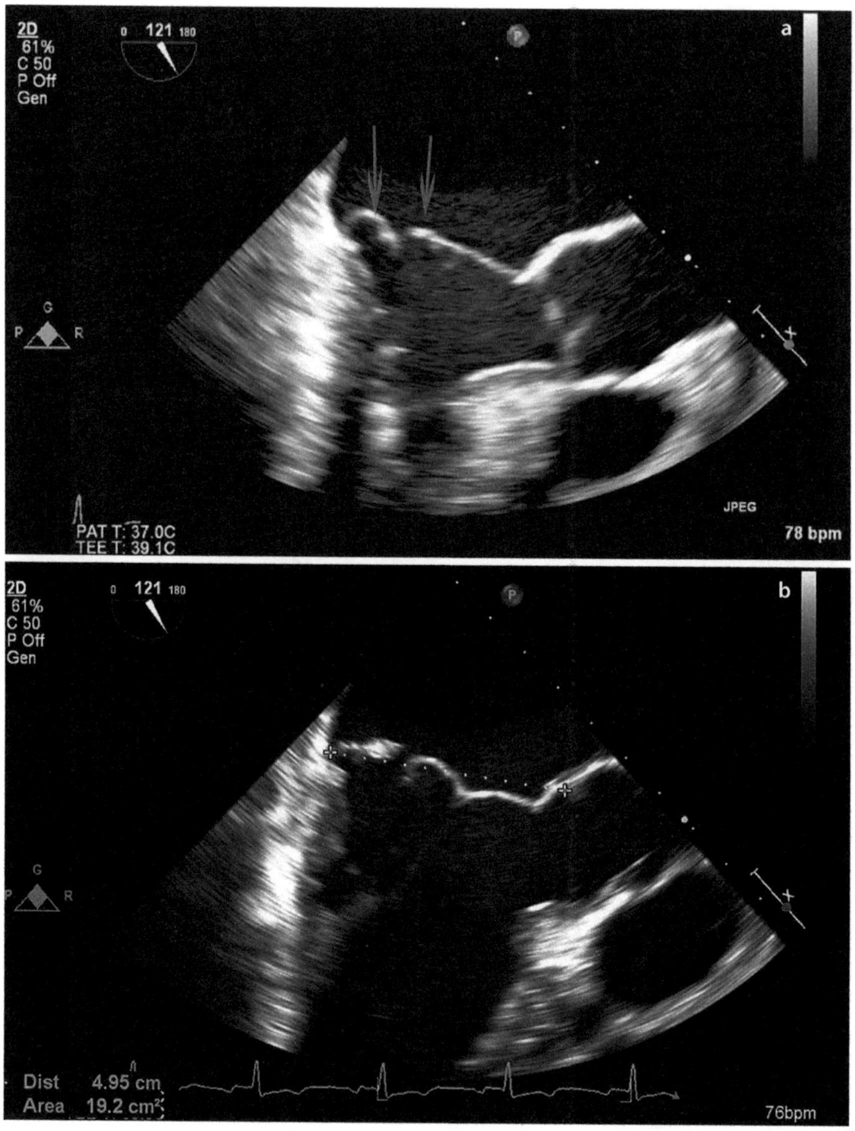

Fig. 1.101 Prolapse of P2 and A2 is evident in TEE long-axis view (*arrow*) **a**. Mitral valve annulus measures 50 mm in this view **b**

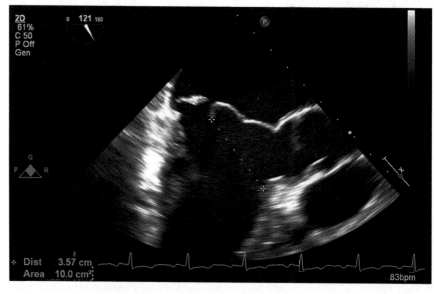

Fig. 1.102 C-Sept measures 36 mm in this TEE long-axis view

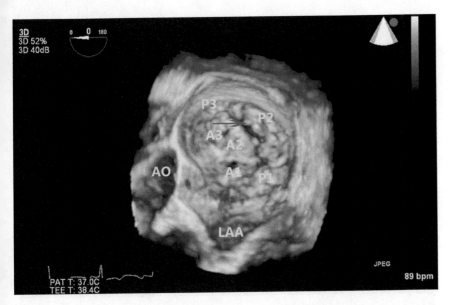

◧ **Fig. 1.103** All MV scallops are evident in this 4-dimensional echocardiography, P1, P2 and P3 and A2 are prolaptic, rupture of chorda of P2 is also evident in this view (*arrow*). *AO* aorta, *LAA* left atrial appendage

This view is a 3D zoom of mitral valve from LA side by TEE before Z rotation, LAA is in 6 o'clock and aortic valve is in 9 o'clock.

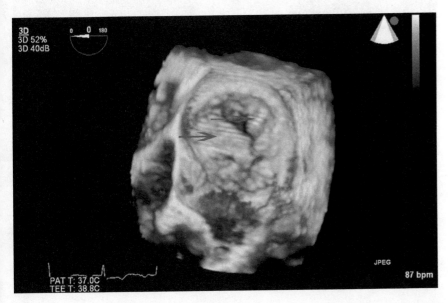

◧ **Fig. 1.104** Stitch effect is seen in this view (*arrow*), it can be resolved by holding the breath

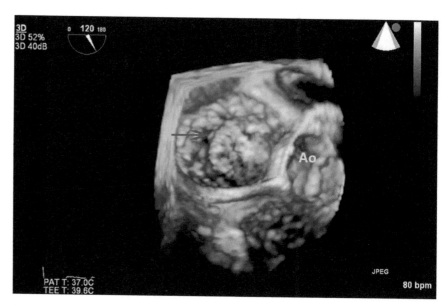

Fig. 1.105 Rupture of P2 is evident by this view (*arrow*), this view is a 3D zoom of mitral valve in 120° view from LA side, aortic valve is in 3 o'clock. *AO*, aortic valve

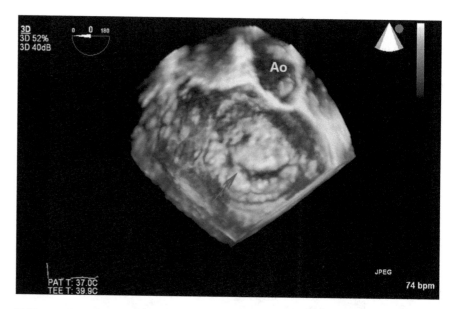

Fig. 1.106 Prolapse of nearly all MV scallops and rupture of chorda of P2 are visible in this view in favor of Barlow disease, 3D zoom of mitral valve from LA, aortic valve is positioned in 12 o'clock. *AO* aortic valve

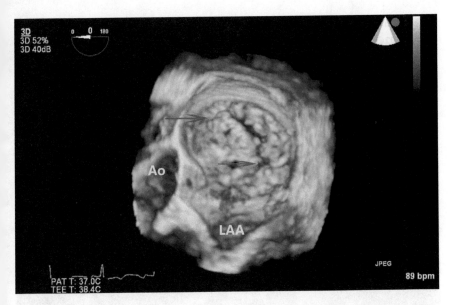

□ **Fig. 1.107** Anterior (*green arrow*) and posterior (*pink arrow*) commissures are shown in 3D zoom from LA side. *LAA* left atrial appendage, *AO* aortic valve

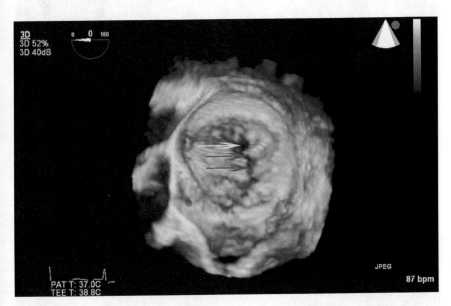

□ **Fig. 1.108** Prolapse and rupture of P2 is fully visualized by 3D zoom (*green arrow*), failure of coaptation of mitral valve leaflets in systole is evident in nearly all mitral valve scallops (*pink arrow*), pseudocleft (*yellow arrow*) is shown between P2 and P3

Diagnosis   Barlow disease and rupture of chorda of P2 producing severe MR.

Comment   Surgery (mitral valve repair).

1.11 Case 10: Barlow Disease, Severe Mitral Regurgitation, and Rupture of Chorda of A2 and A3

A 55-year-old man presented with dyspnea on exertion functional class III of 3 months duration. Transthoracic echocardiography revealed mild left ventricular dilation and lower limit of normal LV systolic function (LVEDd = 60 mm, LVESd = 43 mm, LVEF = 55%, PAPs = 40 mmHg).

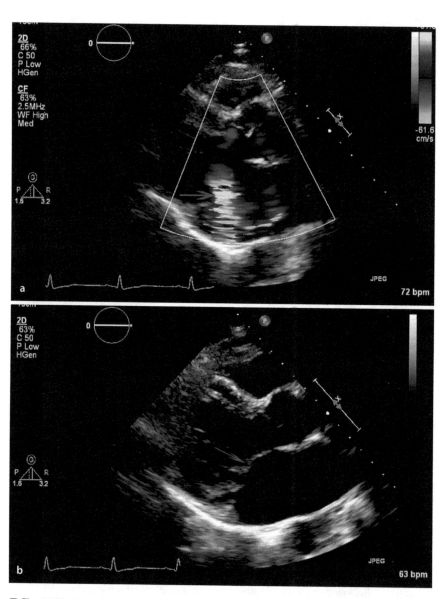

□ **Fig. 1.109**   Parasternal long-axis view shows severe eccentric mitral regurgitation (*arrow*) toward posterior wall **a**, although both mitral leaflets are thick and prolaptic (*arrows*) **b** in this view, but the main mechanism of mitral regurgitation is prolapse of A2, because the regurgitation jet is toward posterior wall

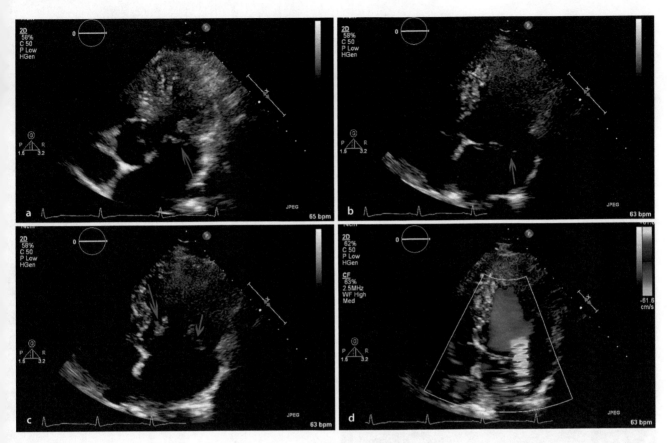

□ Fig. 1.110 Complete flail of anterior mitral leaflet (A2) is evident in apical four-chamber views (*arrows*) **a**, **b**, severe thickening of mitral leaflets is evident in this view (*arrows*) **c**, mitral regurgitation is eccentric toward lateral wall (*arrow*) **d**

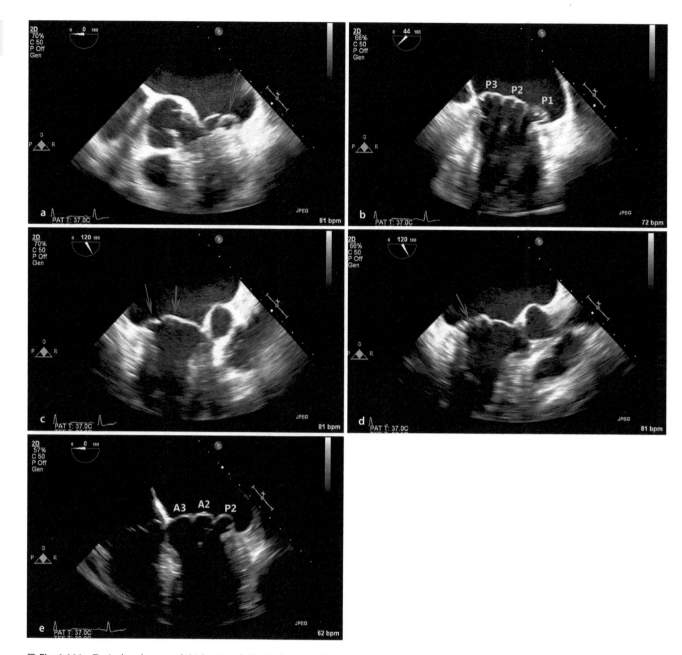

◘ Fig. 1.111   Typical prolapse and thickening of all mitral valve scallops are evident in TEE 0° view **a**, short-axis view **b** and long-axis view **c**, head of ruptured chorda on A2 is evident in TEE long-axis view (*arrow*) **d**, prolapse od P2, A2, and A3 is evident in TEE 0° view **e**

It is of notice that when LAA is closed in TEE short-axis view, the scallops will be P1, P2, and P3.

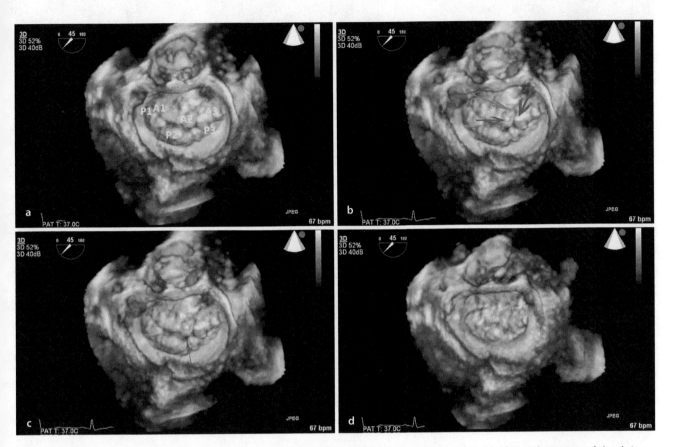

◨ **Fig. 1.112** Prolapse of nearly all mitral valve scallops is evident by 3D zoom of mitral valve from left atrial side in 45° **a**, rupture of chorda is evident in A2 and A3 scallops (*green arrows*) **b**, the indentation between A2 and A3 is marked by a *pink arrow* **b**, failure of coaptation of mitral scallops is more prominent in late systole (*green arrow*) **c** compared to mid systole **d**

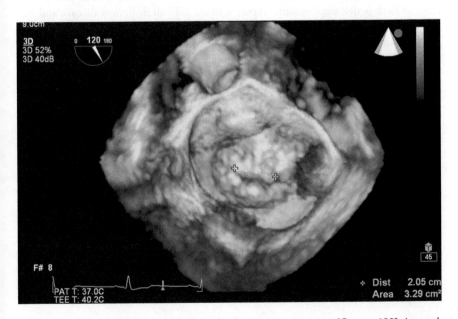

◨ **Fig. 1.113** Flail width measures 20.5 mm by direct measurement on 3D zoom 120° view and is too wide for Mitraclip

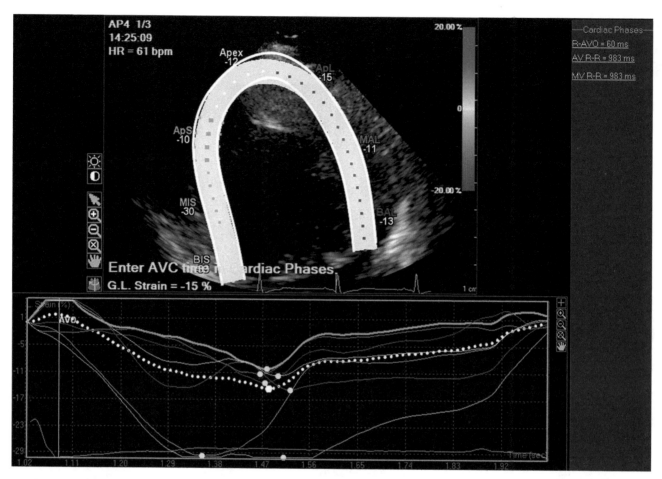

Fig. 1.114   Global longitudinal strain measures −15% in apical two-chamber view

Diagnosis   Severe eccentric mitral regurgitation due to Barlow disease and rupture of chorda of A2 and A3, nearly all mitral valve scallops are thickened and prolaptic in favor of Barlow disease. Although repair is more difficult in Barlow disease and A2, A3 prolapse and rupture, but with respect to patients' symptoms and LVEF = 55% and low values of global longitudinal strain, the patient referred for surgery (mitral valve repair with saddle-shaped ring annuloplasty.

1.12 · Case 11: Severe Functional and Organic MR Due to Prolapse of A2 in a Post CABG Patient (Candidate for Mitraclip)

81

1

1.12 Case 11: Severe Functional and Organic MR Due to Prolapse of A2 in a Post CABG Patient (Candidate for Mitraclip)

A 79-year-old woman presented with dyspnea functional class IV. She underwent CABG 12 years ago. Transthoracic echocardiography showed LVEF about 45%, mild left ventricular dilation (LVEDD = 59 mm), severe organic and functional MR, severe TR and PAPs about 60 mmHg, severe RV systolic dysfunction, and workup for PTE was negative, creatinine = 1.6.

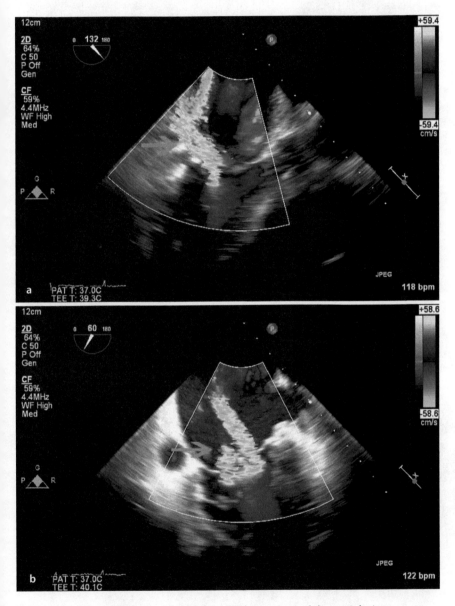

☐ **Fig. 1.115**   Severe MR (*arrows*) is evident by TEE long-axis **a** and short-axis **b** views

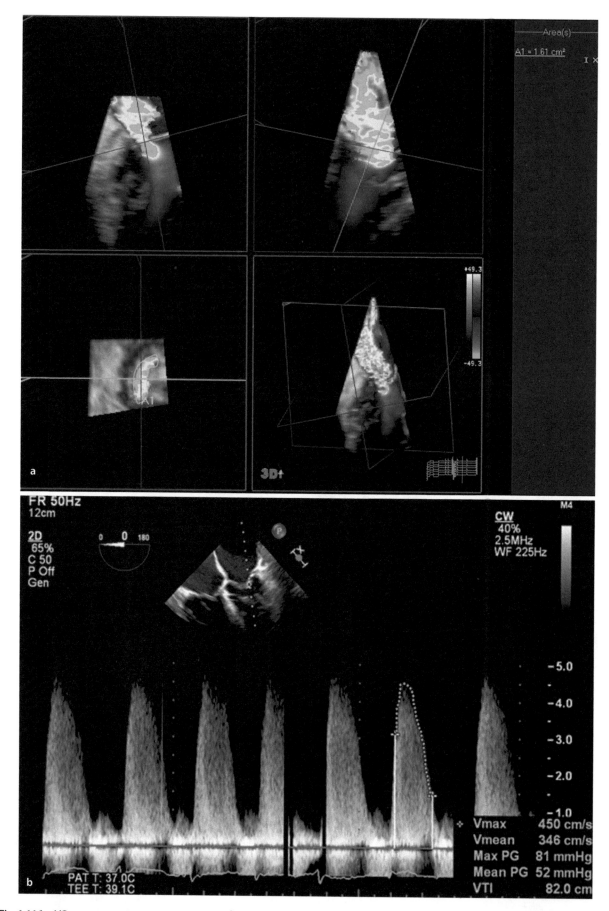

Fig. 1.116   MR vena contracta area measures 1.6 cm² by 3DQ full volume **a** and MR VTI is equal to 82 cm by continuous Doppler study **b**

MR volume is calculated as follows: MR vena contracta area multiply by MR VTI = 1.6*82 = 131 cm³ in favor of severe MR.

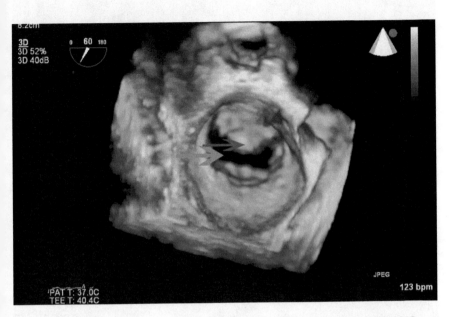

☐ **Fig. 1.117** Failure of coaptation of mitral valve leaflets in systole is evident in TEE 60° 3D zoom from LA side (*green arrow*), besides prolapse of A2 is completely evident in this view (*pink arrow*)

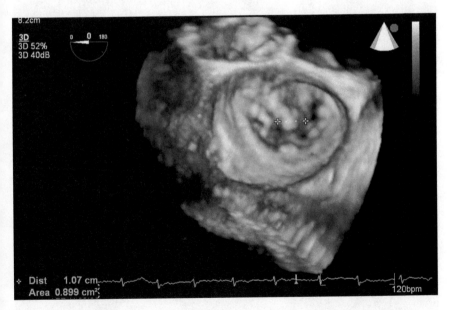

☐ **Fig. 1.118** Flail width measures 11 mm in TEE 0° by 3D zoom from LA side

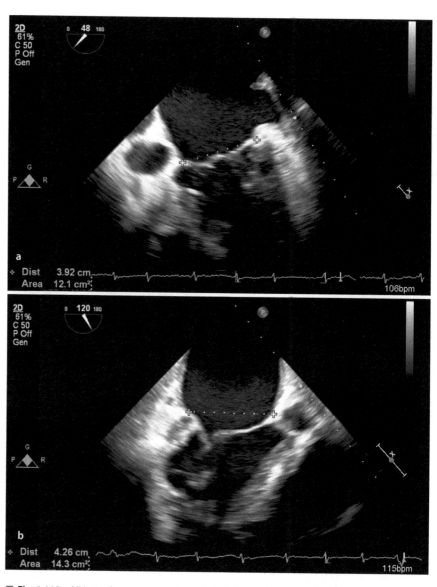

Fig. 1.119 MV annulus measures 39 mm in TEE short-axis view **a** and 43 mm in TEE long-axis view **b** and is dilated. MV annulus is measured in systole

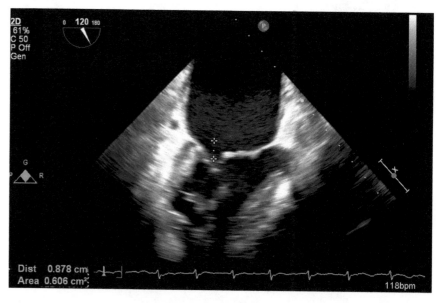

Fig. 1.120 Coaptation depth measures 9 mm in TEE long-axis view

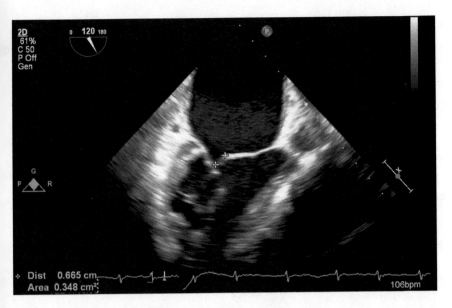

Fig. 1.121 flail gap measures 6.65 mm in TEE long-axis view

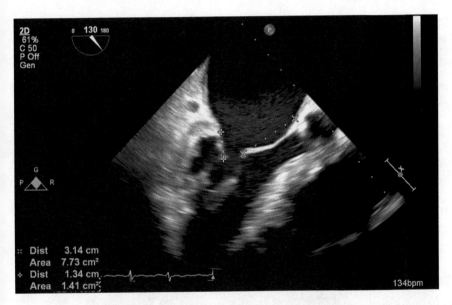

Fig. 1.122 AMVL length measures 31 mm and PMVL length measures 13 mm in TEE long-axis view

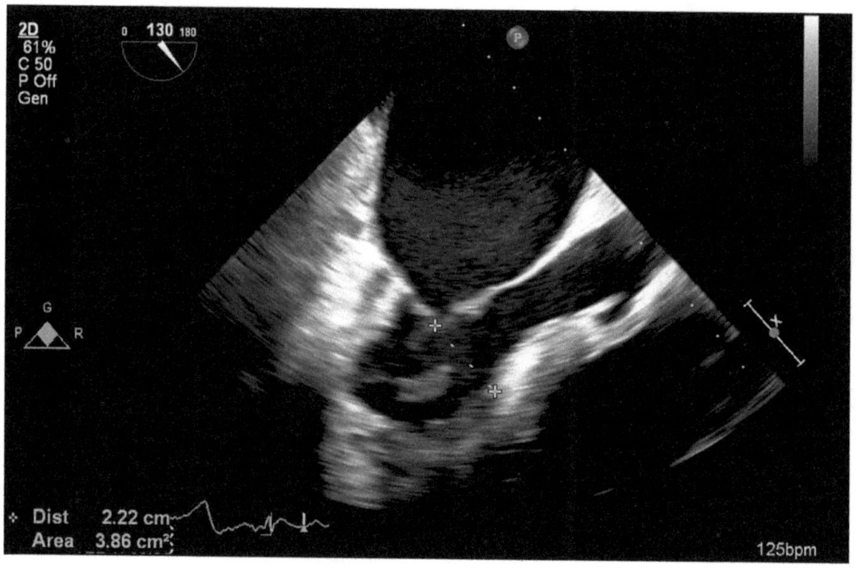

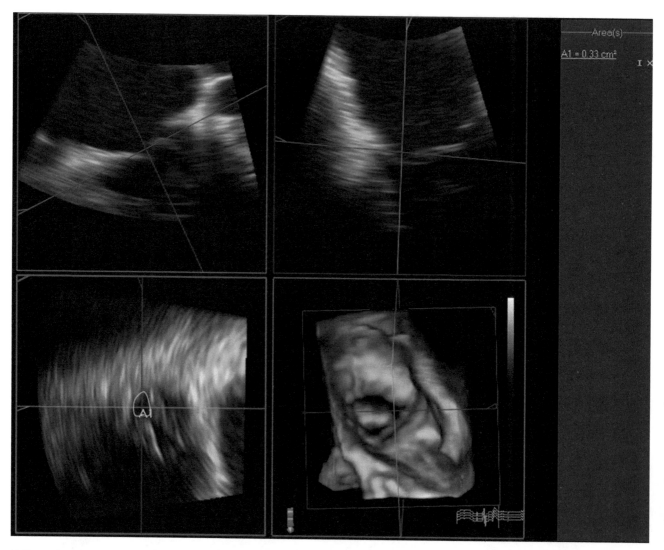

Fig. 1.123   C-sept measures 22 mm in TEE long-axis view

Fig. 1.124   Anatomic regurgitation area of MR measures 0.41 cm² by 3DQ method

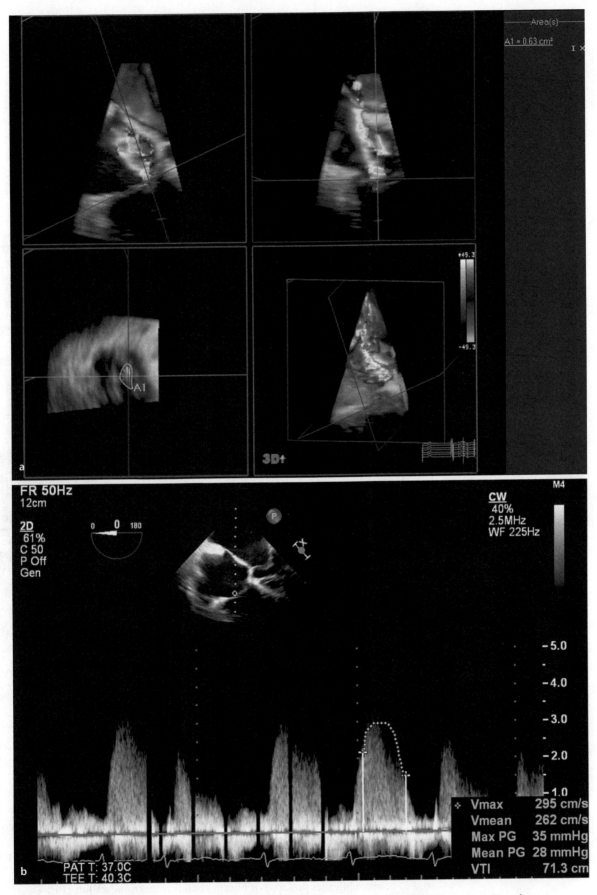

□ **Fig. 1.125** Tricuspid regurgitation vena contracta area measures 0.6 cm² by 3DQ method **a** and TR VTI measures 71 cm **b**

TR volume is calculated as follows: TR vena contracta area multiply by VTI = 0.6*71 = 42 cm³.

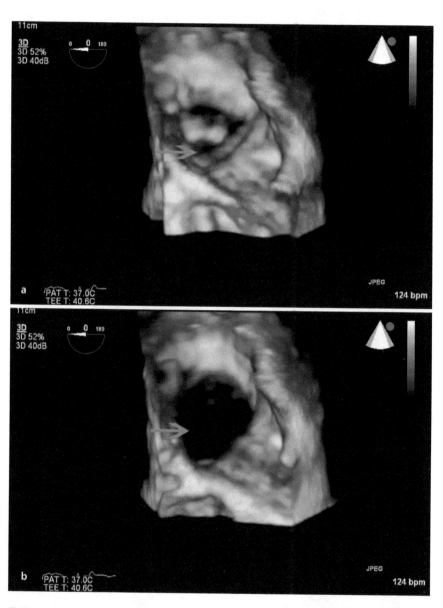

☐ **Fig. 1.126**   Failure of TV leaflet coaptation in systole is shown in TEE 0° view (*arrow*) **a**, TV is also shown in diastole (*arrow*) **b**. Failure of TV leaflet coaptation in systole is shown in TEE 0° view (*arrow*)

Diagnosis   Severe functional and organic MR due to prolapse of AMVL and senile degenerative changes and severe TR.

Comment   Mitraclip.

Lesson   Mitraclip is class IIb recommendation in severe primary MR, but when the surgical risk is high, it should be considered for the patient.

Flail gap should be ≤15 mm and flail width ≤10 mm, coaptation depth <11 mm and zona coapta >2 mm for Mitraclip.

Severe bileaflet prolapse or bileaflet flail is a contraindication [14].

1.13 Case 12: Severe MR Due to Fibroelastic Deficiency and Flail of A2

A 44-year-old man with a history of dyspnea on exertion and easy fatigability for 2 months duration, there was not any history of infection and trauma. In physical examination pan systolic murmur grade IV/VI was heard.

Transthoracic echocardiography revealed normal left ventricular size and function.

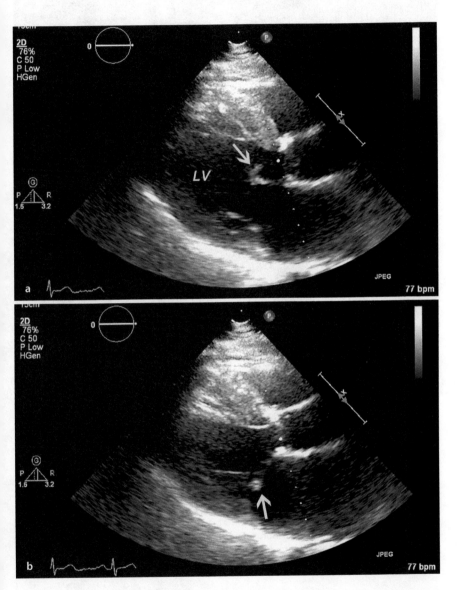

■ **Fig. 1.127** Parasternal long-axis view shows a mobile hyperechogenic mass with attachment to anterior mitral leaflet (**a**, diastole, *arrow*) and mal-coaptation of mitral valve leaflets depicts in systolic time (**b**, *arrow*)

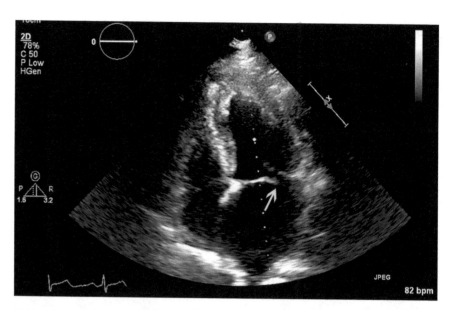

◘ Fig. 1.128 Apical four-chamber view demonstrates nonmyxomatous mitral structure and flail anterior mitral leaflet (*arrow*)

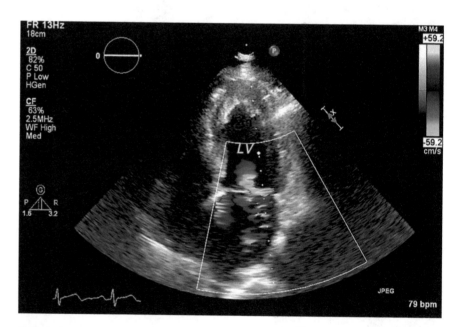

◘ Fig. 1.129 Color Doppler apical four-chamber view shows mitral regurgitation directed to lateral wall of left atrium that it seems highly eccentric

Transesophageal echocardiograph was performed for evaluation of mitral regurgitation severity and assessment of anterior mitral leaflet scallops.

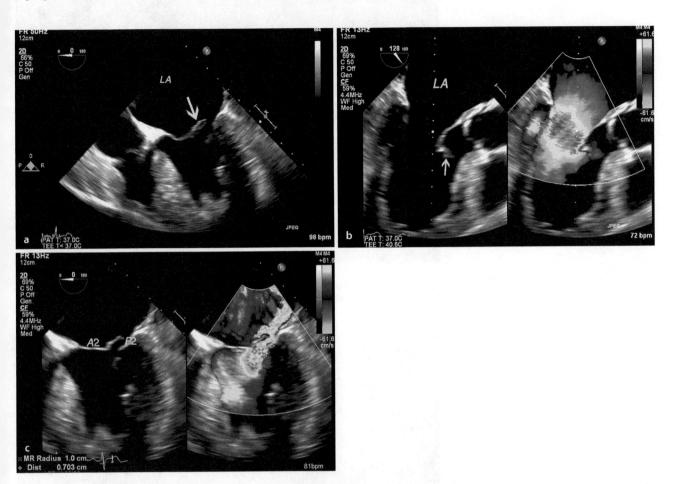

☐ **Fig. 1.130** Mild esophageal 0° view **a** and parasternal 120° view **b** depict flail of anterior mitral leaflet and attachment of a remnant ruptured chordae (*arrow*) to it at the level of A2 scallop **a** and there is not any coaptation between A2, P2 scallop in systolic time (*arrow*, **c**)

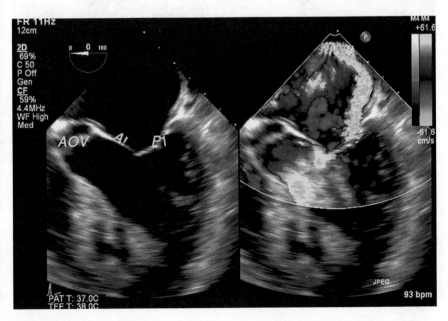

☐ **Fig. 1.131** Mid-esophageal 0° view with 1–2 cm withdrawal of probe depicts good coaptation of A1, P1

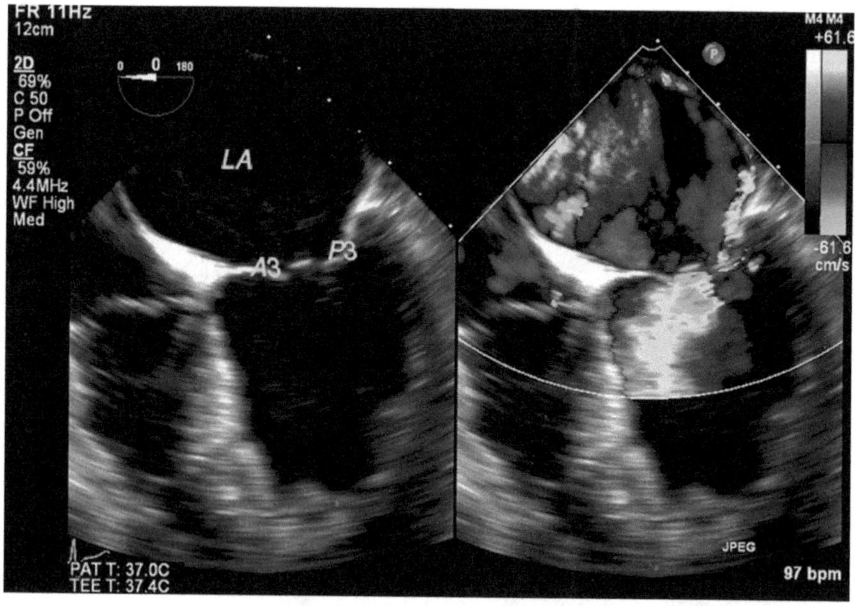

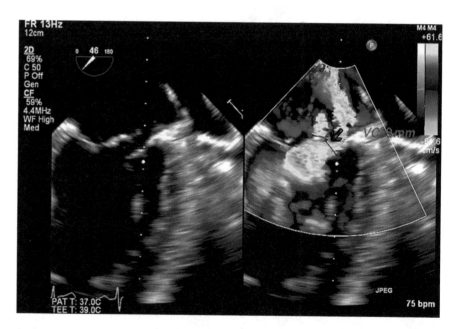

Fig. 1.132 Mid-esophageal 0° view with 1–2 cm advancement of probe in relation to standard view demonstrates good coaptation of A3, P3

Fig. 1.133 Color study shows vena contracta of mitral regurgitation is about 7 mm in favor of severe mitral regurgitation

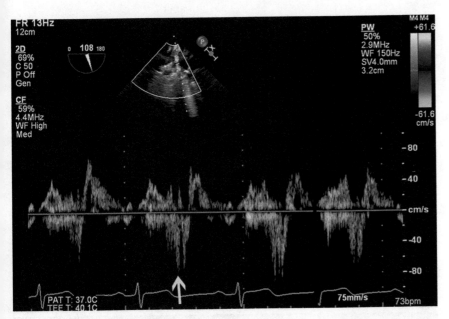

◻ **Fig. 1.134** Color Doppler flow study of left pulmonary veins shows systolic flow reversal in left pulmonary vein suggestive for severe mitral regurgitation

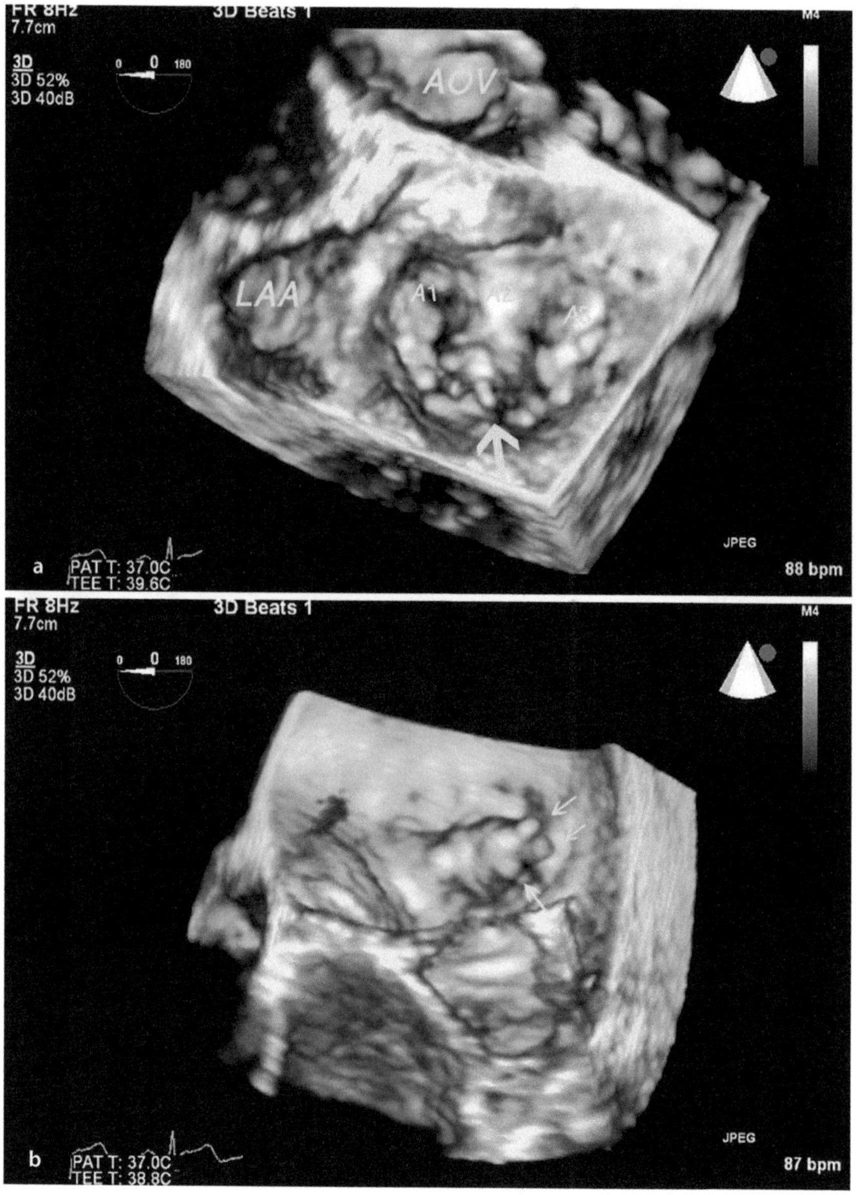

◘ Fig. 1.135 3D zoom view of mitral valve from left atrial side depicts flail of A2 scallop **a** with 3 remnant chordae attachment to it **b**

Diagnosis   Severe mitral regurgitation with flail A2 scallop due to fibroelastic deficiency (FED).

Recommendation   The patient referred for mitral valve repair.

1.14   Case 13: Severe MR Due to Barlow Disease

A 45-year-old woman with a history of easy fatigability and dyspnea on exertion (functional class III). Physical examination revealed pan systolic murmur in mitral area and other systolic murmur grade III in left sternal border.

Transthoracic echocardiography showed mild left ventricular dilation with normal systolic function.

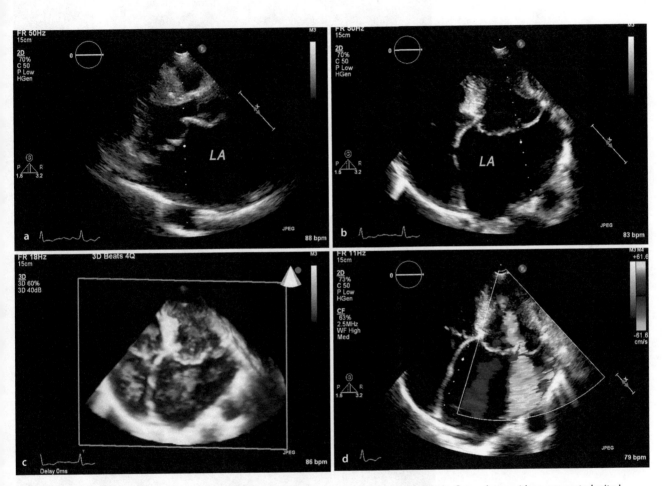

■ **Fig. 1.136**   Parasternal long-axis view **a** and apical four-chamber view 2D and 3D **b**, **c** reveal bi-leaflet prolapse with severe central mitral regurgitation **d** Transesophageal echocardiography was done for full evaluation of scallops

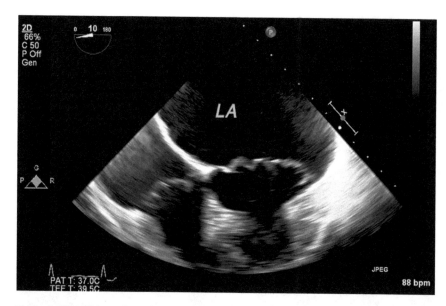

Fig. 1.137 Mid-esophageal 0° view depicts myxomatous mitral valve structure with prolapse of A2, P2 scallops

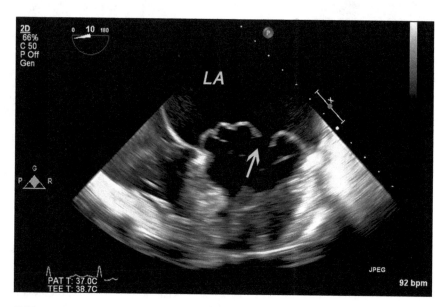

Fig. 1.138 Advancement of TEE probe reveals that A3, P3 scallops are prolaptic and there is a noncooptation point at the level of A3, P3 scallop (*arrow*) and tip of scallops are toward left ventricle in favor of partial flail of mitral valve due to elongation of mitral valve chordae

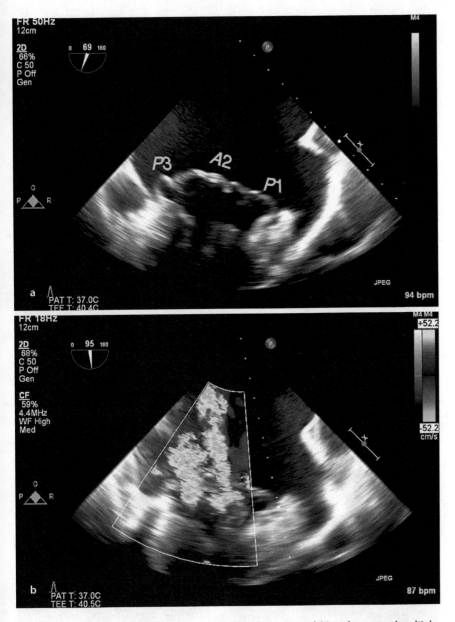

Fig. 1.139 Mid-esophageal commissural view shows P1, P3, and A2 prolapse **a** and multiple commissural jets of mitral regurgitation **b**

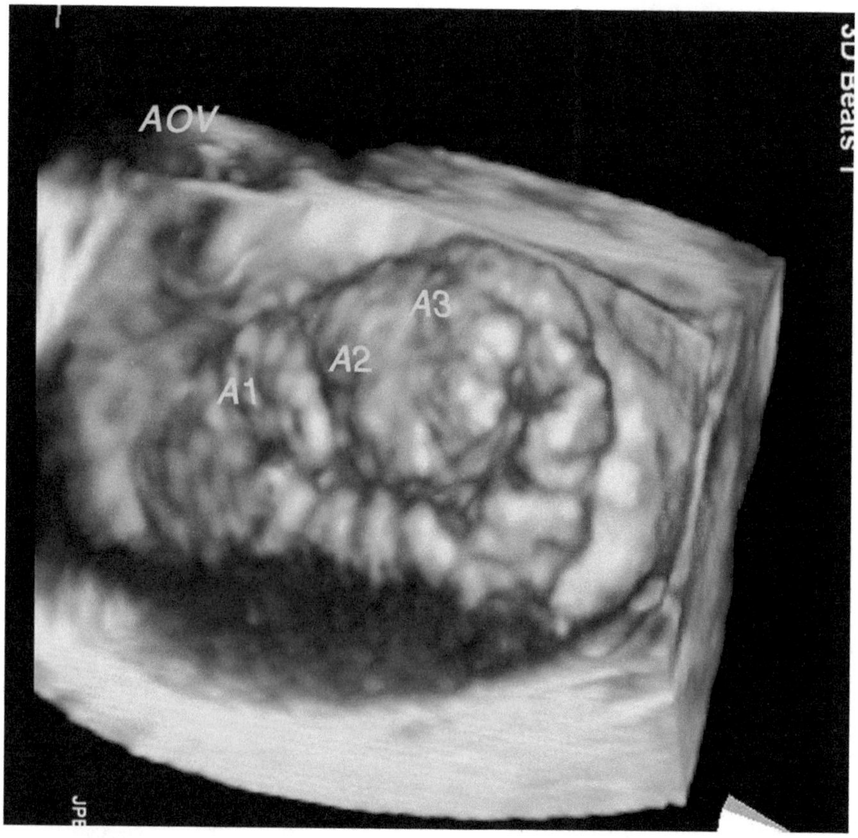

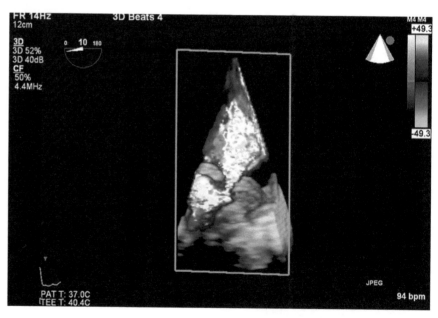

□ **Fig. 1.140**   3D enface view of mitral valve from left atrial side shows size of affected leaflets (all scallops especially A2, P2 and A3, P3 scallops) in relation to total valve area as well as neighboring anatomic structure

□ **Fig. 1.141**   Color full volume view of mitral valve shows a large PISA along the commissure

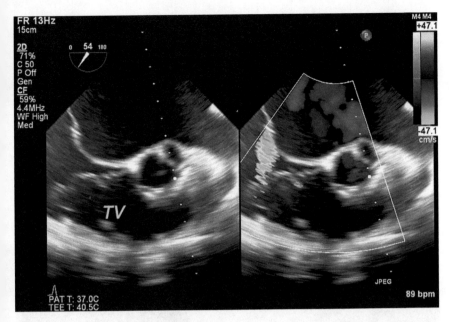

◼ **Fig. 1.142** Mid-esophageal 54° depicts tricuspid valve is also myxomatous and prolaptic with moderate tricuspid regurgitation and annular dilation up to 38 mm

Diagnosis Myxomatous mitral valve with prolapse of all scallops and severe mitral regurgitation and prolapse of tricuspid valve with moderate tricuspid regurgitation.

Recommendation Patient was sent for MV repair and TV repair.

What is the indication of TV repair at the time of left-sided valve surgery?

Even mild TR should be recommended for TV repair at the time of left-sided valve surgery if TV annulus is significantly dilated (>40 mm).

What are the criteria for successful MV repair?

1. No more than mild MR.
2. No more than mild MS
3. No systolic anterior motion and no LVOT gradient.

1.15   Case 14: Severe Mitral Regurgitation Due to Flail of P3 (Forme Fruste)

A 58-year-old man presented with a history of dyspnea and easy fatigability from 2 weeks previously after a chest trauma. In physical examination a pan systolic murmur IV/VI in mitral area and S4 was heard. Patient doesn't have any history of chills and fever.

Transthoracic echo reveals normal left ventricle size and functions.

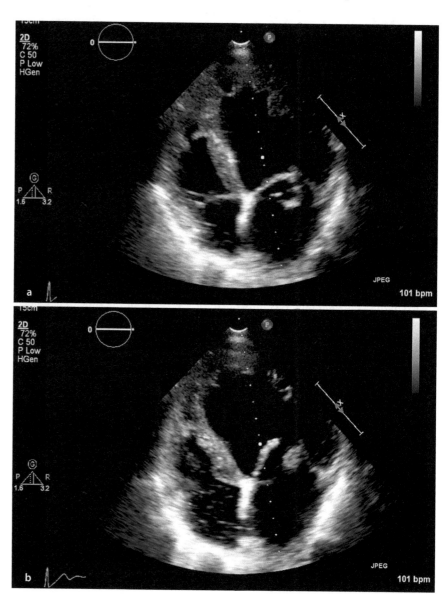

■ **Fig. 1.143**   Apical four-chamber view shows a long mobile particle attached to posterior mitral leaflet (**a**, diastole and **b**, systole)

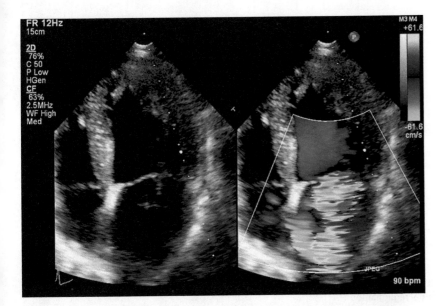

Fig. 1.144 Color Doppler flow study of apical four-chamber view demonstrates severe mitral regurgitation (*arrow*). Transesophageal echocardiography was performed for further evaluation of mitral valve

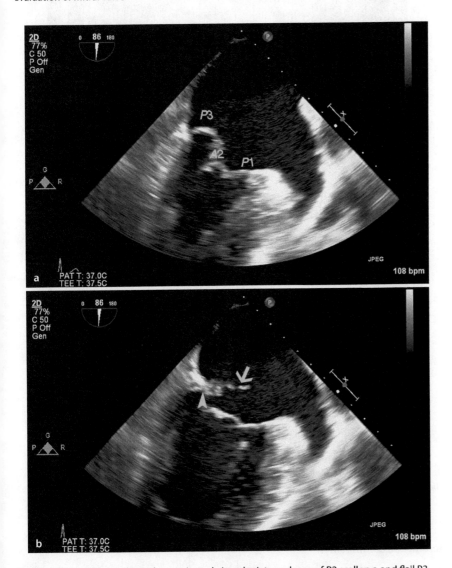

Fig. 1.145 Mid-esophageal commissural view depicts prolapse of P3 scallop **a** and flail P3 scallop (*arrow head*) and a remnant chordal rupture attached to it (**b**, *arrow*)

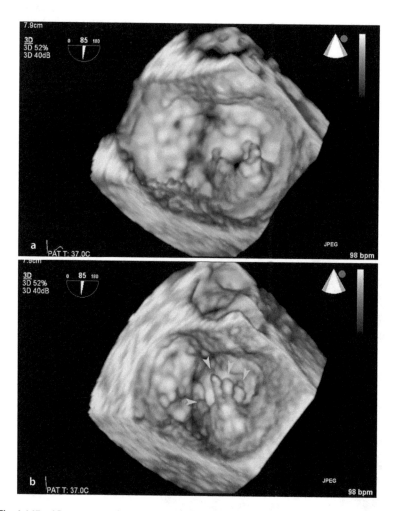

☐ **Fig. 1.146**   Color Doppler study of mid-esophageal long-axis view demonstrates severe mitral regurgitation

☐ **Fig. 1.147**   3D zoom view from left atrial side shows flail P3 scallop reached to posterome-dial commissure **a**, 4 remnants of chordal rupture attached to the P3 scallop (*arrow heads*) **b**

Diagnosis   Severe mitral regurgitation and flail P3 scallop with extension to posteromedial commissure.

Comment   The patient sent for mitral valve repair.

1.16   Case 15: Severe MR Due to Flail P2 (FED+)

A 40-year-old man with a history of chest trauma 6 months ago and recent dyspnea on exertion and easy fatigability. In physical examination a systolic murmur grade IV/VI in mitral area was heard.

Transthoracic echo shows mild left ventricular dilation and mild left ventricular dysfunction.

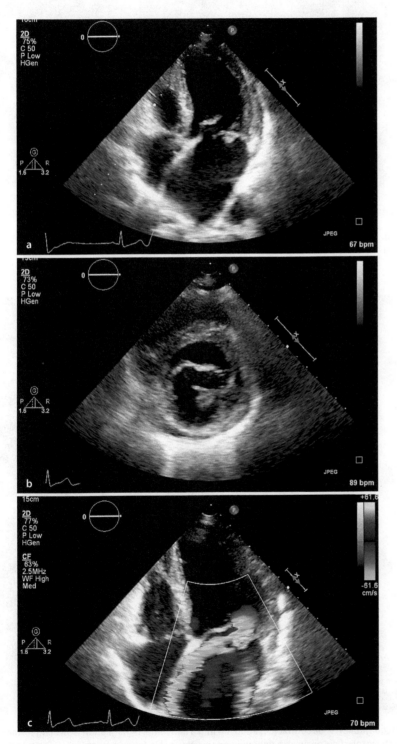

■ **Fig. 1.148**   Apical four-chamber view **a** and short-axis view of left ventricle **b** show a long hyperechogenic mobile mass attached to posterior mitral leaflet indicative for rupture of chorda with severe MR **c**

Transesophageal echo performed for evaluation of the cause of posterior mitral valve rupture and determination of exact involved scallops:

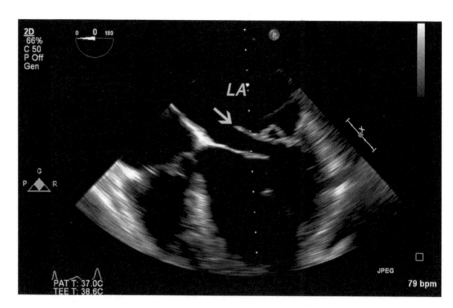

Fig. 1.149   Mid-esophageal degree view shows that mitral leaflets are not myxomatous and a long chordal rupture attached to P2 (*arrow*)

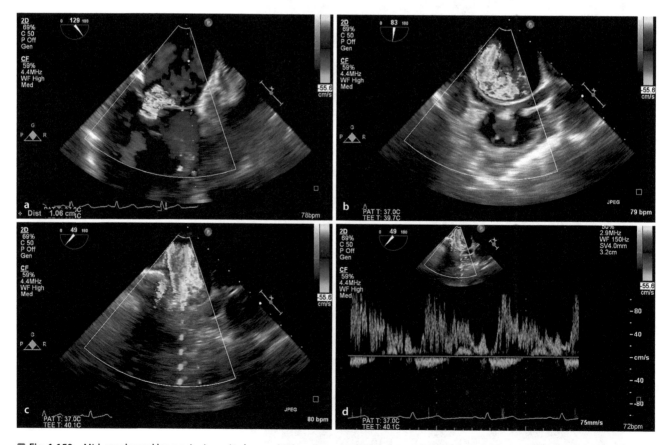

Fig. 1.150   Mid-esophageal long-axis view mitral regurgitation vena contracta is about 10 mm **a** and mitral regurgitation is swirling toward the inter-atrial septum **b** and mid-esophageal 49 depicts systolic flow reversal in right pulmonary veins **c, d** in favor of severe mitral regurgitation

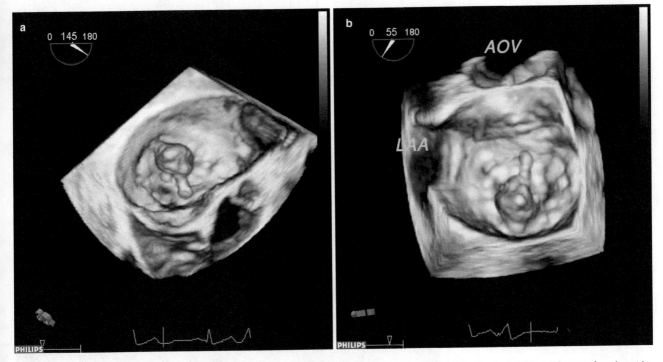

◘ **Fig. 1.151** 3D zoom view of mitral valve in 70° view **a** and anatomic view **b** (aortic valve is put in 12 o'clock and left atrial appendage is put in the 9 o'clock) show a long chordal remnant attached to tip of P2 scallop (*arrow*, **b**)

Diagnosis With respect to the fact that mitral leaflets were not myxomatous, chest trauma and chordal rupture were considered as the cause of chordal rupture.

Comment The patient was referred for MV repair.

1.17   Case 16: Severe MR Due to Flail of P2 (FED+)

A 65-year-old man with a history of atypical chest pain and easy fatigability of recent duration. Physical examination showed pan systolic murmur in mitral area.

Transthoracic echocardiography showed normal left ventricular size and function.

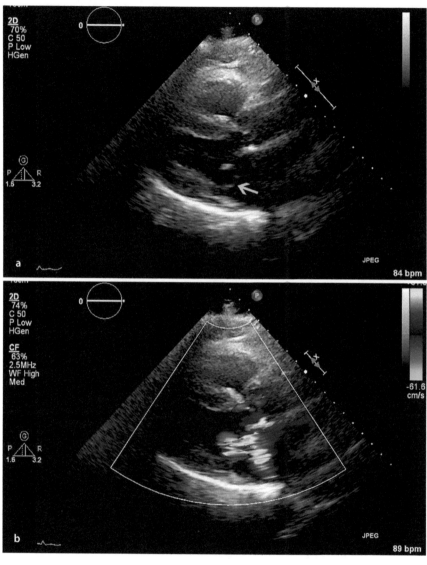

Fig. 1.152 Parasternal long-axis view shows posterior mitral leaflet is positioned above annulus so it seems prolaptic (*arrow*, **a**) with severe mitral regurgitation **b**

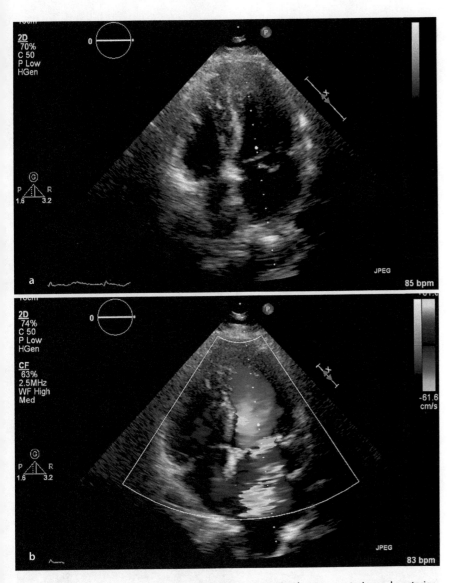

◻ Fig. 1.153 Apical four-chamber view depicts no coaptation between anterior and posterior mitral leaflets during systolic time and tip of posterior mitral leaflet is located in left atrial side (*arrow*) in favor of flail of posterior mitral leaflet **a** with severe mitral regurgitation **b**. Transesophageal echocardiography was performed for full evaluation of mitral valve

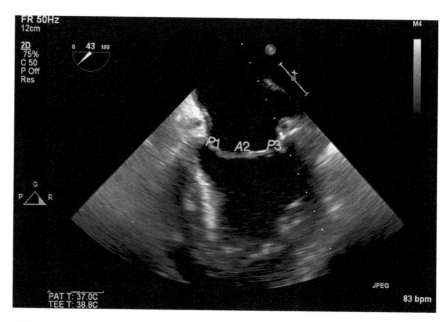

☐ **Fig. 1.154**   Mid-esophageal 0° view at the level of A2, P2 shows flail P2 scallop (*arrow head*) and remnant chordal rupture that it is attached to tip of P2 scallop (*arrow*)

☐ **Fig. 1.155**   Mid-esophageal commissural view doesn't show any evidence of flail scallop (this view shows clearly P1, A2, P3 scallops)

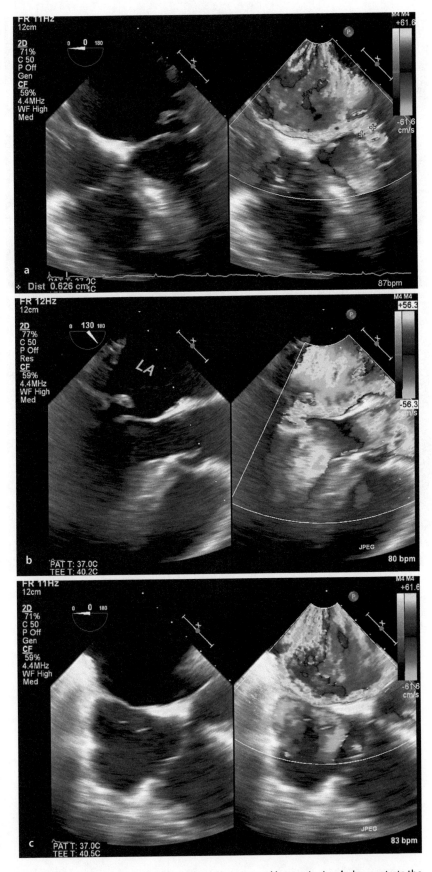

■ Fig. 1.156 Color Doppler mid-esophageal 0° view **a** and long-axis view **b** demonstrate the jet of mitral regurgitation directs anteriorly (away from flail P2 scallop) and it is toward the interatrial septum **c** in favor of severe mitral regurgitation

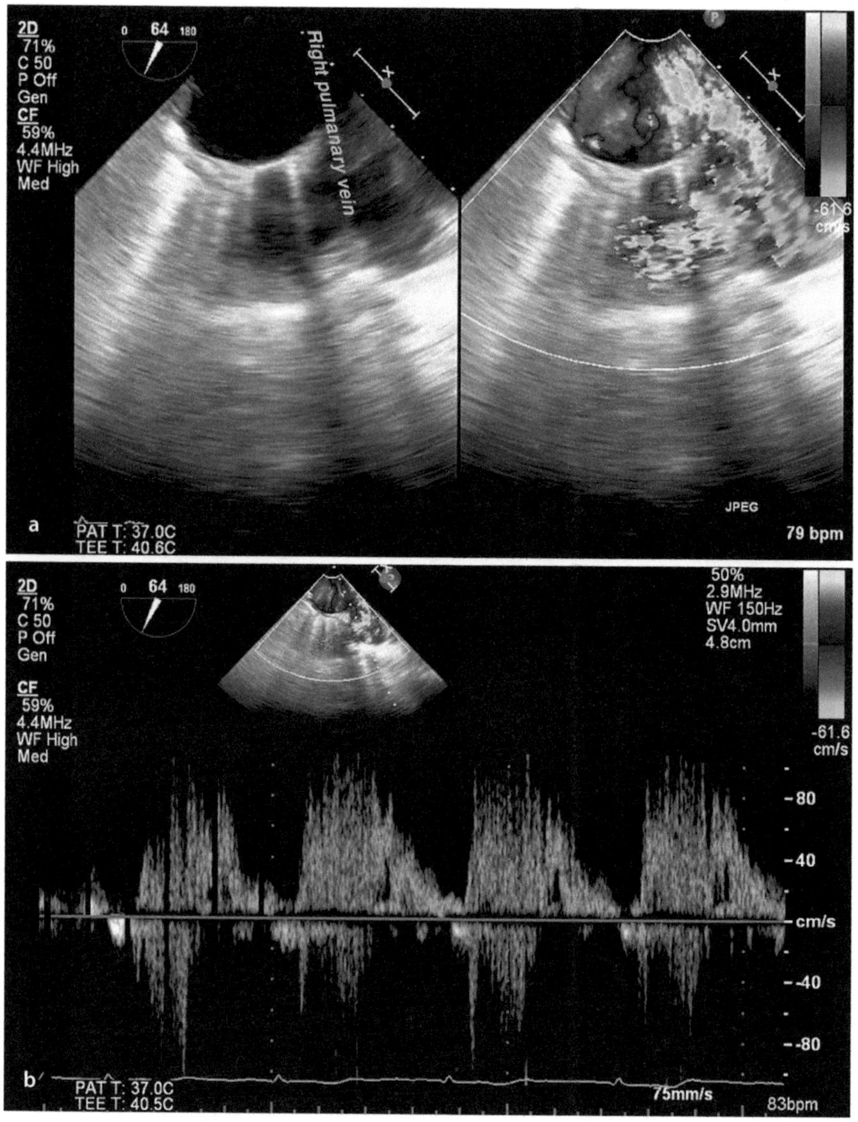

Fig. 1.157 Mid-esophageal short-axis view with slightly pullback and counterclockwise rotation shows right pulmonary veins (**a**, *right side*) and color study (**a**, *left side*) and Doppler study **b** depict systolic flow reversal in right pulmonary veins in favor of severe mitral regurgitation

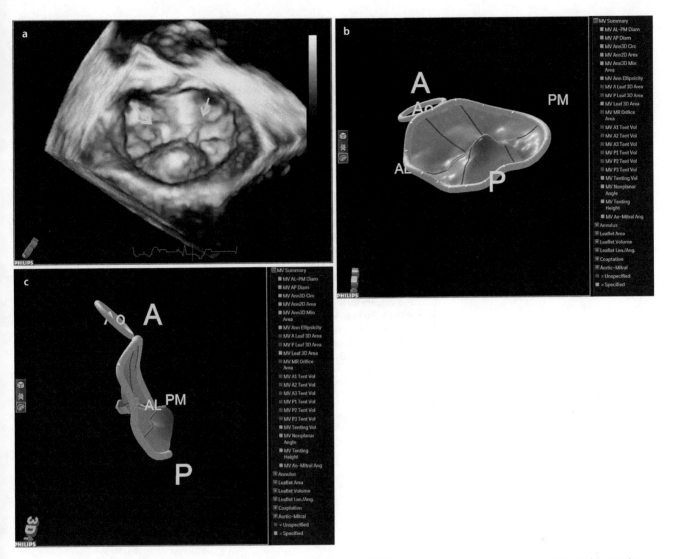

Fig. 1.158 3D zoom view surgical view of mitral valve from atrial side shows flail P2 scallop and two remnant chordae (*arrows*) that attach to P2 scallop **a** and mitral valve navigator shows clearly flail parameters in detail **b, c**

Diagnosis   Severe MR due to flail P2.

Recommendation   The patient was sent to operation room for mitral valve repair.

References

1. Adams DH, Rosenhek R, Falk V. Degenerative mitral valve regurgitation: best practice revolution. Eur Heart J. 2010;31(16):1958–66.
2. Anyanwu AC, Adams DH. Etiologic classification of degenerative mitral valve disease: Barlow's disease and fibroelastic deficiency. Semin Thorac Cardiovasc Surg. 2007;19(2):90–6.
3. Clavel MA, Francesca M, Vatury O, Suri R, Mankad S, Sarano M. Fibroelastic deficiency versus barlow's disease: differences in mitral annular dynamics by 3-dimensional echocardiography. J Am Coll Cardiol. 2014;63(12):A1985.
4. Chandra S, Salgo IS, Sugeng L, Weinert L, Tsang W, Takeuchi M, et al. Characterization of degenerative mitral valve disease using morphologic analysis of real-time three-dimensional echocardiographic images: objective insight into complexity and planning of mitral valve repair. Circ Cardiovasc Imaging. 2011;4(1):24–32.
5. Kovalova S, Necas J, Mikula O. Discrimination between fibroelastic deficiency and Barlow disease using parameters of mitral annulus derived from real-time three-dimensional echocardiography. J Echocardiogr. 2013;11(3):83–8.

6. Kovalova S, Necas J. RT-3D TEE: characteristics of mitral annulus using mitral valve quantification (MVQ) program. Echocardiography. 2011;28(4):461–7.

7. Delling FN, Vasan RS. Epidemiology and pathophysiology of mitral valve prolapse: new insights into disease progression, genetics, and molecular basis. Circulation. 2014;129(21):2158–70.

8. Kumar N, Kumar M, Duran CM. A revised terminology for recording surgical findings of the mitral valve. J Heart Valve Dis. 1995;4(1):70–5. discussion 6–7

9. Shah PM. Current concepts in mitral valve prolapse–diagnosis and management. J Cardiol. 2010;56(2):125–33.

10. Devereux RB, Kramer-Fox R, Shear MK, Kligfield P, Pini R, Savage DD. Diagnosis and classification of severity of mitral valve prolapse: methodologic, biologic, and prognostic considerations. Am Heart J. 1987;113(5):1265–80.

11. Avierinos JF, Detaint D, Messika-Zeitoun D, Mohty D, Enriquez-Sarano M. Risk, determinants, and outcome implications of progression of mitral regurgitation after diagnosis of mitral valve prolapse in a single community. Am J Cardiol. 2008;101(5):662–7.

12. Avierinos JF, Gersh BJ, Melton 3rd LJ, Bailey KR, Shub C, Nishimura RA, et al. Natural history of asymptomatic mitral valve prolapse in the community. Circulation. 2002;106(11):1355–61.

13. Ling LH, Enriquez-Sarano M, Seward JB, Tajik AJ, Schaff HV, Bailey KR, et al. Clinical outcome of mitral regurgitation due to flail leaflet. N Engl J Med. 1996;335(19):1417–23.

14. Mauri L, Garg P, Massaro JM, Foster E, Glower D, Mehoudar P, et al. The EVEREST II trial: design and rationale for a randomized study of the evalve mitraclip system compared with mitral valve surgery for mitral regurgitation. Am Heart J. 2010;160(1):23–9.

15. Kahlert P, Plicht B, Schenk IM, Janosi RA, Erbel R, Buck T. Direct assessment of size and shape of noncircular vena contracta area in functional versus organic mitral regurgitation using real-time three-dimensional echocardiography. J Am Soc Echocardiogr. 2008;21(8):912–21.

16. Lange A, Palka P, Donnelly J, Burstow D. Quantification of mitral regurgitation orifice area by 3-dimensional echocardiography: comparison with effective regurgitant orifice area by PISA method and proximal regurgitant jet diameter. Int J Cardiol. 2002;86(1):87–98.

Rheumatic Mitral Stenosis

Videos can be found in the electronic supplementary material in the online version of the chapter.
On http://springerlink.com enter the DOI number given on the bottom of the chapter opening page.
Scroll down to the Supplementary material tab and click on the respective videos link.

© Springer International Publishing AG 2017
H. Sadeghian, Z. Savand-Roomi, *3D Echocardiography of Structural Heart Disease*,
DOI 10.1007/978-3-319-54039-9_2

2.1   Introduction

Mitral stenosis (MS) is often due to rheumatic fever; about 25% of patients with rheumatic heart disease have isolated MS, 40% have MS and MR, and 38% have multivalve involvement; involvement of pulmonary valve is rare [1].

Mitral valve area ≤ 1.5 cm^2 is considered as severe mitral stenosis and ≤ 1 cm^2 as very severe MS [2].

Mitral valve area ≤ 1.5 cm^2 usually corresponds to mean transmitral gradient between 5 and 10 mmHg, but the gradient depends on flow and heart rate [2].

Planimetry is the gold standard method for evaluation of mitral valve area [3]; mitral pressure half-time depends on left ventricular and atrial compliance [2].

PTMC is indicated in symptomatic patients with severe mitral stenosis (MVA $\leq$ 1.5 cm^2) (class I) or in asymptomatic patients with very severe MS (MVA $\leq$ 1 cm^2) (class IIa) [2]. Besides, PTMC is indicated in asymptomatic patients with severe MS and PAPs > 50 mmHg at rest who are candidate for noncardiac surgery or pregnancy (IIa) [4].

Severe MS and new onset atrial fibrillation is class IIb for PTMC; moderate MS with hemodynamically significant stenosis during ETT is class IIb for PTMC [2].

Before percutaneous mitral valve commissurotomy, TEE is needed for rule out of left atrial thrombosis and sometimes for careful evaluation of severity of MR and other valvular heart diseases. TEE is also needed after embolic events [4]. Moderate mitral regurgitation is a controversial issue for PTMC; in some centers, more than mild MR is a contraindication for PTMC [4], while, in other centers, moderate to severe MR is a contraindication for PTMC [2]. PTMC is contraindicated in the presence of severe aortic valve disease or combined severe tricuspid stenosis and regurgitation [4]. Severe TR in a patient with rheumatic heart disease is commonly due to annulus dilation in consequence of elevated systolic pulmonary arterial pressure, and sometimes there is rheumatic involvement of tricuspid valve; usually after a successful balloon dilation of mitral valve, severity of TR will reduce due to decrease in PAPs.

LA clot is a contraindication for PTMC, but in case of LAA clot, it is usually possible to try intensive anticoagulant therapy for 2–6 months and repeat TEE. It is of notice that if there is a mobile clot in LAA with protrusion to the left atrium, surgery is mandatory for the removal of clot and correction of valvular heart disease.

Severe or bicommissural calcification or splitting of both commissures is a contraindication for PTMC [4]; if commissural calcification is not present, commissural calcification score will be 0; if entire of both commissures are calcified, score will be 4; and if less than one half of a commissure is calcified, score will be one. Commissural calcification score is a strong predictor of outcome of PTMC and MR; mitral valve area will be greater after PTMC with commissural scores 0 and 1 compared to scores 2 and 3 [5].

2.2   Case 1: Severe Mitral Stenosis, Mild MR, Mild AS, Moderate AI, No LA, and LAA Clot Suitable for PTMC

A 55-year-old man presented with dyspnea on exertion functional class II of recent duration.

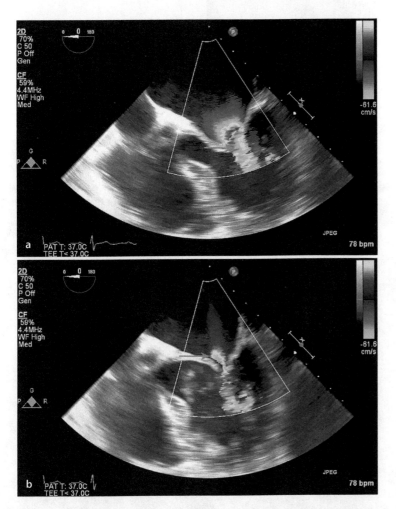

◘ Fig. 2.1   Severe mitral stenosis (diastolic turbulency across mitral valve) and mild mitral regurgitation are seen in TEE 0° view (*arrows*) **a, b**

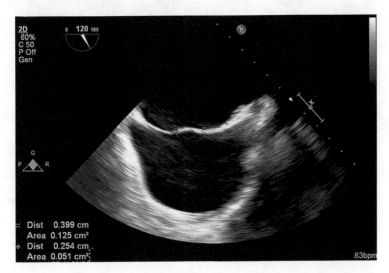

◘ Fig. 2.2   Interatrial septum measures 2.5 mm in foramen ovale and up to 4 mm in other sites

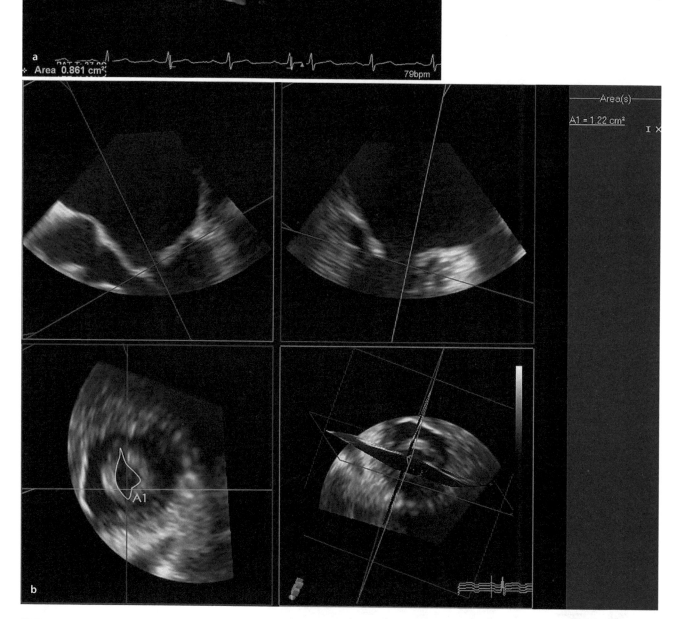

Fig. 2.3   Mitral valve area measures 0.86 cm² by direct planimetry with 3D zoom **a** and 1.22 cm² by 3DQ **b** and 1.08 cm² by 3D zoom by MPR mode **c** [5]

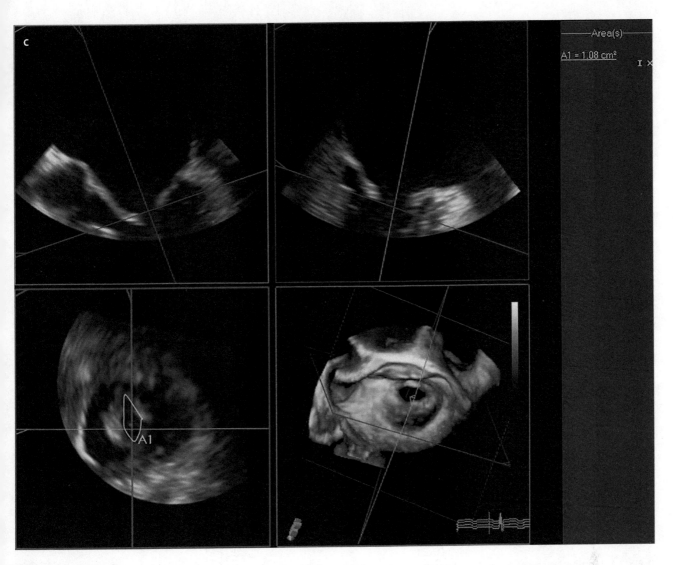

◻ **Fig. 2.3** (continued)

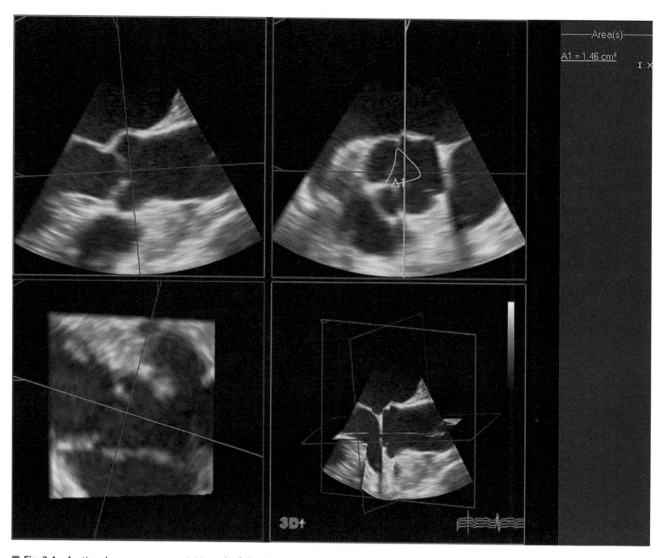

□ Fig. 2.4   Aortic valve area measures 1.46 mm by full volume in mid-systole in tip of leaflets

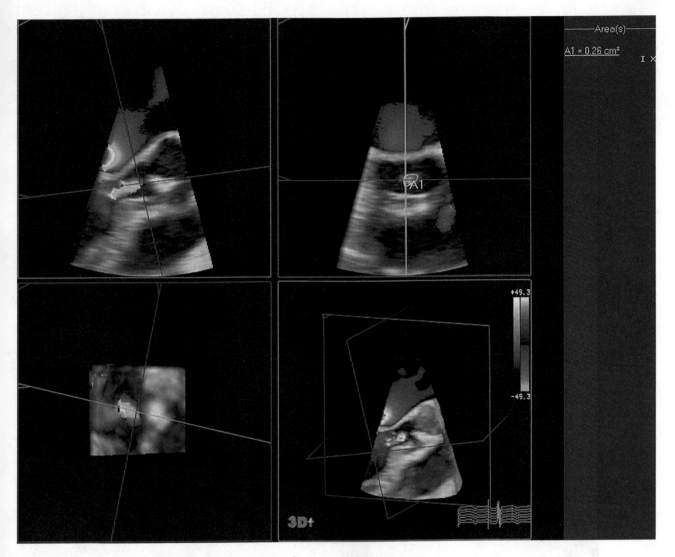

◘ **Fig. 2.5** Aortic valve vena contracta area measures 2.6 mm² in favor of moderate AI

It is of notice that in conventional method for measuring aortic annulus by 3DQ, in short-axis view of aortic valve (red plane), green plane passes between left and noncoronary cusp and through right coronary cusp, so in green plane (left upper view), red plane crosses the right coronary cusp, and then aortic annulus is measured in two diameters (D1 = 25.6 mm, D2 which is the larger diameter = 26.4 mm; in this case, mean diameter is 26 mm) [6]. By recently introduced coaxial orthogonal method, in sagittal and coronal views, two other planes are put orthogonal and in base of aortic leaflets, and it is also called double oblique method (25.8 mm in this case, B); this cross-sectional 3D sizing of aortic annulus offers a discrimination of post-TAVI paravalvular leak which is significantly superior to 2D TEE but inferior to CT scan and should be considered when CT scan is not possible for the patient [7].

According to some studies, mean diameter and annular cross-sectional area measured by CT scan for TAVI are 1.3 mm and about 10% greater than the values by 3D echocardiography [7].

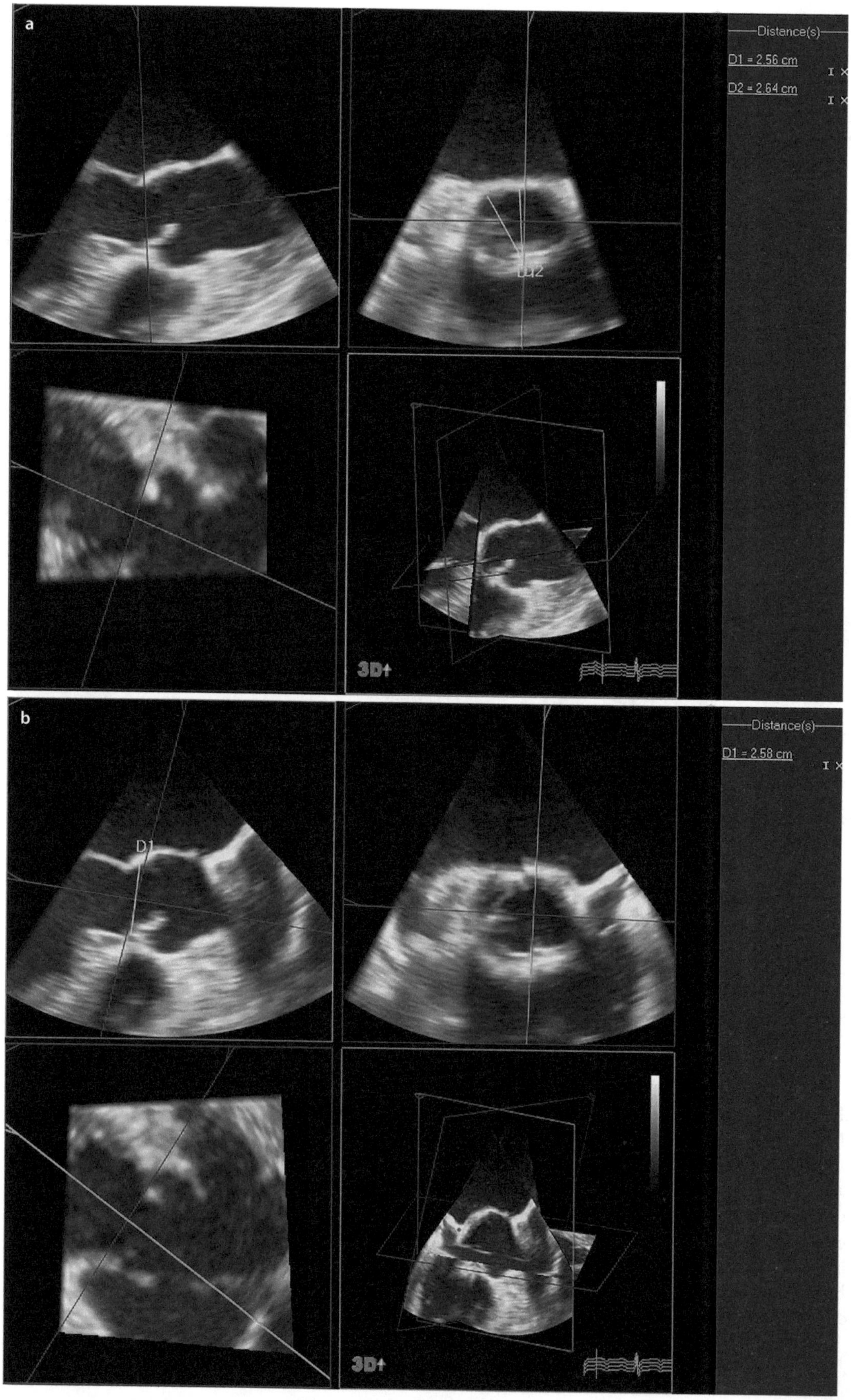

Fig. 2.6 Aortic annulus measures 25.6 by conventional method, 26.4 mm in its larger diameter **a**, and 25.8 mm by double oblique method **b** by 3DQ

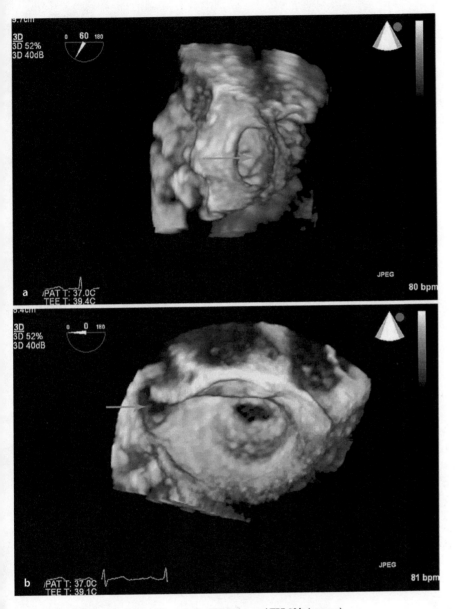

▪ **Fig. 2.7**　LAA has no clot by 3D zoom by TEE 60° **a** and TEE 0° **b** (*arrows*)

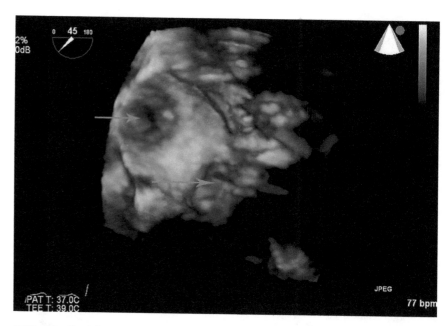

☐ Fig. 2.8 Two left pulmonary veins are visualized in TEE short-axis view (*arrow*) by 3D zoom from LA side

Diagnosis   Severe MS, mild MR, mild AS, moderate AI, no LA, and LAA clot.

Comment   The patient is referred for PTMC.

2.3 Case 2: Severe MS, No MR, Mild AS, Mild to Moderate AI, and LAA Clot

A 53-year-old woman presented with dyspnea on exertion functional class II of recent exacerbation.

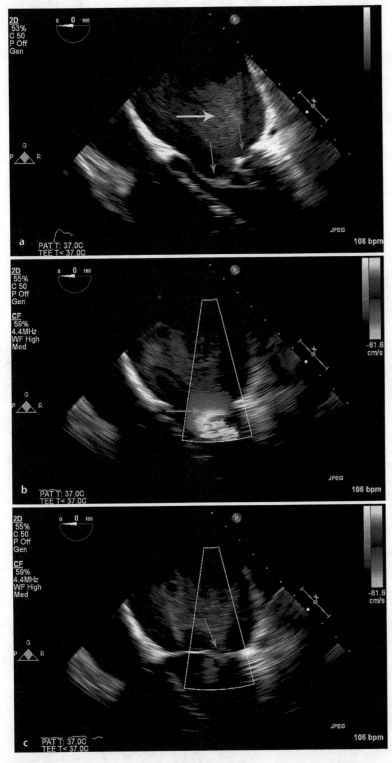

◘ **Fig. 2.9** Thickening and doming of anterior mitral leaflet (*green arrow*) and restriction of posterior mitral leaflet (*pink arrow*) are evident in TEE 0° view in favor of severe MS **a**, severe spontaneous contrast (*yellow arrow*) is also evident in this view **a**, and diastolic turbulency (*arrow*) in favor of severe MS and nearly no MR (*arrow*) **b**, **c** are evident in this view

2

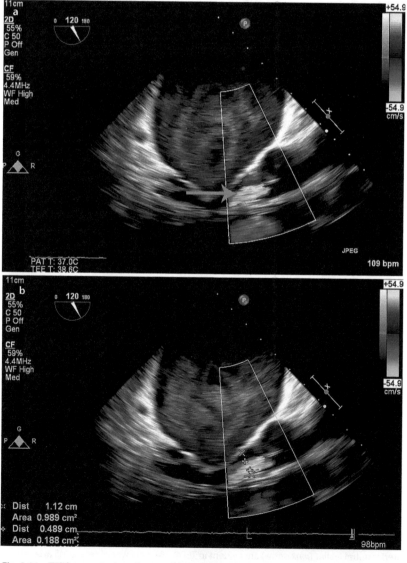

☐ **Fig. 2.10**   Spontaneous contrast grade III in left atrium (*green arrow*) and fresh clot formation in LAA (*pink arrow*) in TEE short-axis view

☐ **Fig. 2.11**   TEE long-axis view shows mild to moderate AI (*arrow*) **a**, width of AI/ LVOT = 4.9/11 mm **b**

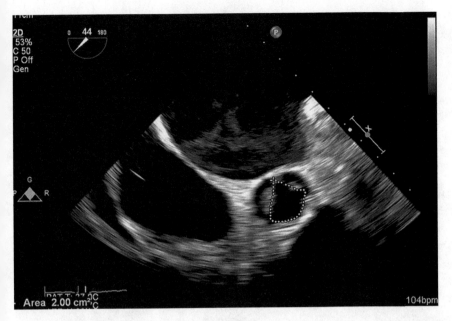

☑ **Fig. 2.12** Aortic valve area measures 2 cm² by TEE short-axis view

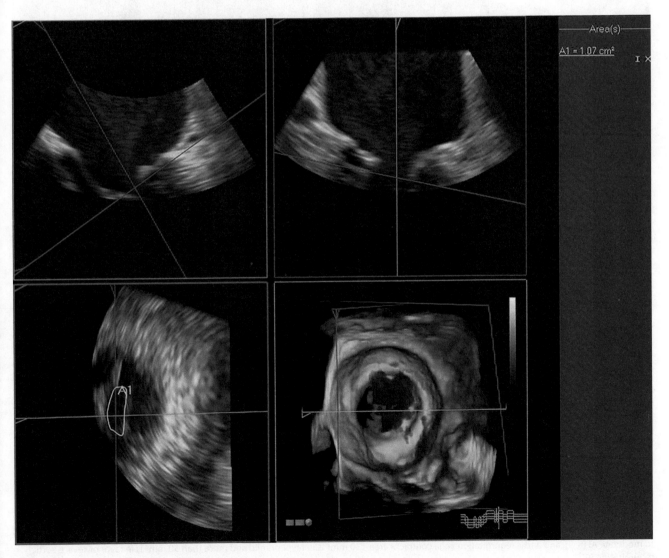

☑ **Fig. 2.13** Mitral valve area measures 1.07 cm² by 3DQ measurement

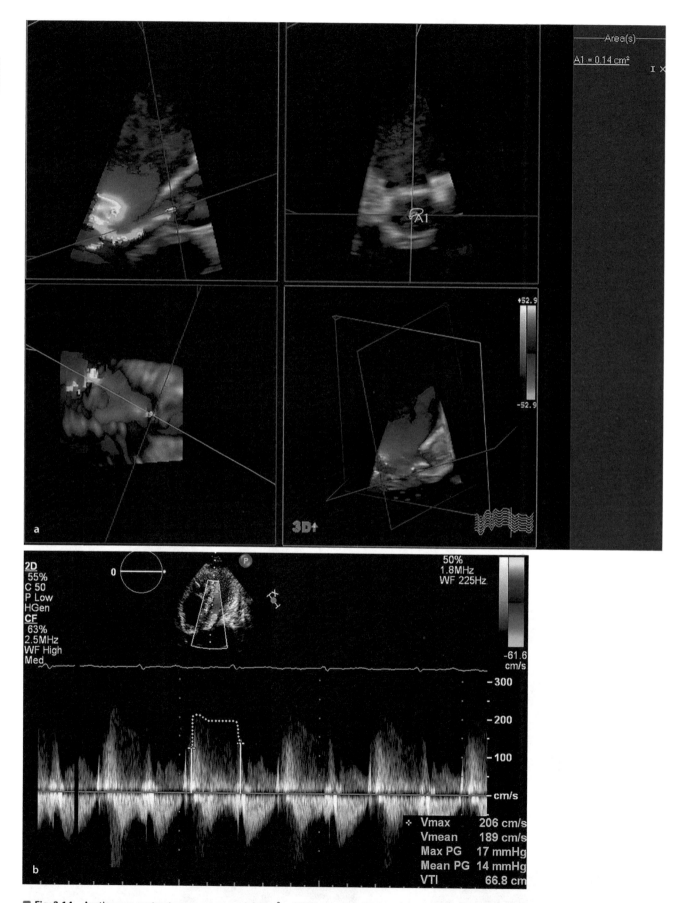

■ **Fig. 2.14** Aortic vena contracta area measures 0.14 cm² **a**, AI VTI measures 66.8 cm **b** and AI volume = 9.5 cm³ (0.14*66.8) in favor of mild to moderate AI [8, 9], and aortic regurgitation vena contracta area <30 mm² is in favor of mild and more than 50 mm² is in favor of severe aortic regurgitation [9]

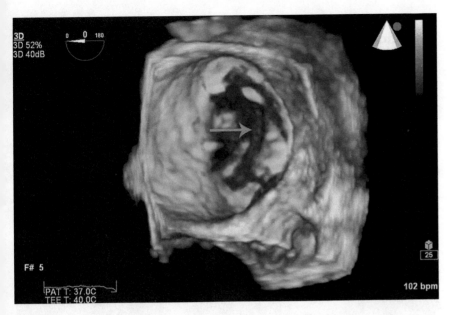

■ **Fig. 2.15** Severe spontaneous contrast (*arrow*) is evident in LA by 3D zoom

Diagnosis Severe MS, no MR, mild AS, mild to moderate AI, severe spontaneous contrast in LA, and LAA impending to fresh clot formation in LAA.

Comment Anticoagulant therapy for 3 months and TEE after that.

2.4   Case 3: Severe MS, Mild MR, Mild AI, No LAA, and LAA Clot Suitable for PTMC

A 44-year-old woman presented with dyspnea on exertion functional class III with recent exacerbation.

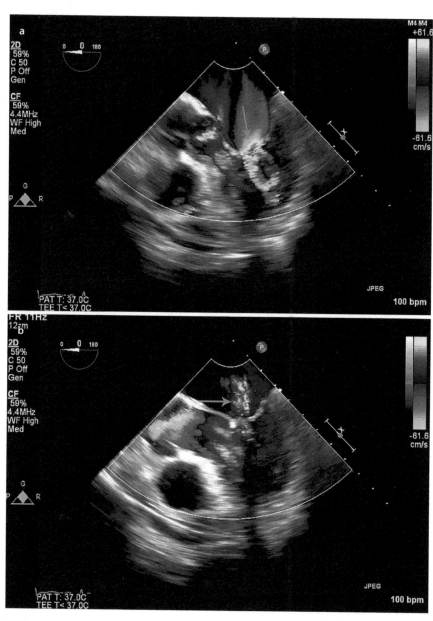

◻ **Fig. 2.16**   Diastolic turbulency across mitral valve in favor of mitral stenosis (*arrow*) **a** and mild mitral regurgitation (*arrow*) are evident in TEE long-axis view **b**

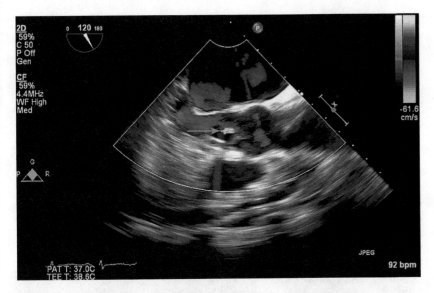

☐ **Fig. 2.17** Mild aortic regurgitation (*arrow*) is also evident in TEE long-axis view

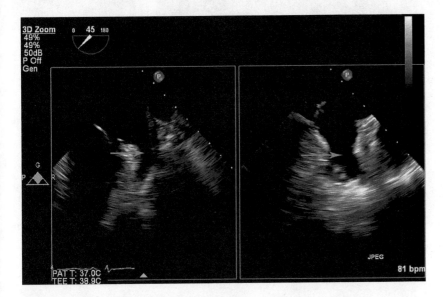

☐ **Fig. 2.18** No clot is seen in LAA (*arrows*) in TEE 45° and its orthogonal view

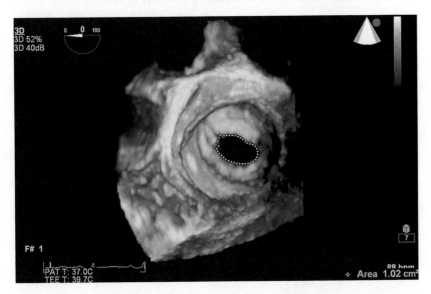

☐ **Fig. 2.19** Mitral valve area measures 1.02 by direct planimetry by 3D echo

2

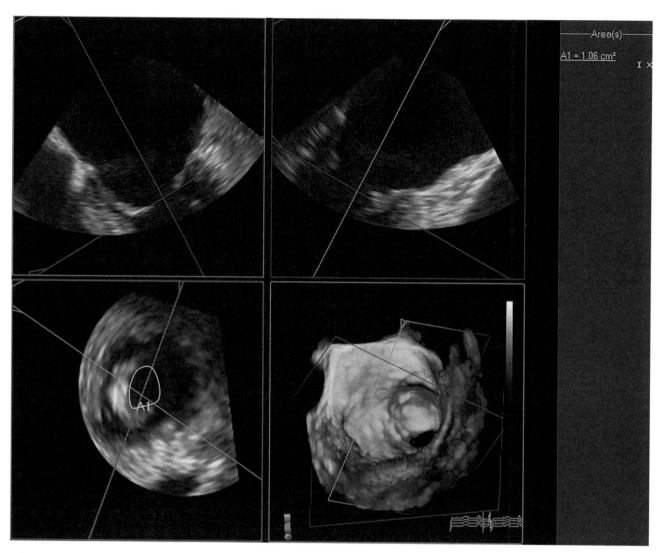

Fig. 2.20   Mitral valve area measures 1.06 cm² by 3DQ method

Diagnosis   Severe MS, mild MR, mild AI, no LA, and LAA clot.

Comment   PTMC.

2.5 Case 4: Severe MS, Severe Spontaneous Contrast in LA, and LAA Clot

A 41-year-old woman presented with dyspnea on exertion functional class III of recent exacerbation.

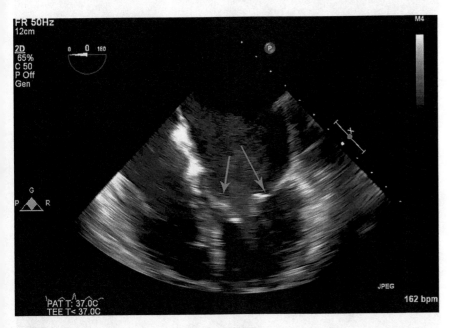

Fig. 2.21 Severe spontaneous contrast is seen in TEE 0°, and mitral valve is domed, thick, and calcified and has restricted motion (*arrows*)

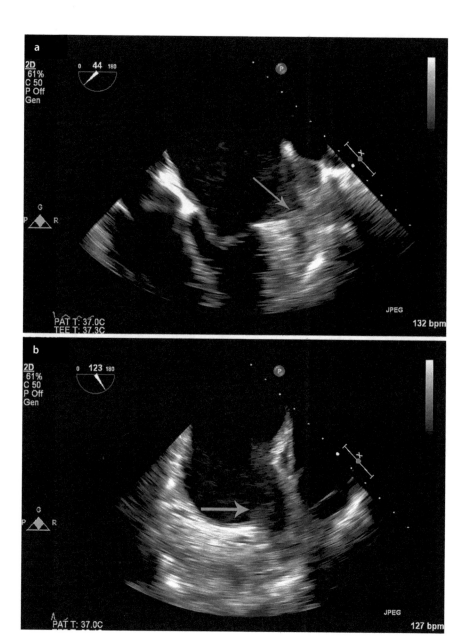

☐ **Fig. 2.22**   Fresh clot is seen in LAA in TEE 46° (*arrow*) **a**, and the clot protrudes into left atrium (*arrow*) by TEE 123° view **b**

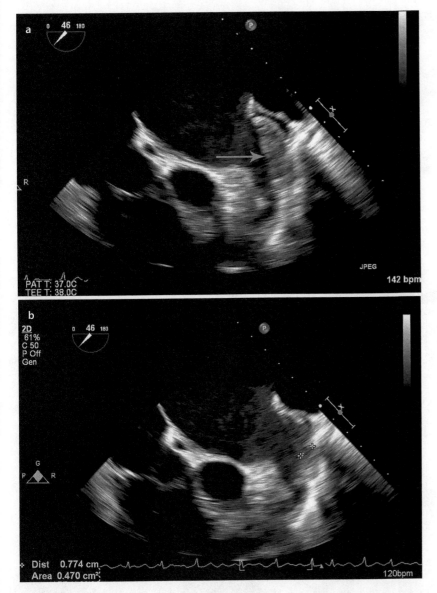

☐ **Fig. 2.23** Thickening of LAA wall in TEE short-axis view (*arrow*) **a**; in favor of clot formation, there is a clot in lateral wall of LAA that measures up to 8 mm in this view **b**

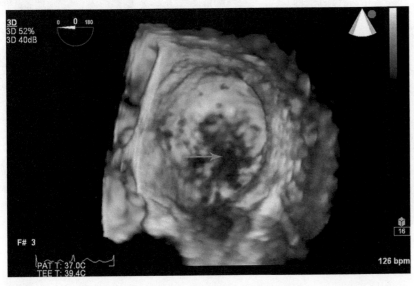

☐ **Fig. 2.24** Severe spontaneous contrast is seen in LA with 3D zoom from LA side (*arrow*)

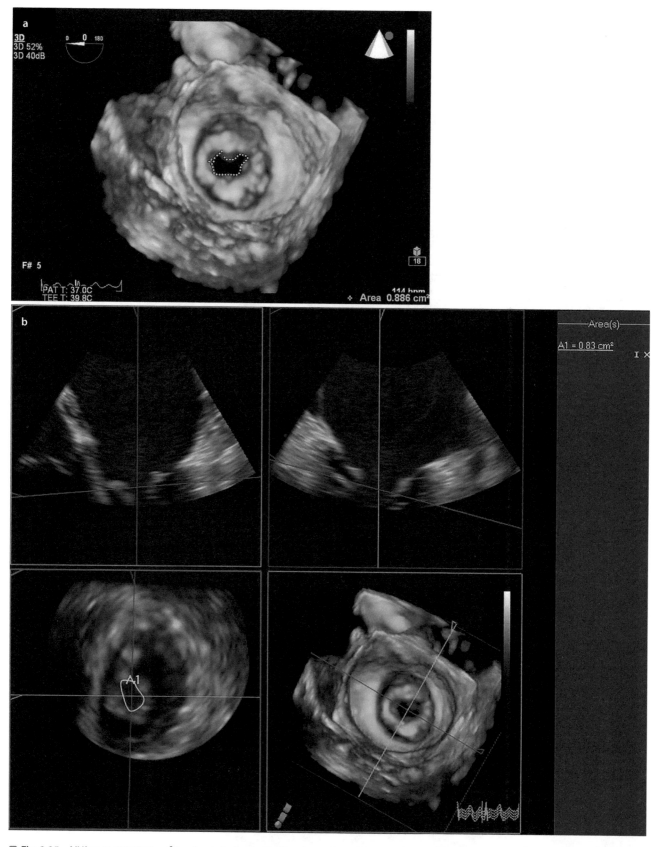

Fig. 2.25   MVA measures 0.86 cm² by direct planimetry by 3D echocardiography **a** and 0.83 cm² by 3DQ **b**

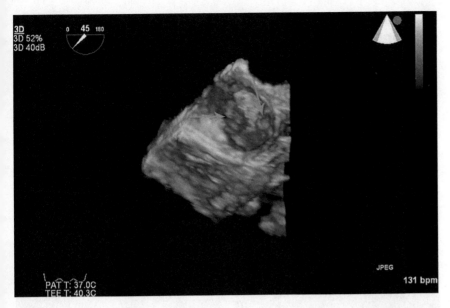

◘ Fig. 2.26   Clot in LAA is seen by 3D zoom

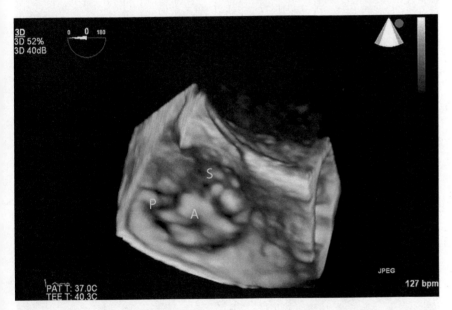

◘ Fig. 2.27   Three leaflets of tricuspid valve are seen by 3D zoom from right atrial side. *A*, anterior tricuspid leaflet; *S*, septal tricuspid leaflet; and *P*, posterior tricuspid leaflet

Diagnosis   Severe MS and LAA clot.

Comment   Anticoagulant therapy for 3 months and TEE after that.

2.6   Case 5: Severe MS, Severe MR, Severe TR, and Severe Spontaneous Contrast in LA

A 55-year-old woman presented with dyspnea on exertion functional class III of recent exacerbation.

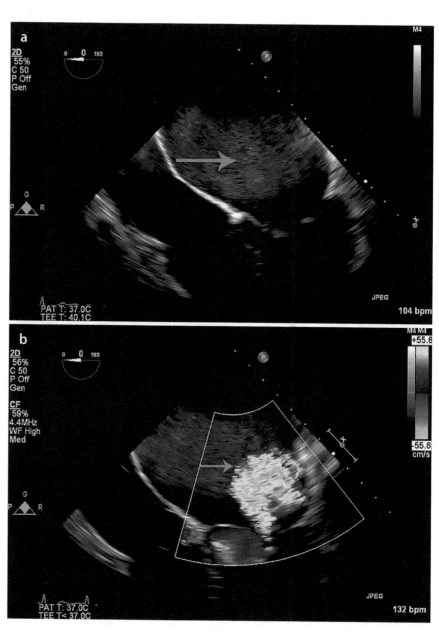

☐ **Fig. 2.28**   Severe spontaneous contrast is seen in TEE 0° view (*arrow*) **a**, and severe MR is seen in this view (*arrow*) **b**

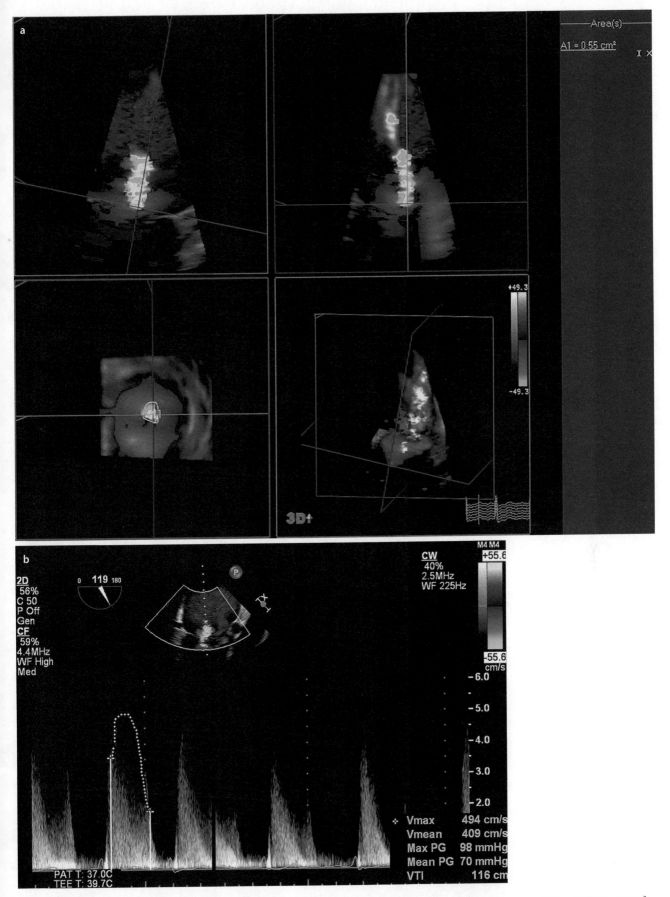

◻ **Fig. 2.29** MR VC area measures 0.55 cm² by 3DQ full volume **a**, VTI of MR measures 116 cm **b**, and MR volume measures as follow: 0.55*116 = 64 cm³ indicative of severe MR, and mitral regurgitation vena contracta area more than 0.41 cm² can discriminate moderate from severe mitral regurgitation [10]

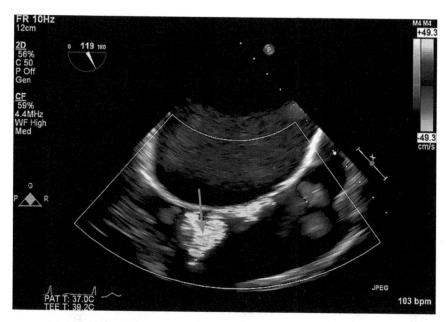

Fig. 2.30 Severe TR is evident in TEE long-axis view (*arrow*)

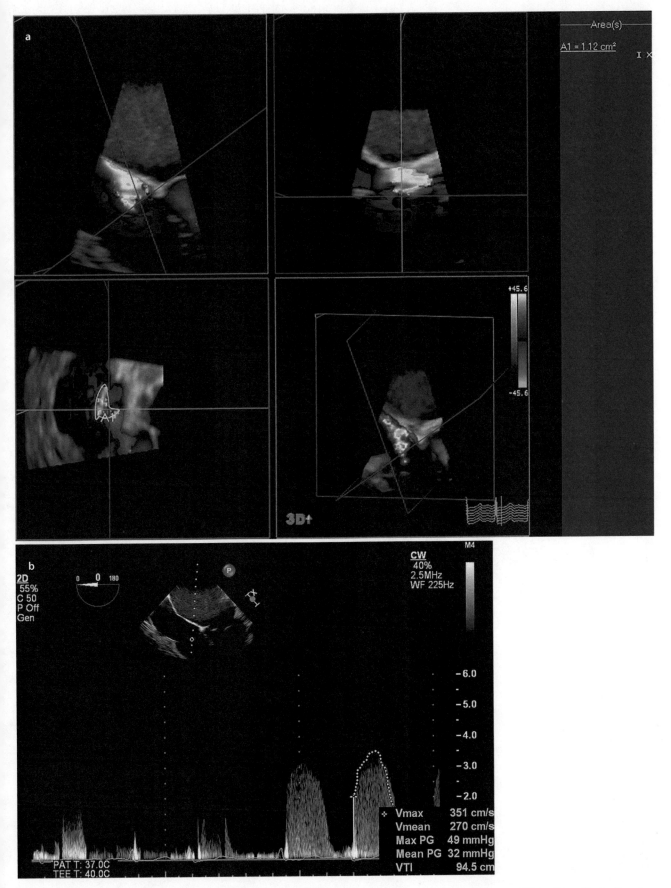

◘ Fig. 2.31 TR VC area measures 1.12 cm² **a**, and TR VTI is equal to 95 cm **b**, so TR volume measures as follows: 1.12*95 = 106 cm³ indicative of severe TR [11]

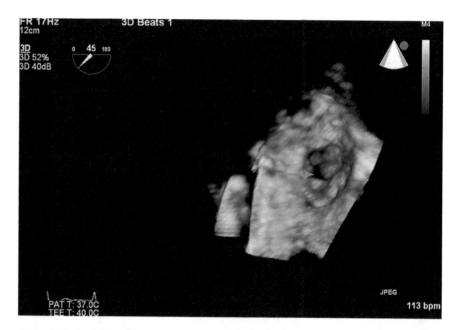

Fig. 2.32 No LAA colt by 3D zoom from LA (*arrow*)

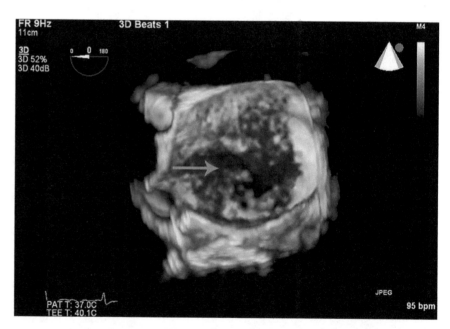

Fig. 2.33 Severe spontaneous contrast (*arrow*) is seen by 3D zoom from left atrial side and makes it impossible to measure mitral valve area by direct planimetry by 3D zoom

Diagnosis   Severe MS, severe MR, and severe TR due to annulus dilation and mild thickening of leaflets.

Comment   MVR + TV annuloplasty.

2.7 Case 6: Severe MS, Moderate MR, and a Mobile Mass on Ventricular Side of Aortic Valve

A 62-year-old woman was referred for transthoracic echocardiography before CABG. TTE showed severe MS and moderate MR, and the patient underwent TEE for decision making about OMVC or MVR in the time of CABG.

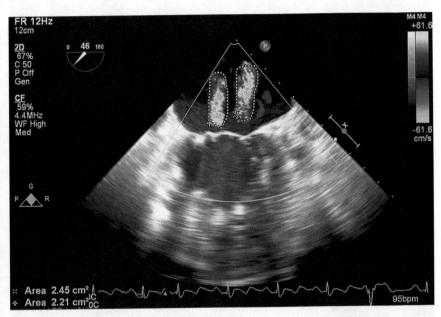

Fig. 2.34 Moderate MR is evident in TEE 45° view, and there are two jets of MR, surface of one 2.2 cm² and another one 2.5 cm²

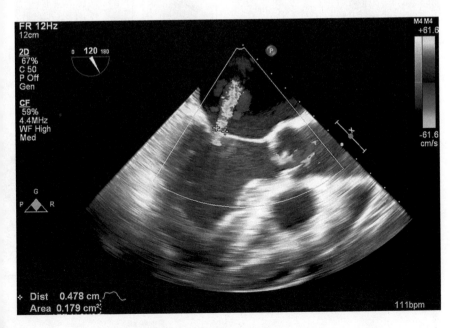

Fig. 2.35 MR VC measures 4.8 mm in TEE long-axis view

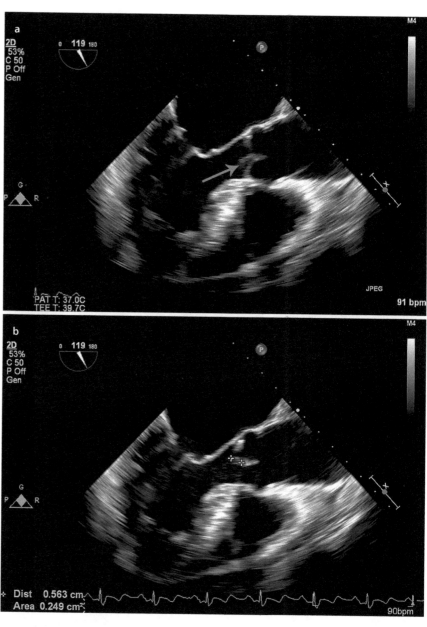

■ **Fig. 2.36** TEE long-axis view shows a mobile mass on ventricular side of NCC (*arrow*) **a**. This mass measures about 5 mm **b**

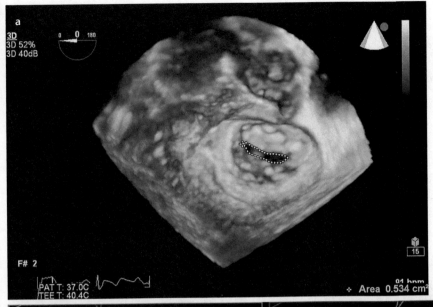

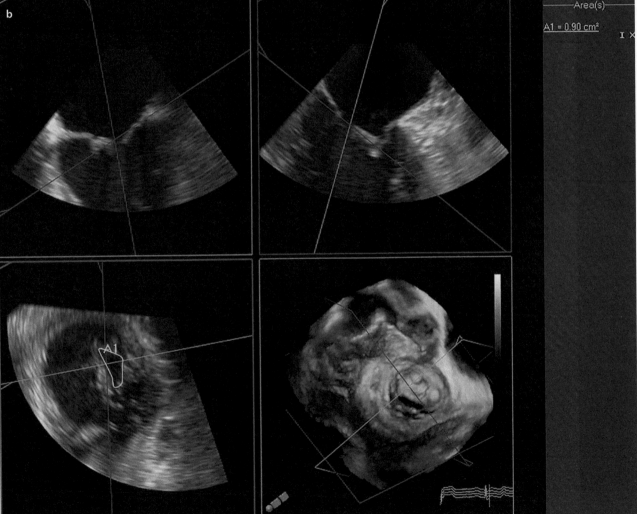

☐ **Fig. 2.37** MVA is 0.53 by direct planimetry by 3D echocardiography **a** and 0.9 cm² by 3DQ **b**

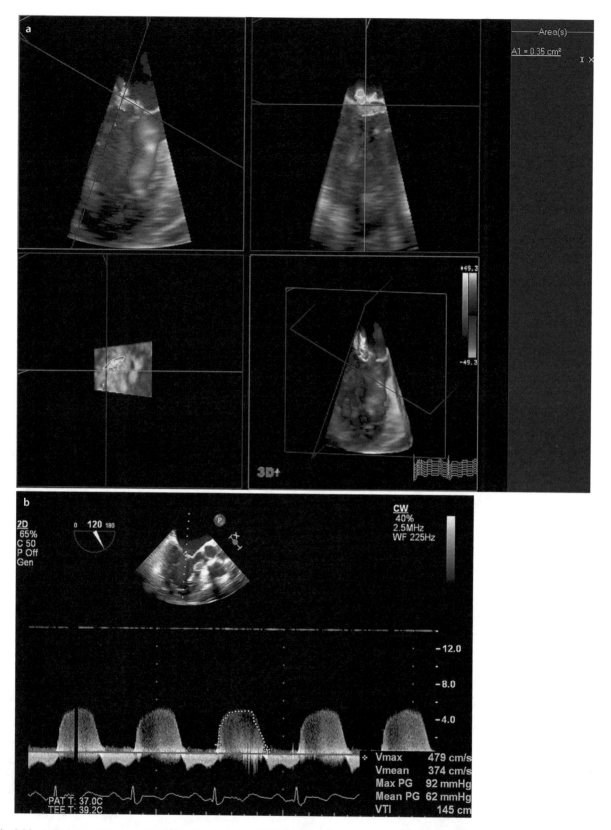

□ **Fig. 2.38** MR VC area measures 0.35 cm² by full volume **a** and MR VTI measures 145 cm **b**, MR RV = 0.35*145 = 50 cm³ indicative of moderate MR

Diagnosis Severe MS, moderate MR, and a mobile mass on ventricular side of NCC in favor of vegetation or Lambl's excrescence.

Comment MVR, work-up for IE, and repeat TEE.

2.8   Case 7: Severe MS, Mild MR, No LA, and LAA Clot

A 55-year-old woman presented with dyspnea on exertion functional class III of recent exacerbation.

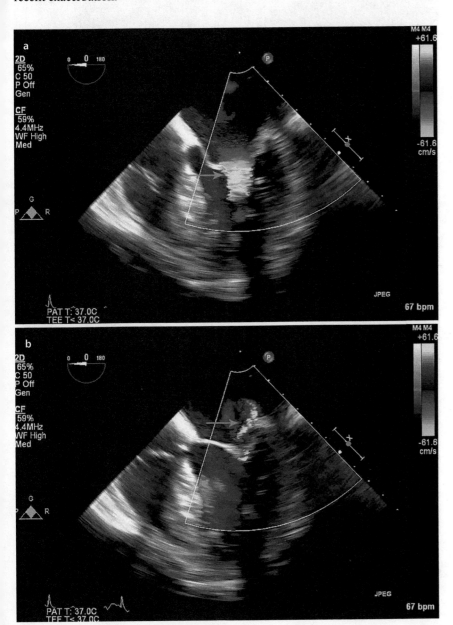

◼ **Fig. 2.39**   TEE 0° shows diastolic turbulency (*arrow*) across mitral valve in favor of mitral stenosis **a**, and mild mitral regurgitation is evident in this view (*arrow*) **b**

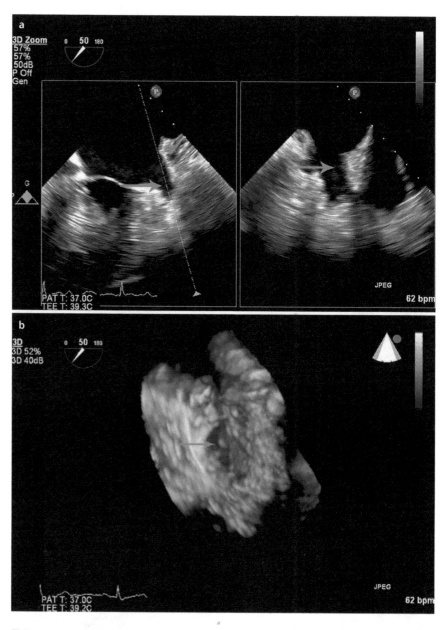

Fig. 2.40 No LA and LAA (*arrows*) clot is seen in TEE short-axis and its orthogonal view **a** with 3D zoom **b** (*arrows*)

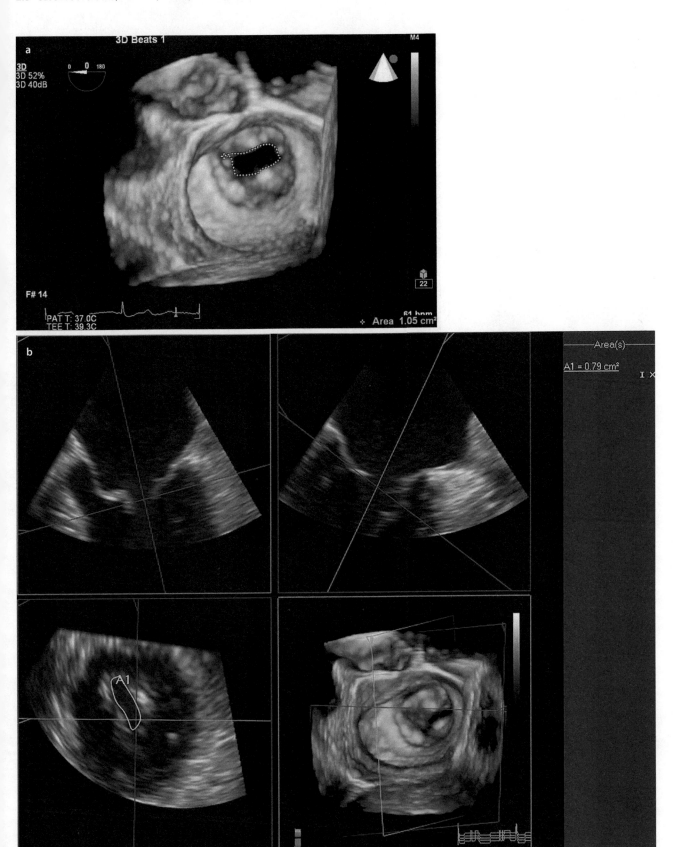

◨ **Fig. 2.41** Mitral valve area measures 1.05 cm² by direct planimetry by 3D zoom from LA side **a** and 1.29 cm² by 3DQ method **b**

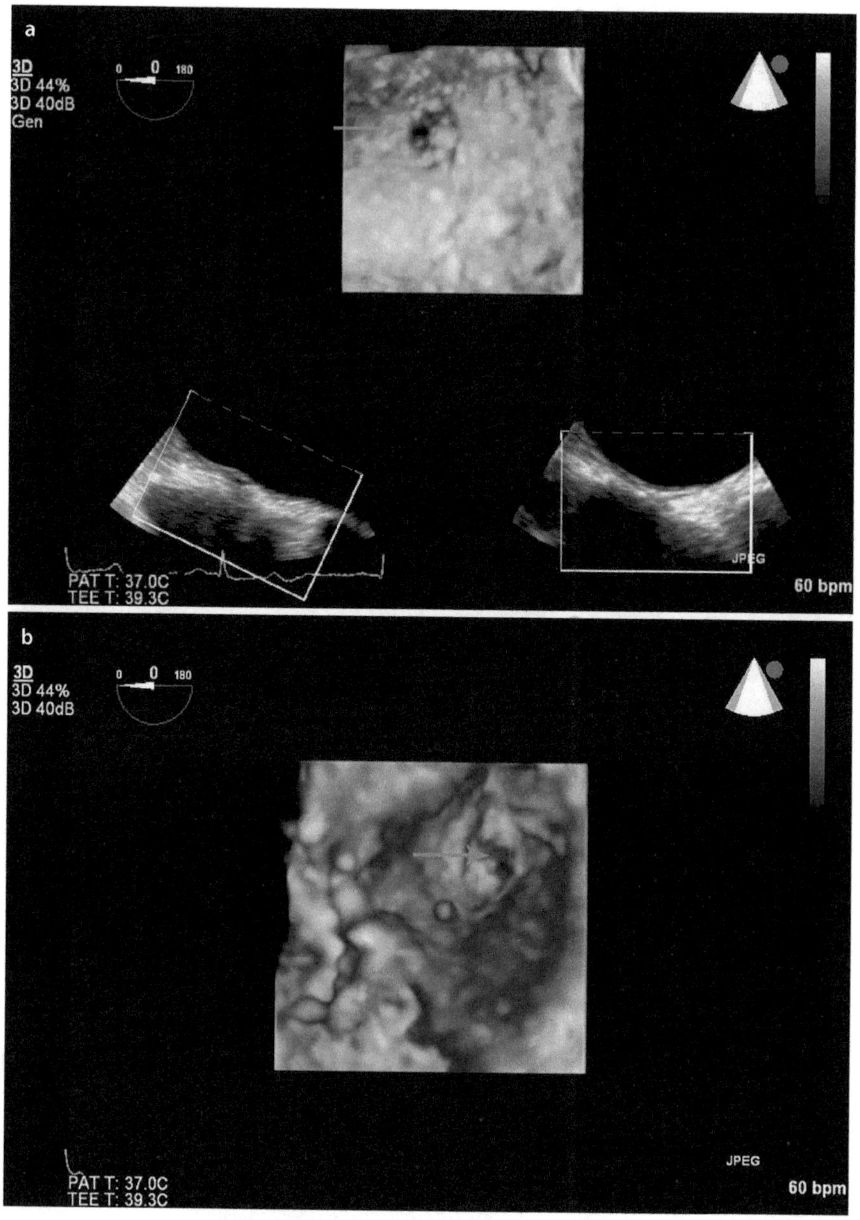

Fig. 2.42 Interatrial septum in site of foramen ovale with 3D zoom from LA side by I crop (*arrow*) **a** and from right atrial side (*arrow*) **b**

Diagnosis   Severe MS, mild MR, no LA, and LAA clot.

Comment   PTMC.

2.9 Case 8: Severe MS, Mild MR, Moderate AS, Moderate AI, No LA, and LAA Clot

A 45-year-old woman presented with dyspnea functional class III of recent exacerbation.

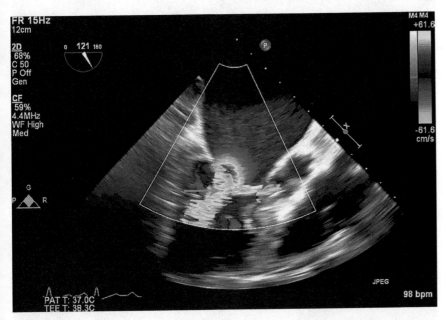

◨ **Fig. 2.43** Diastolic turbulency across mitral valve in favor of severe mitral stenosis (*green arrow*); moderate AI is also evident in this TEE long-axis view (*pink arrow*)

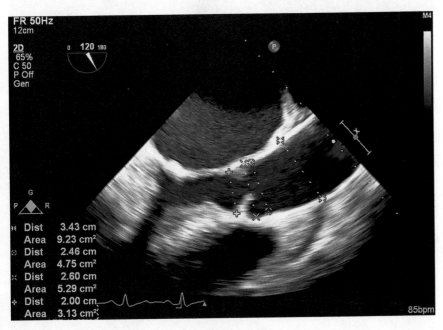

◨ **Fig. 2.44** Aortic annulus, sinus of Valsalva, sinotubular junction, and ascending aorta measure 20, 26, 24.6, and 34 mm, respectively, in TEE long-axis view

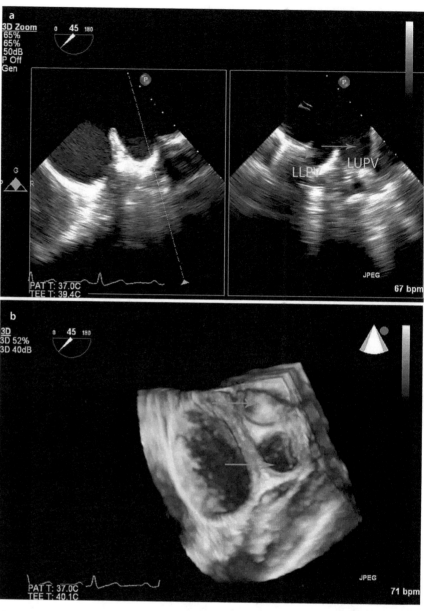

Fig. 2.45 Left pulmonary veins are visualized in TEE 45° and its orthogonal view (*arrows*) **a** and by 3D zoom (*arrows*) **b**. *LUPV*, left upper pulmonary vein; *LLPV*, left lower pulmonary vein

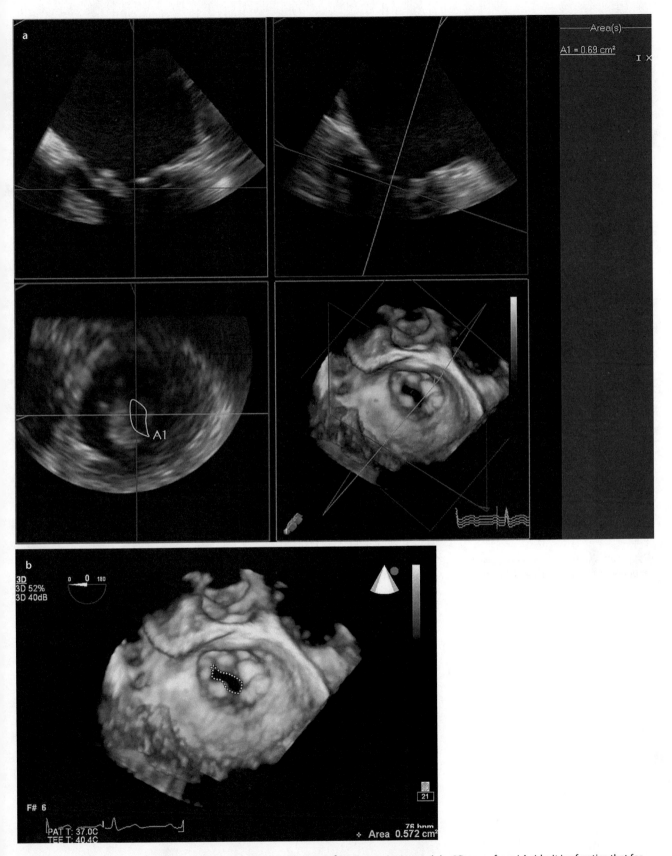

◻ **Fig. 2.46** Mitral valve area measures 0.69 cm² by 3DQ **a** and 0.57 cm² by direct planimetry **b** by 3D zoom from LA side. It is of notice that for measuring mitral valve area, the planes should be put at the tip of mitral leaflets in upper images and then the mitral valve area can be measured in left lower image

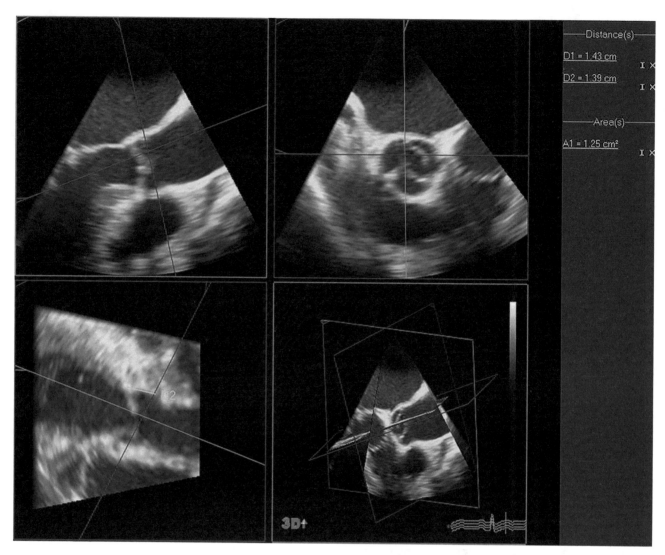

Distance(s)

D1 = 1.43 cm

D2 = 1.39 cm

Area(s)

A1 = 1.25 cm²

Fig. 2.47 Aortic valve area measures 1.25 cm² by planimetry by 3DQ. It is of notice that the planes should be put at the tip of aortic leaflets in left upper and lower images and then the aortic valve area can be measured in right upper image

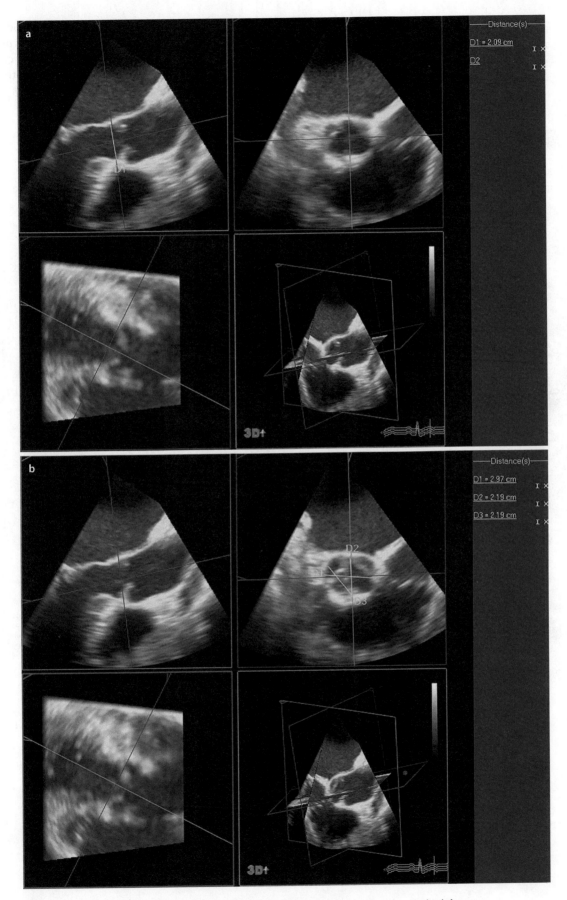

Distance(s)
D1 = 2.09 cm
D2

Distance(s)
D1 = 2.97 cm
D2 = 2.19 cm
D3 = 2.19 cm

D2
D3

3D+

3D+

Fig. 2.48 Aortic annulus measures 21 mm by double oblique method **a** and 22 mm by the other methods **b**

For measuring aortic annulus, we can use double oblique method; in this method, three planes are put in the lower insertion point of aortic leaflets in sagittal view (left upper quadrant, base of noncoronary cusp, and right coronary cusp) and coronal view (left lower quadrant, left and right coronary cusps). In transverse view (right upper quadrant), usually two measurements are done [7, 12].

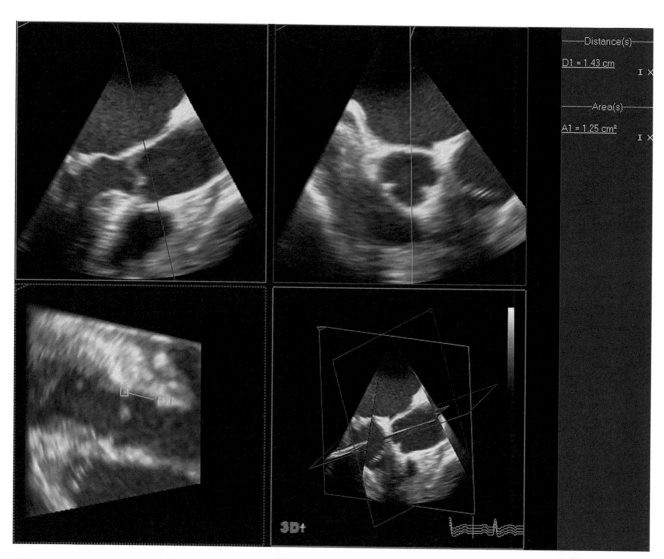

Fig. 2.49   Distance of left main from aortic annulus measures 14.3 mm by 3DQ in coronal view

Diagnosis   Severe MS, mild MR, moderate AS, moderate AI, no LA, and LAA clot.

Comment   PTMC.

Lesson   The distance of left main from left coronary cusp is 12.6 ± 2.6 in a postmortem study and 14.4 ± 2.9 by multislice computed tomography [6].

2.10   Case 9: Severe MS, Mild MR, Moderate AI, No LA, and LAA Clot

A 45-year-old man presented with dyspnea on exertion functional class III of recent exacerbation.

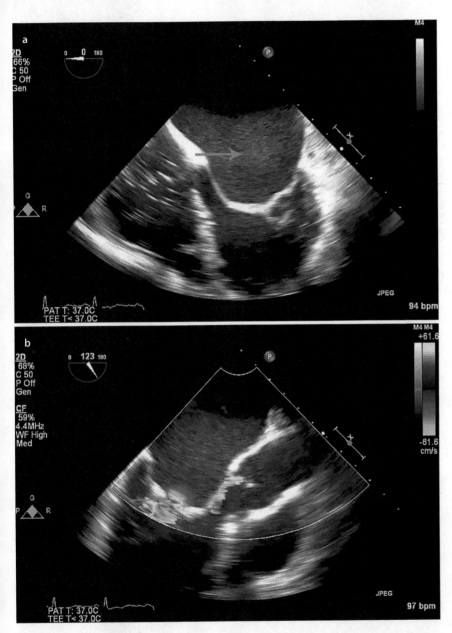

Fig. 2.50   Severe mitral stenosis and severe spontaneous contrast (*arrow*) in LA are seen in TEE 0° view **a**, and diastolic turbulency across mitral valve (*green arrow*) in favor of severe mitral stenosis and moderate aortic regurgitation (*pink arrow*) are evident in TEE long-axis view **b**

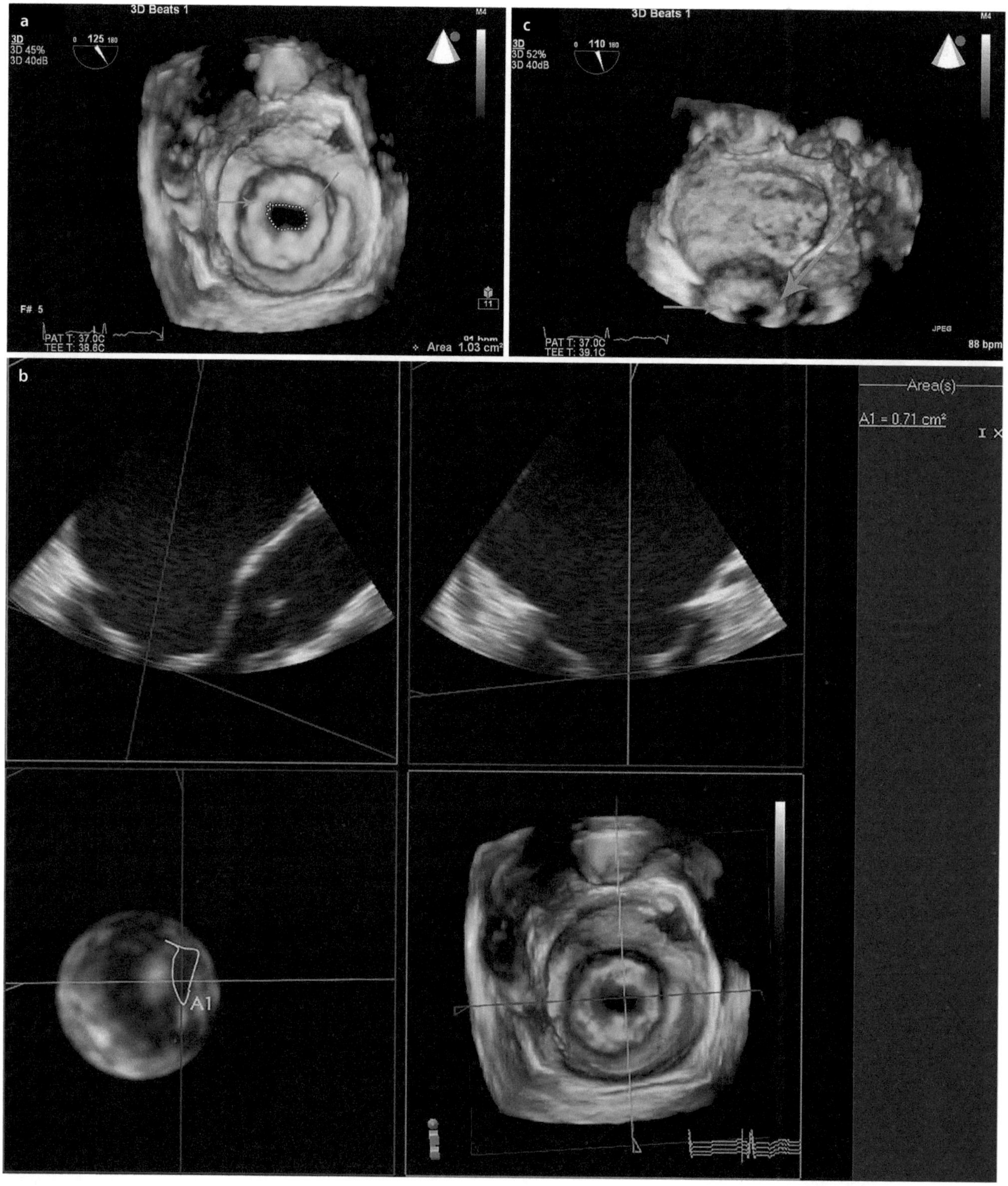

■ Fig. 2.51   MVA measures 1 cm² by direct planimetry by 3D zoom of mitral valve in 120° **a** and 0.71 cm² by 3DQ **b**, and both commissures are fused (*arrows*) **a, c**

2.10 · Case 9: Severe MS, Mild MR, Moderate AI, No LA, and LAA Clot

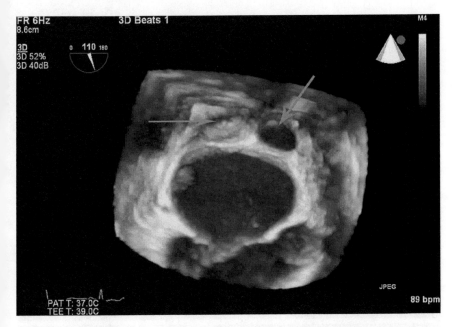

◻ **Fig. 2.52** Upper pulmonary veins are visualized posterior of LA (*arrows*) by TEE 3D zoom in 110° view

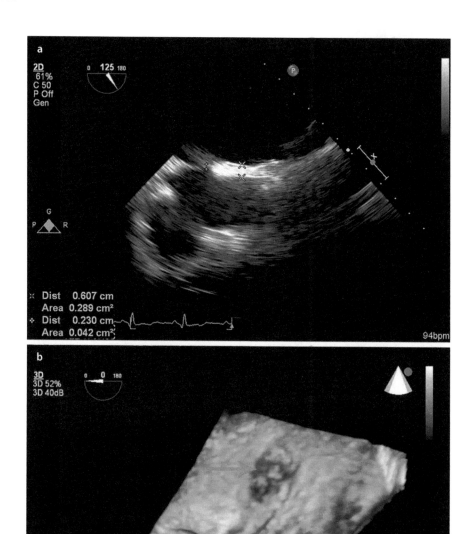

Fig. 2.53 Interatrial septum measures 2.3 mm in foramen ovale and 6 mm in other sites **a**, and foramen ovale is visualized by 3D zoom of interatrial septum from left atrial side (*arrow*) **b**

Diagnosis   Severe MS, mild MR, moderate AI, no LA, and LAA clot.

Comment   PTMC.

Lessons

Mitral valve area can be measured by direct planimetry [5] on 3D zoom or by 3DQ.

Mitral valve area by 3D echo is less than MVA by 2D echocardiography and PHT [13].

2.11 Case 10: Mild Mitral Stenosis due to Severe Mitral Annulus Calcification and Senile Degenerative Changes of Mitral Valve

A 65-year-old woman presented with dyspnea on exertion functional class II to III with recent exacerbation.

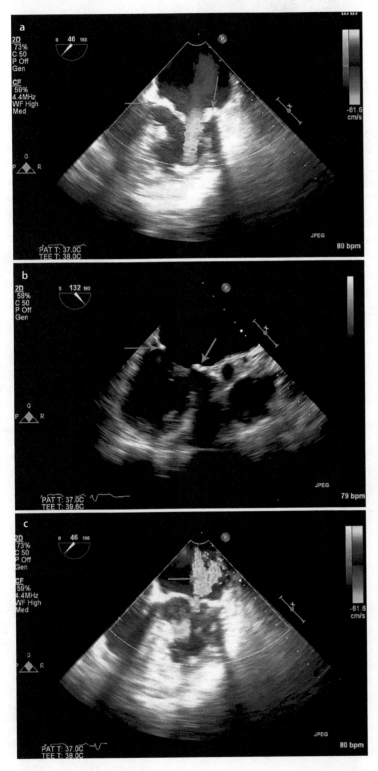

◻ **Fig. 2.54** Severe mitral annular calcification (*green arrows*) is seen in TEE short-axis **a** and TEE long-axis **b** views; this calcification produces turbulency across mitral valve (*pink arrow*) **a** and mitral stenosis, and moderate mitral regurgitation is also evident in TEE short-axis view (*arrow*) **c**

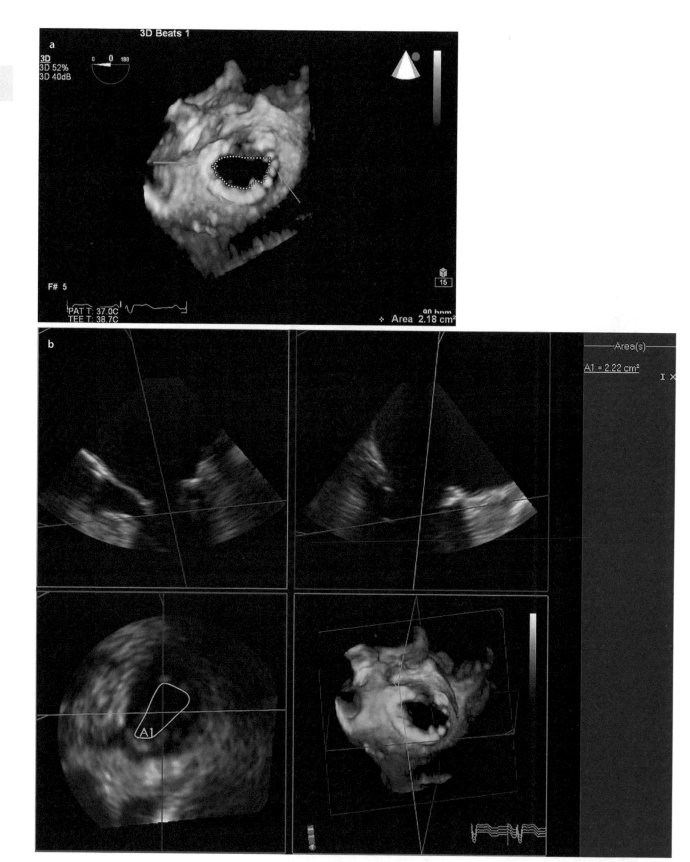

◘ Fig. 2.55   Mitral valve area measures 2.1 cm² by direct planimetry on 3D zoom **a**, severe calcification of posterior mitral annulus is evident in this view (*arrows*) **a**, and mitral valve area measures 2.2 cm² by 3DQ **b**

Diagnosis   Moderate mitral stenosis and moderate mitral regurgitation due to senile degenerative changes of mitral valve and severe posterior mitral annular calcification.

Comment   Follow-up.

Lesson   Senile degenerative changes of mitral valve usually produce mild mitral stenosis, and severe mitral stenosis occurs in about one-fourth of patients [14].

2.12 Case 11: Severe Mitral Stenosis, Severe Mitral Regurgitation, Severe Tricuspid Regurgitation, No LA, and LAA Clot

A 35-year-old woman presented with dyspnea on exertion functional class III of recent exacerbation.

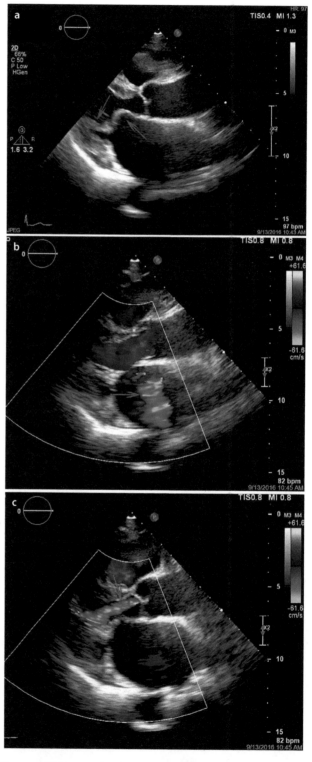

Fig. 2.56 Parasternal long-axis view shows thickening and doming of mitral leaflets (*green arrow*) **a**, thickening of subvalvular apparatus is also apparent in this view (*pink arrow*) **a**, and severe mitral regurgitation (*arrow*) **b** and moderate aortic regurgitation are also evident in this view **b, c**

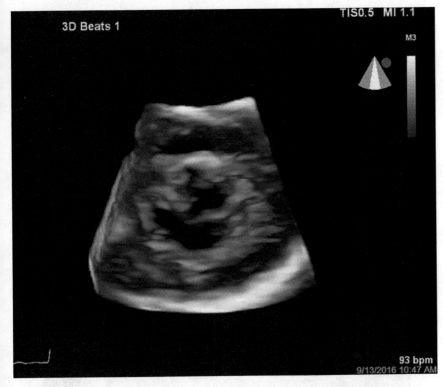

Fig. 2.57   3D zoom of mitral valve from LA side in parasternal long-axis view

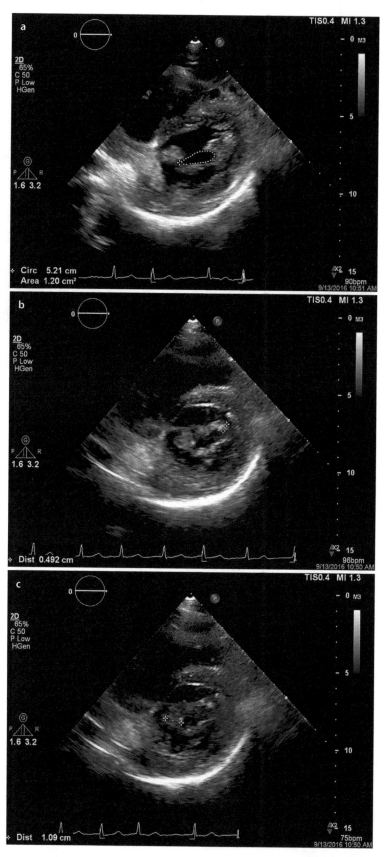

■ **Fig. 2.58**   Mitral valve area measures 1.2 cm² by direct planimetry **a** [15], and anterior and posterior commissural thickness measures 5 mm and 11 mm, respectively **b**, **c**, so commissural score will be 4 [16]

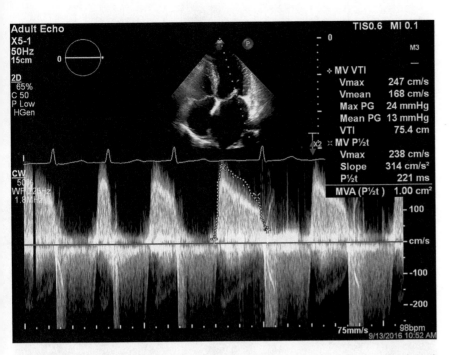

Fig. 2.59 Peak and mean mitral valve gradients measure 24 and 13 mmHg, respectively, and mitral valve measures 1 cm² by PHT

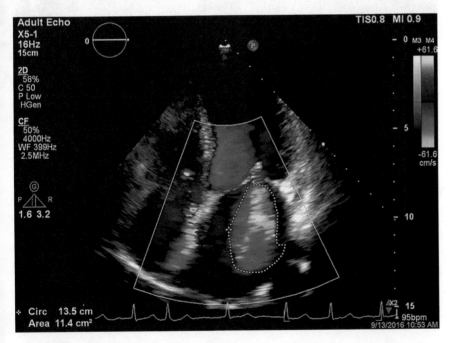

Fig. 2.60 Severe mitral regurgitation is seen in apical four-chamber view, and surface of mitral regurgitation measures 11cm²

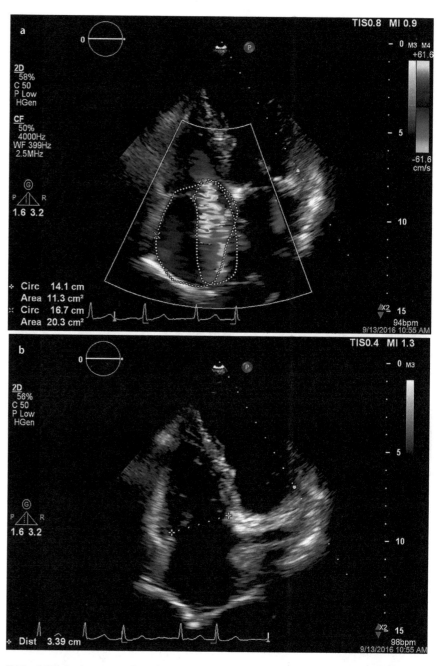

Fig. 2.61 Severe tricuspid regurgitation (TR) is seen in apical four-chamber view **a**, surface of TR/RA = 11/20 cm² **a**, TV annulus measures 34 mm in apical four-chamber view (mildly dilated) **b**

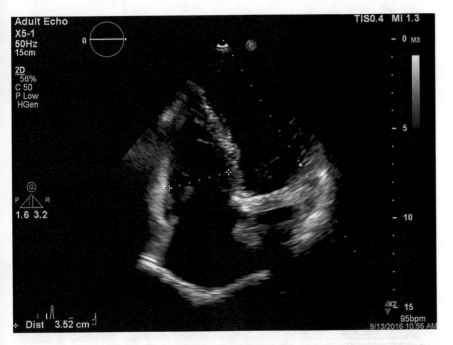

Fig. 2.62 The right ventricle measures 35 mm in apical four-chamber view (mildly dilated)

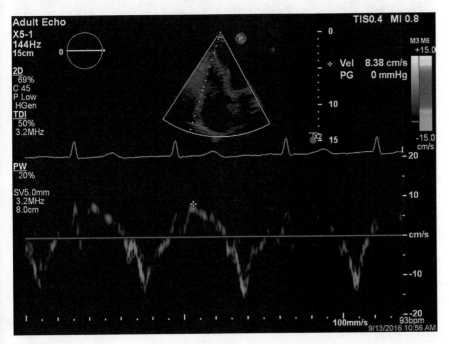

Fig. 2.63 Right ventricular Sm measures 8 cm/s in favor of mild right ventricular systolic dysfunction

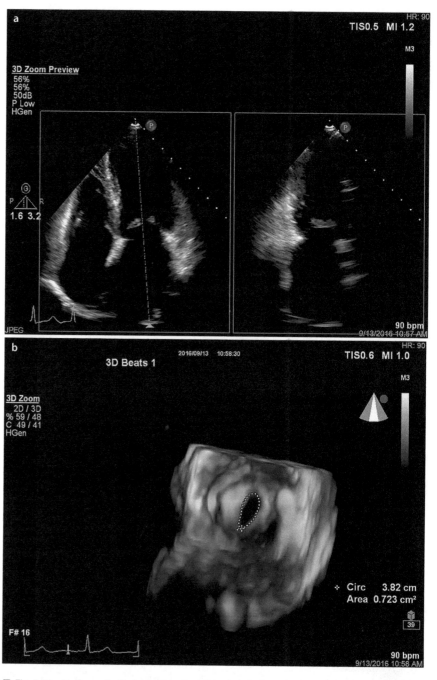

Fig. 2.64 X-plane of mitral valve in apical four-chamber view **a** and then 3D zoom of mitral valve **b**, mitral valve area measures 0.7 cm² by direct planimetry from left ventricular side **b** and 0.7 cm² by3DQ method **c**

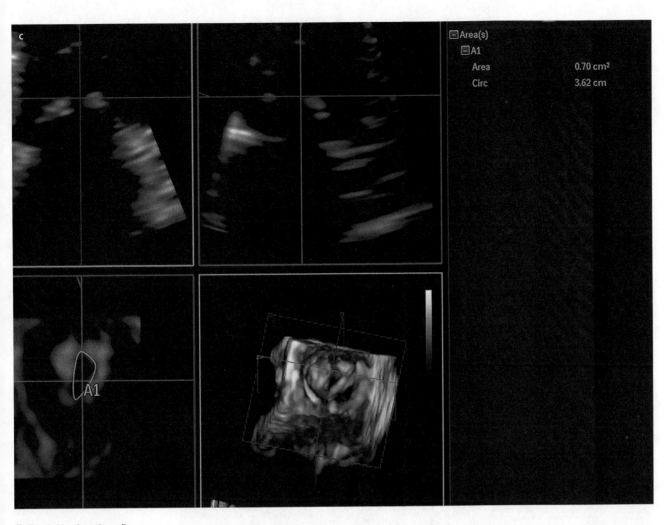

Fig. 2.64 (continued)

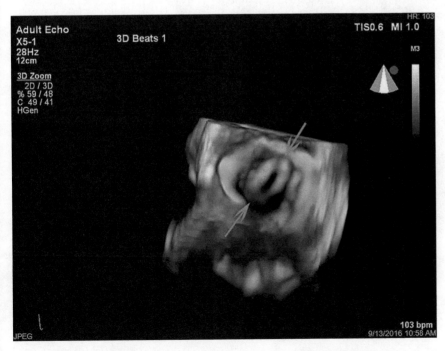

Fig. 2.65 Both commissures are fused by 3D zoom from left ventricular side (*arrows*)

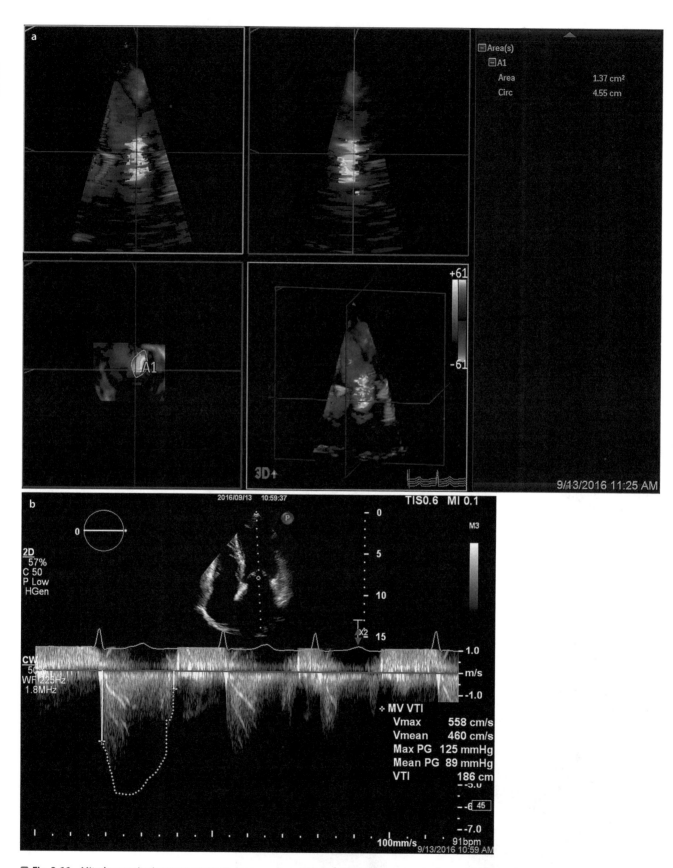

□ **Fig. 2.66**   Mitral regurgitation vena contracta area measures 1.37 cm² by full volume **a**, mitral regurgitation VTI measures 186 cm **b**, and MR volume will be calculated as follows: 1.37*186 = 254 cm³ in favor of severe mitral regurgitation

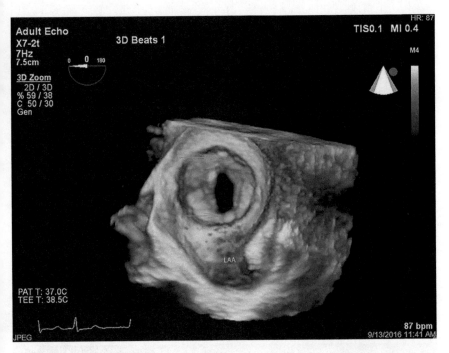

Fig. 2.67 3D zoom of mitral valve from left atrial side shows fusion of both commissures (*arrows*), and left atrial appendage (LAA) is visualized in this view in 6 o'clock (before Z rotation)

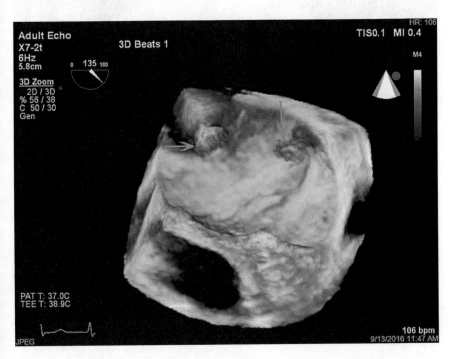

Fig. 2.68 Flow from left pulmonary veins is well visualized by 3D zoom 130° (*arrows*)

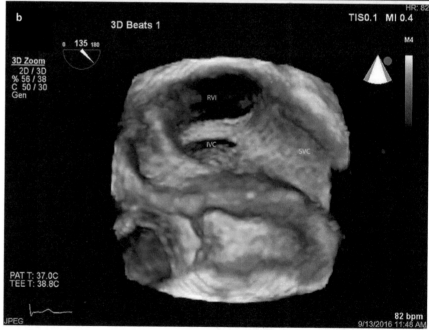

Fig. 2.69 3D zoom of interatrial septum from right atrial side reveals superior and inferior vena cava (SVC and IVC) in 0° **a** and 130° **b**, right ventricular inflow (RVI) tract is well visualized in this view **b** and is located in anterior side, and IVC and SVC are in posterior side like anatomic position

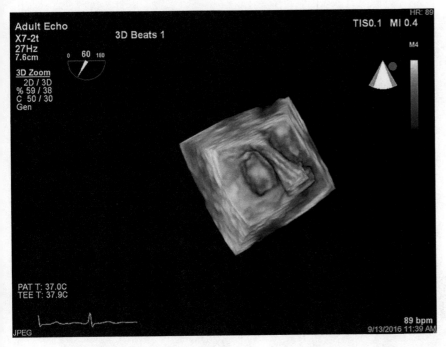

■ **Fig. 2.70** Left atrial appendage is visualized by 3D zoom from left atrial side in 60°

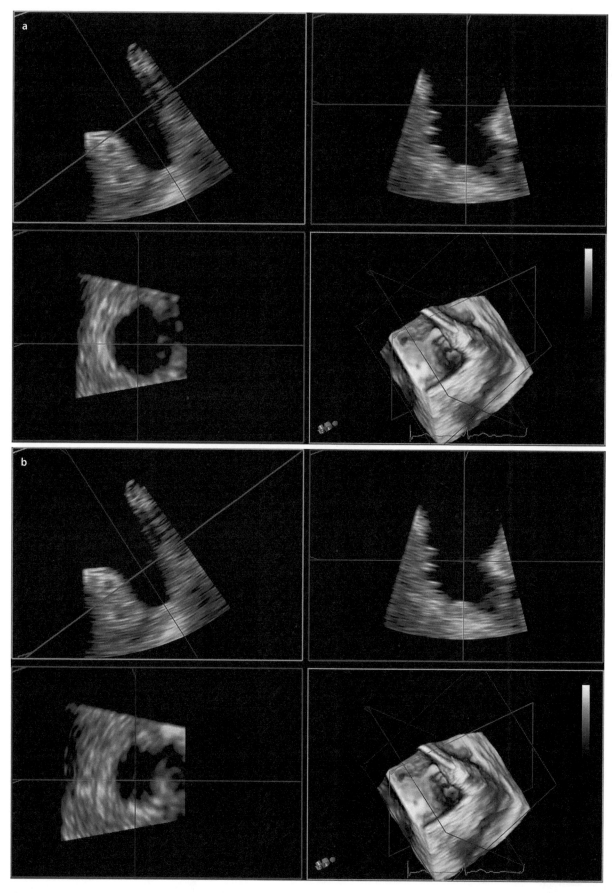

■ **Fig. 2.71**   No clot in left atrial appendage by 3DQ from base to apex **a–e**

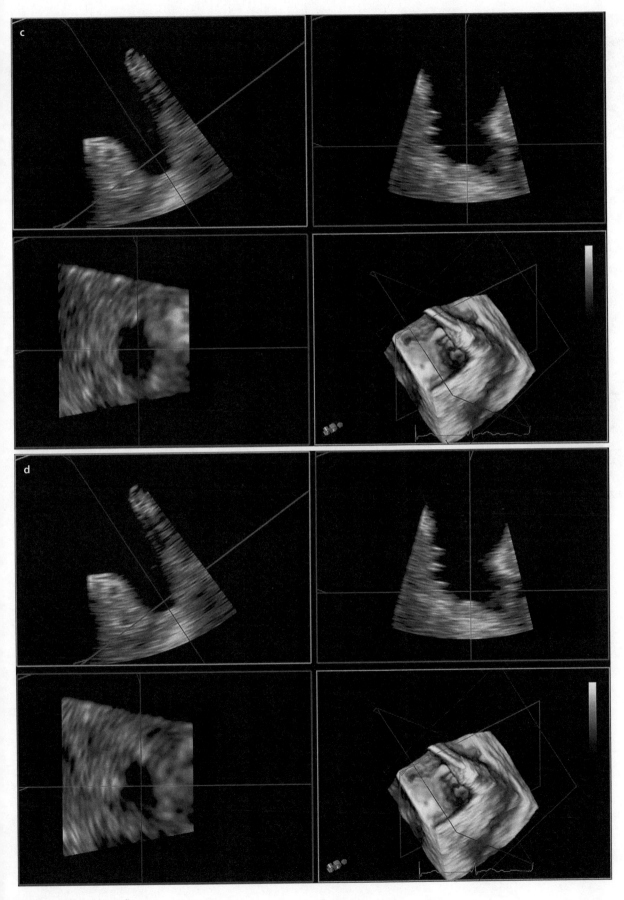

◘ Fig. 2.71   (continued)

2

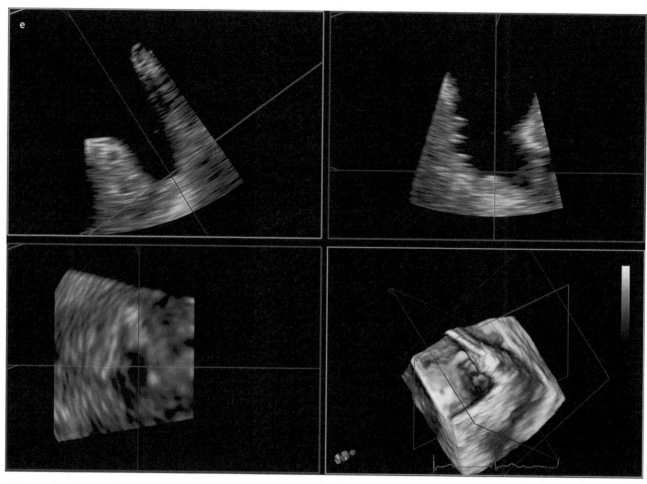

❑ **Fig. 2.71**   (continued)

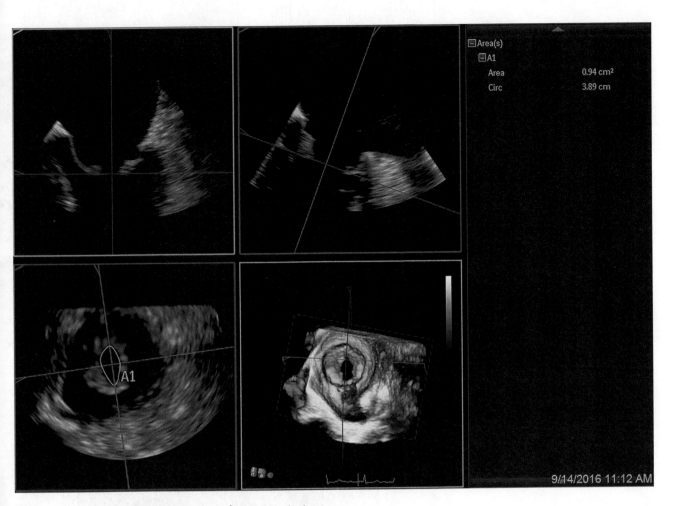

Fig. 2.72 Mitral valve area measures 0.94 cm² by 3DQ method

Diagnosis Severe mitral stenosis, severe mitral regurgitation, severe tricuspid regurgitation, no LA, and LAA clot.

Comment The patient is referred for surgery (MVR + Tricuspid valve annuloplasty).

Lesson

Commissural score before PTMC:

Commissural thickness <5 for each commissure: 1

Commissural thickness >5 for each commissure: 2, in the absence of severe commissural calcification or splitting of commissures [16, 17].

2.13   Case 12: Severe Mitral Stenosis, Mild Mitral Regurgitation, Severe Tricuspid Regurgitation, and Severe Spontaneous Contrast Impending to Fresh Clot Formation in LAA

A 45-year-old woman presented with cerebrovascular accident 1 month ago; she had atrial fibrillation.

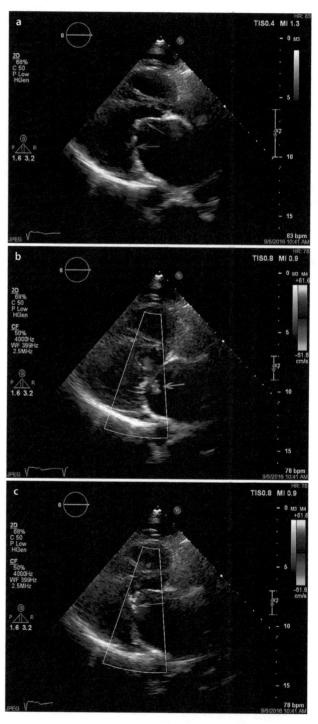

☐ **Fig. 2.73**   Thickening and doming of anterior mitral leaflet (*green arrow*) and restricted posterior mitral leaflet motion in diastole (*pink arrow*) are evident in parasternal long-axis view **a**, mild mitral regurgitation (*green arrow*) is evident in this view **b**, and turbulency across mitral valve in diastole (*green arrow*) **c** in favor of mitral stenosis is also evident in this view

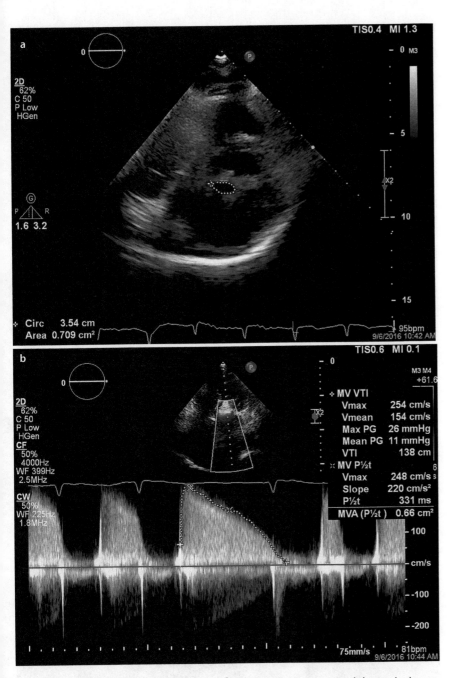

Fig. 2.74 Mitral valve area measures 0.7 cm² by planimetry in parasternal short-axis view **a**; peak and mean mitral gradient measures 26 and 11 mmHg, respectively; and mitral valve area measures 0.66 cm² by pressure half-time **b** by continuous wave Doppler in apical four-chamber view

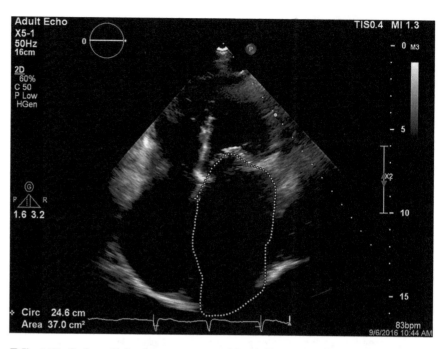

Fig. 2.75 Surface of left atrium measures 37 cm² in apical four-chamber view in favor of moderate left atrial enlargement

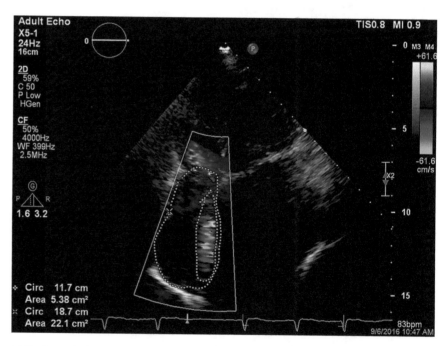

Fig. 2.76 Surface of tricuspid regurgitation measures 11 cm² indicative of severe tricuspid regurgitation, and surface of right atrium measures 22 cm² in favor of mild right atrial enlargement

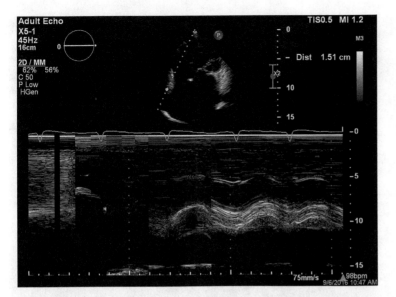

Fig. 2.77 Tricuspid annulus posterior systolic excursion measures 15 cm in favor of moderate right ventricular systolic dysfunction in the presence of severe tricuspid regurgitation

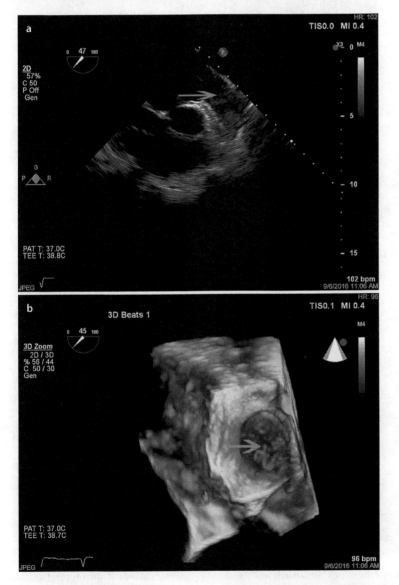

Fig. 2.78 Severe spontaneous contrast impending to fresh clot formation in left atrial appendage (LAA) is evident in TEE short-axis view (*arrow*) **a** and by 3D zoom of LAA from left atrium (*arrow*) **b**

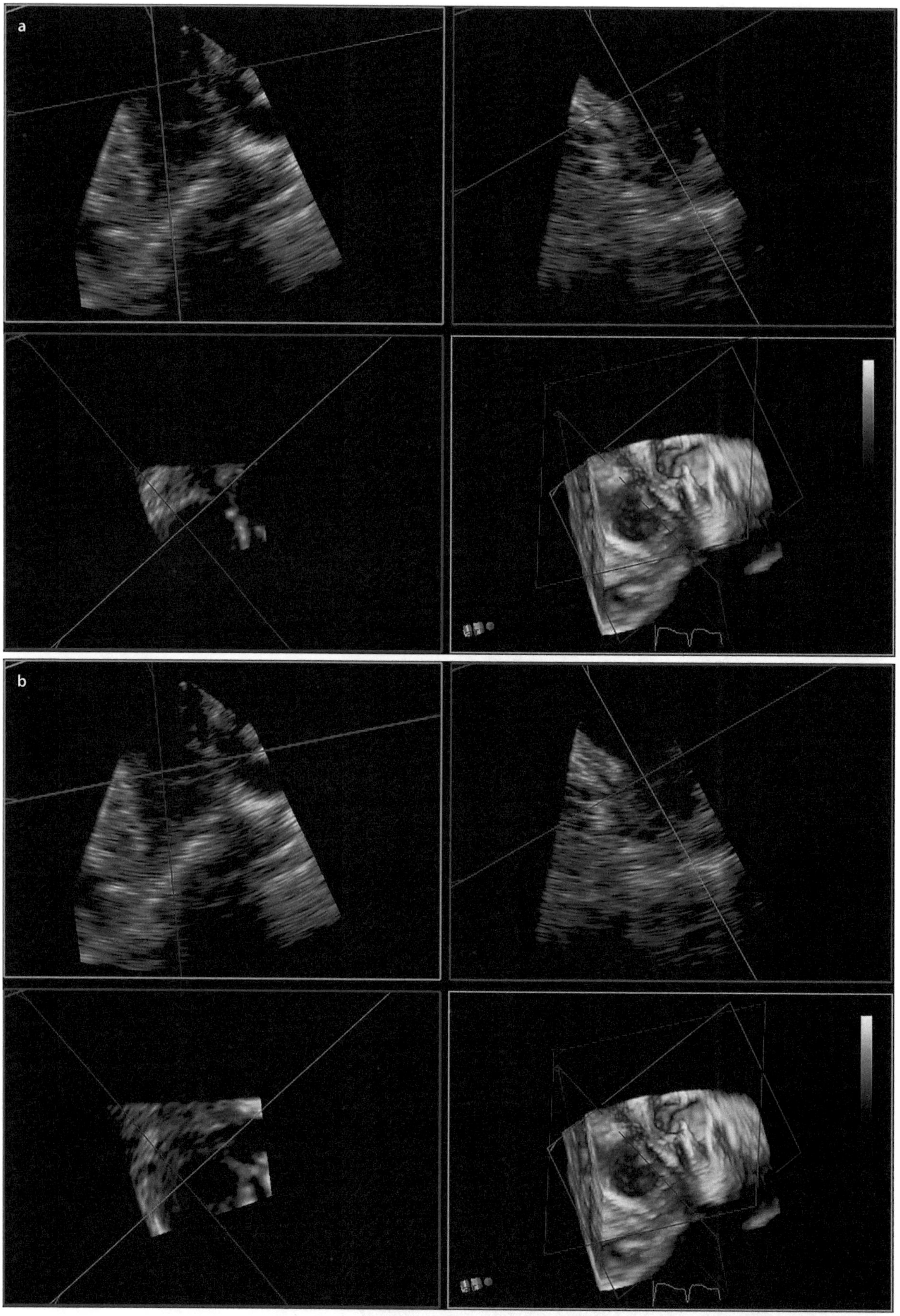

2

■ **Fig. 2.79** Spontaneous contrast grade III impending to fresh clot formation is well visualized in different cuts of left atrial appendage from base to apex **a–e**

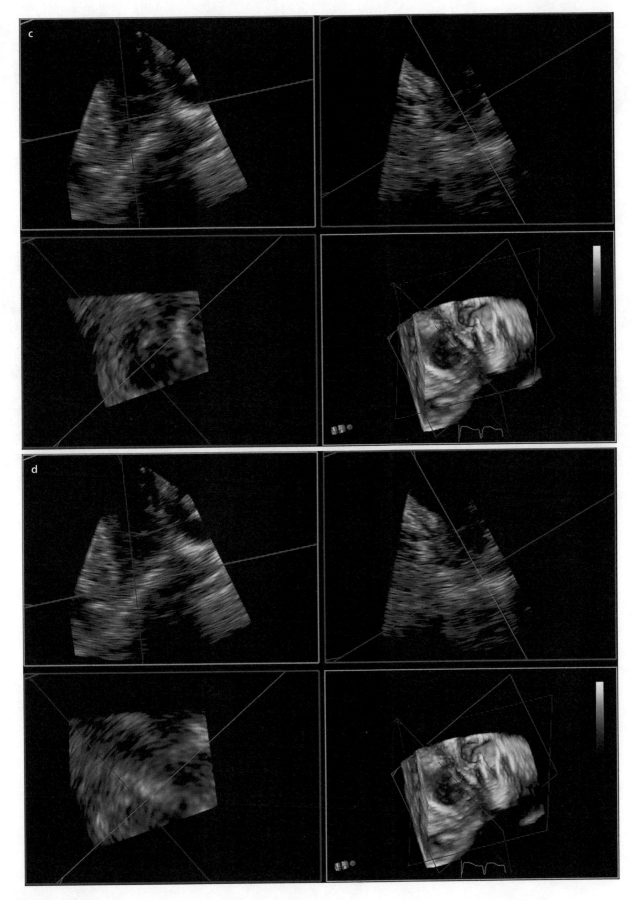

■ Fig. 2.79 (continued)

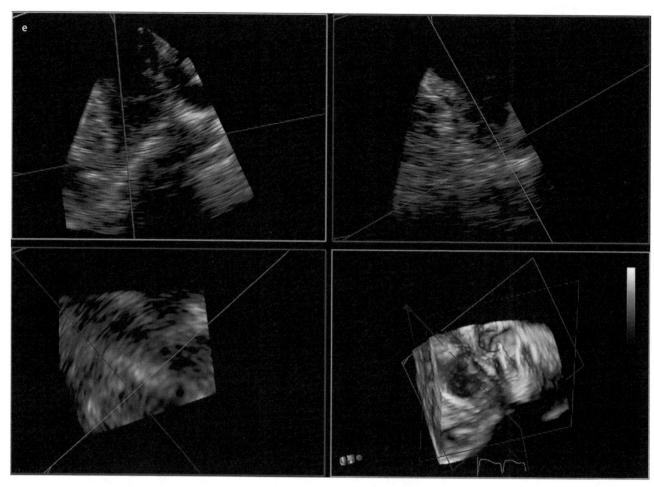

◻ **Fig. 2.79**   (continued)

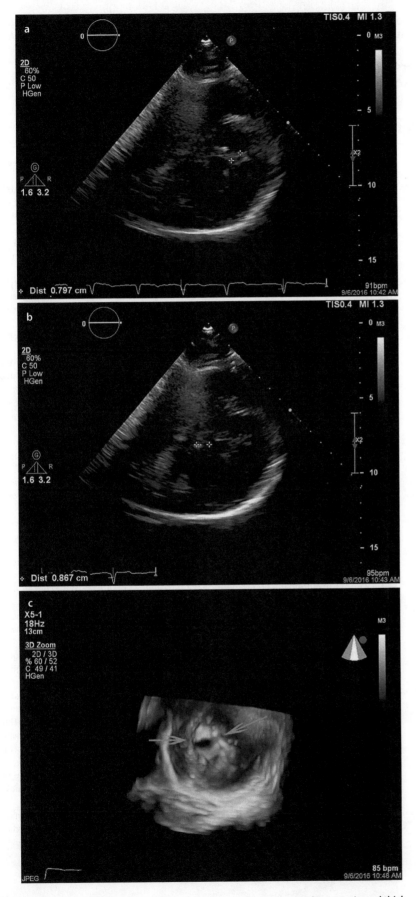

■ Fig. 2.80   Anterior commissural thickness measures 9 mm **a**, posterior commissural thickness measures 8 mm **b**, and 3D zoom of mitral valve from left ventricular side shows fusion of both commissures (*arrows*) **c**

Diagnosis   Severe mitral stenosis, mild mitral regurgitation, severe tricuspid regurgitation, and severe spontaneous contrast impending to fresh clot formation in LAA.

Recommendation   Full anticoagulant therapy for 3 months and TEE after that. LAA clot is a contraindication for PTMC [5].

References

1. Otto CM, Bownow RO, et al. Braunwald's heart disease. 10th ed. Philadelphia, PA: Elsevier Saunders; 2015.
2. Nishimura RA, Otto CM, Bonow RO, Carabello BA, Erwin 3rd JP, Guyton RA, et al. 2014 AHA/ACC guideline for the management of patients with valvular heart disease: a report of the American College of Cardiology/American Heart Association task force on practice guidelines. J Am Coll Cardiol. 2014;63(22):e57–185.
3. Baumgartner H, Hung J, Bermejo J, Chambers JB, Evangelista A, Griffin BP, et al. Echocardiographic assessment of valve stenosis: EAE/ASE recommendations for clinical practice. Eur J Echocardiogr. 2009;10(1):1–25.
4. Joint Task Force on the Management of Valvular Heart Disease of the European Society of Cardiac, European Association for Cardio-Thoracic Surgery, Vahanian A, Alfieri O, Andreotti F, Antunes MJ, et al. Guidelines on the management of valvular heart disease (version 2012). Eur Heart J. 2012;33(19):2451–96.
5. Wunderlich NC, Beigel R, Siegel RJ. Management of mitral stenosis using 2D and 3D echo-Doppler imaging. JACC Cardiovasc Imaging. 2013;6(11):1191–205.
6. Piazza N, de Jaegere P, Schultz C, Becker AE, Serruys PW, Anderson RH. Anatomy of the aortic valvar complex and its implications for transcatheter implantation of the aortic valve. Circ Cardiovasc Interv. 2008;1(1):74–81.
7. Jilaihawi H, Doctor N, Kashif M, Chakravarty T, Rafique A, Makar M, et al. Aortic annular sizing for transcatheter aortic valve replacement using cross-sectional 3-dimensional transesophageal echocardiography. J Am Coll Cardiol. 2013;61(9):908–16.
8. Fang L, Hsiung MC, Miller AP, Nanda NC, Yin WH, Young MS, et al. Assessment of aortic regurgitation by live three-dimensional transthoracic echocardiographic measurements of vena contracta area: usefulness and validation. Echocardiography. 2005;22(9):775–81.
9. Chin CH, Chen CH, Lo HS. The correlation between three-dimensional vena contracta area and aortic regurgitation index in patients with aortic regurgitation. Echocardiography. 2010;27(2):161–6.
10. Zeng X, Levine RA, Hua L, Morris EL, Kang Y, Flaherty M, et al. Diagnostic value of vena contracta area in the quantification of mitral regurgitation severity by color Doppler 3D echocardiography. Circ Cardiovasc Imaging. 2011;4(5):506–13.
11. Chen TE, Kwon SH, Enriquez-Sarano M, Wong BF, Mankad SV. Three-dimensional color Doppler echocardiographic quantification of tricuspid regurgitation orifice area: comparison with conventional two-dimensional measures. J Am Soc Echocardiogr. 2013;26(10):1143–52.
12. Khalique OK, Kodali SK, Paradis JM, Nazif TM, Williams MR, Einstein AJ, et al. Aortic annular sizing using a novel 3-dimensional echocardiographic method: use and comparison with cardiac computed tomography. Circ Cardiovasc Imaging. 2014;7(1):155–63.
13. Schlosshan D, Aggarwal G, Mathur G, Allan R, Cranney G. Real-time 3D transesophageal echocardiography for the evaluation of rheumatic mitral stenosis. JACC Cardiovasc Imaging. 2011;4(6):580–8.
14. Iwataki M, Takeuchi M, Otani K, Kuwaki H, Yoshitani H, Abe H, et al. Calcific extension towards the mitral valve causes non-rheumatic mitral stenosis in degenerative aortic stenosis: real-time 3D transoesophageal echocardiography study. Open Heart. 2014;1(1):e000136.
15. Mannaerts HF, Kamp O, Visser CA. Should mitral valve area assessment in patients with mitral stenosis be based on anatomical or on functional evaluation? A plea for 3D echocardiography as the new clinical standard. Eur Heart J. 2004;25(23):2073–4.
16. Sutaria N, Shaw TR, Prendergast B, Northridge D. Transoesophageal echocardiographic assessment of mitral valve commissural morphology predicts outcome after balloon mitral valvotomy. Heart. 2006;92(1):52–7.
17. Sadeghian H, Salarifar M, Rezvanfard M, Nematipour E, Lotfi Tokaldany M, Safir Mardanloo A, et al. Percutaneous transvenous mitral commissurotomy: significance of echocardiographic assessment in prediction of immediate result. Arch Iran Med. 2012;15(10):629–34.

Aortic Valve Disease

Videos can be found in the electronic supplementary material in the online version of the chapter.
On http://springerlink.com enter the DOI number given on the bottom of the chapter opening page.
Scroll down to the Supplementary material tab and click on the respective videos link.

© Springer International Publishing AG 2017
H. Sadeghian, Z. Savand-Roomi, *3D Echocardiography of Structural Heart Disease*,
DOI 10.1007/978-3-319-54039-9_3

3.1   Aortic Stenosis

The most common cause of aortic stenosis (AS) in developing countries is rheumatismal involvement of aortic valve often in association with involvement of other valves, while in developed countries, AS is often due to senile degenerative changes.

Bicuspid aortic valve is other congenital aortic valve disease which produces various degrees of AS and AI.

3.1.1   Definition

Normal aortic velocity is 1.64 m/s. Mild AS is defined as mean aortic gradient below 20 mmHg, moderate AS is defined with mean aortic gradient between 20 and 39 mmHg, and severe AS is as mean aortic gradient ≥40 mmHg or peak aortic velocity ≥4 m/s or aortic valve area ≤1 cm^2 or ≤0.6 cm^2/m^2 [1]. Critical AS is defined as aortic valve area <0.6 cm^2 or less than 0.4 cm^2/m^2 or mean gradient ≥60 mmHg or peak aortic velocity ≥5 m/s [1]. All of these definitions are with normal LVEF.

There are two other conditions of severe AS: (1) Low flow low gradient AS and (2) Paradoxical low gradient AS.

Low flow low gradient AS occurs when LVEF is less than 50%, aortic valve area measures ≤1 cm^2 but mean aortic gradient <40 mmHg.

Paradoxical low flow AS occurs when in the presence of normal LVEF, aortic valve area is ≤1 cm^2 but mean aortic gradient is <40 mmHg.

3.1.2   How to Approach

Severe symptomatic AS should be referred for surgery (AVR), severe asymptomatic AS should be followed up carefully. ETT is class IIa indication in asymptomatic severe As [1]. AVR is class IIa recommendation for asymptomatic patients with very severe AS [1].

For low flow low gradient AS, dobutamine stress echocardiography is recommended, when mean gradient achieved to more than 40 mmHg and stroke volume increases more than 20% without significant increase in aortic valve area, the patient should be referred for surgery.

In paradoxical low flow AS, TEE 3D is very helpful for precise aortic valve area measurement.

TAVI is indicated in patients with high Euroscore >15–20% or STS >10% score when survival of patients is considered more than 1 year [2].

3.2   Aortic Regurgitation

Aortic regurgitation may be due to rheumatismal involvement, bicuspid aortic valve, or dilation of ascending aorta and aortic root.

Severe asymptomatic chronic aortic regurgitation should be referred for surgery if there is LVEF <50% [1, 3], LVEDD >70 mm [3], and LVESD >50 mm [1, 3]. LVEDD >65 mm is class IIb indication for AVR according to ACC/AHA guidelines [1].

Patients with moderate AR undergoing other cardiac surgery, AVR is class IIa recommendation [1].

Patients with bicuspid aortic valve who are candidate for AVR, aortic root replacement is indicated with ascending aorta >45 mm [1].

3.3   Case 1: Severe Aortic Regurgitation

A 30-year-old man presented by dyspnea on exertion functional class III of recent duration.

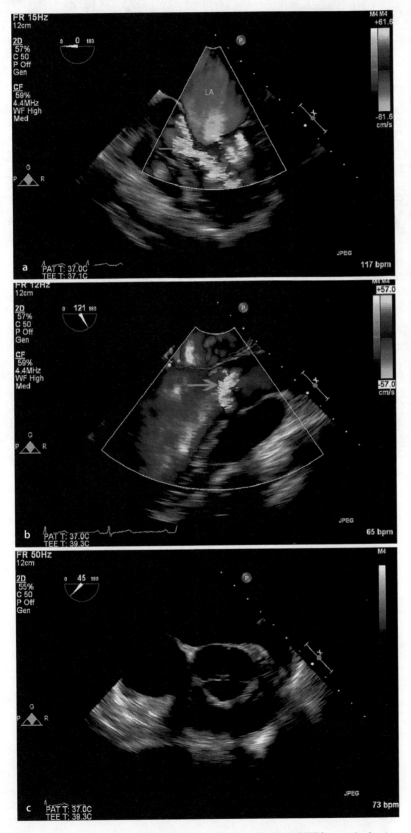

■ **Fig. 3.1**   Severe aortic regurgitation is seen in TEE 0° (*arrow*) **a** and TEE long-axis views (*arrow*) **b**, aortic valve is thick and tricuspid by TEE short-axis view **c**. *LA* left atrium

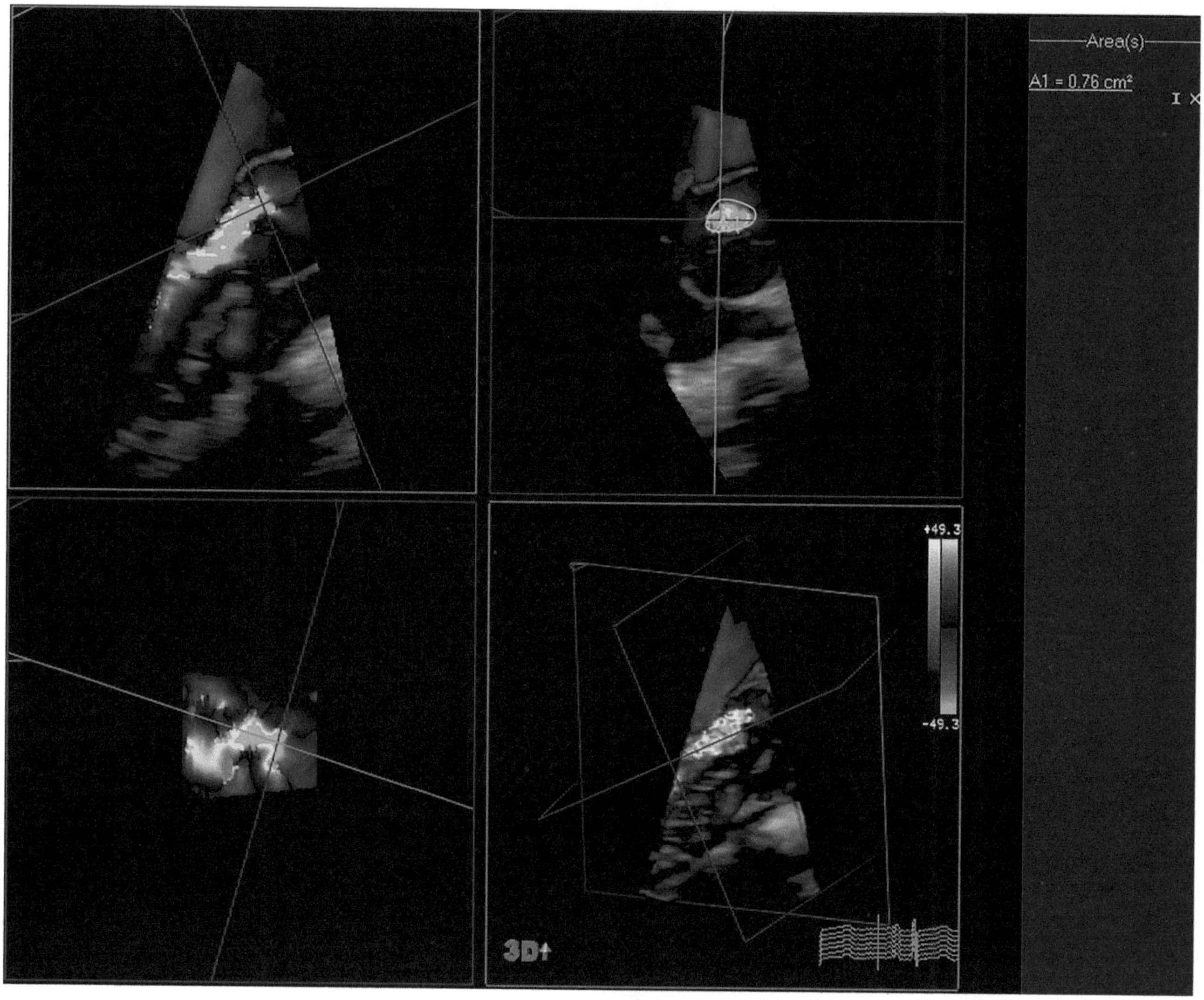

Fig. 3.2 AI vena contracta area measures 0.76 cm² by full volume 3D echocardiography [4]

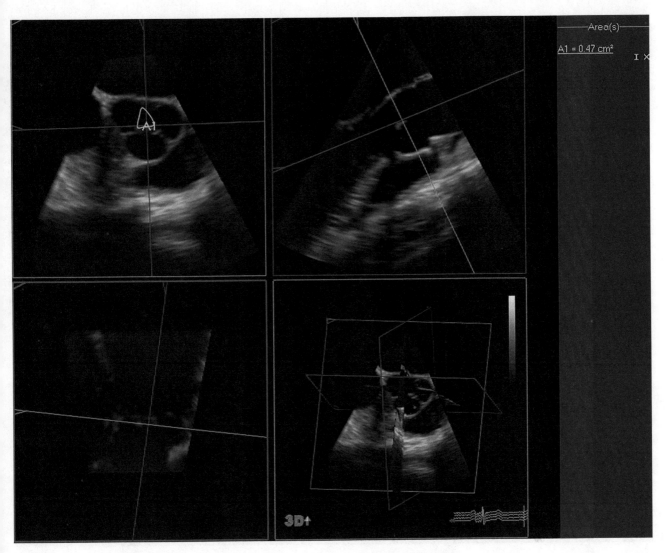

☐ **Fig. 3.3** AI anatomic regurgitation surface area measures 0.47 cm² by full volume of aortic valve

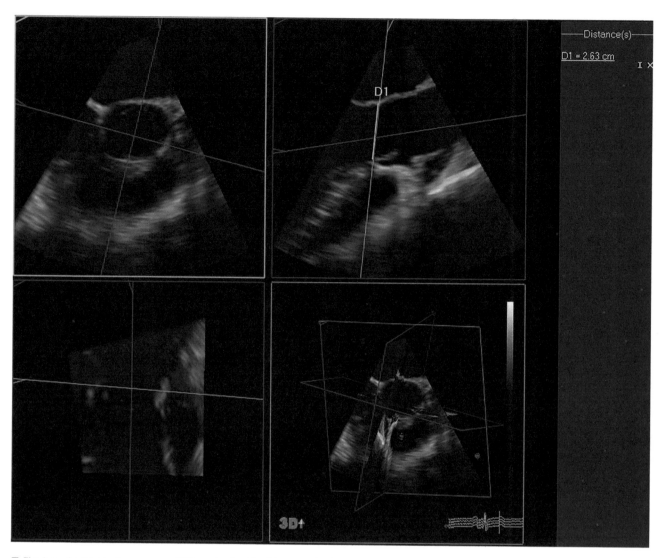

Fig. 3.4 Aortic annulus measures 26.3 mm by double oblique method

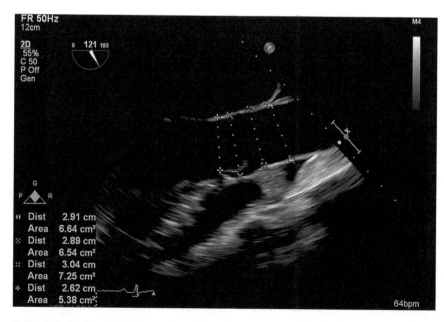

Fig. 3.5 Aortic annulus, sinus of valsalva, sinotubular junction, and ascending aorta measure 26.2, 30.4, 28.9, and 29 cm, respectively

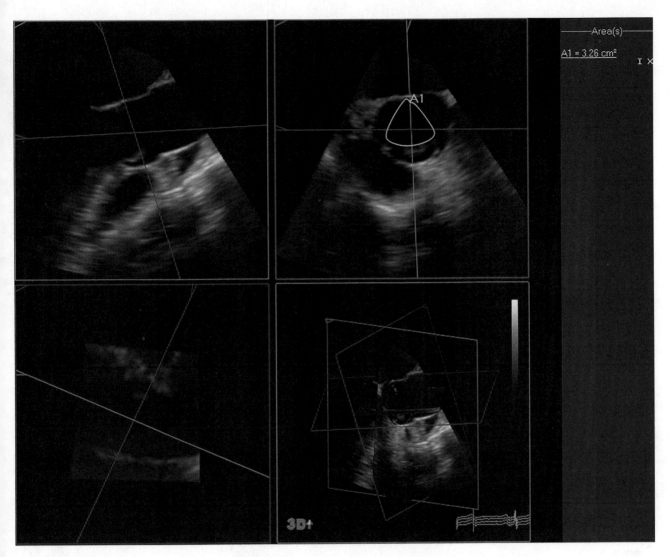

Area(s)

A1 = 3.26 cm²

Fig. 3.6   Aortic valve area measures 3.26 cm² by planimetry by 3DQ method at tip of leaflets in systole

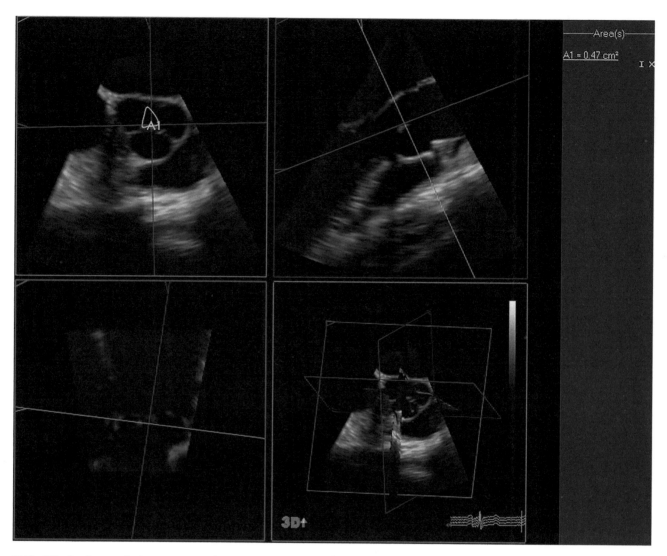

Fig. 3.7   Aortic regurgitation anatomic surface area measures 4.7 mm² by 3DQ method in diastole

Diagnosis   Severe rheumatismal AI, three cuspid aortic valve.

Lesson   Vena contracta area <30 mm² has a sensitivity about 90% for predicting mild aortic regurgitation and >50 mm² has a sensitivity and specificity about 90% for predicting severe aortic regurgitation [5].

Comment   AVR.

3.4   Case 2: Critical AS, Severe AI

A 44-year-old athlete man presented by dyspnea on exertion functional class I. His BSA was 2 m².

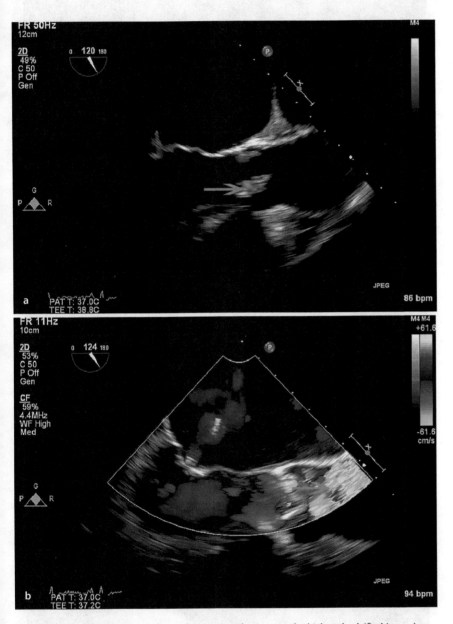

☐ **Fig. 3.8**   TEE long-axis view shows that aortic valve is severely thick and calcified (*arrow*) **a**, severe systolic turbulency by color Doppler in ascending aorta in favor of severe valvular AS (*arrow*) **b**

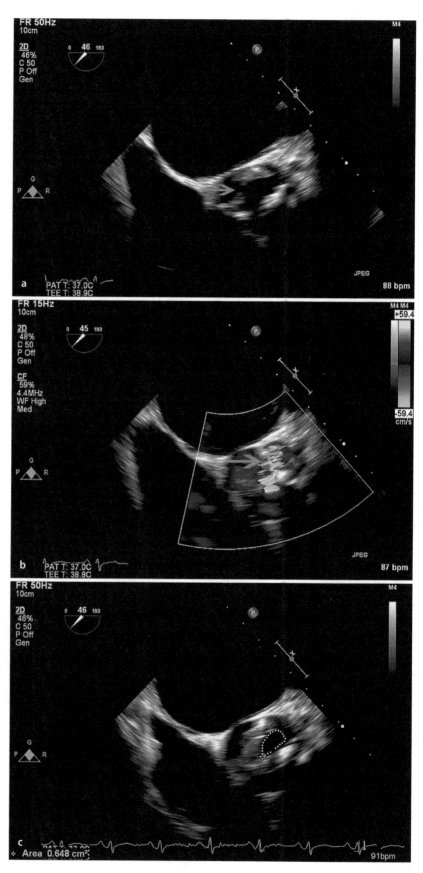

◼ Fig. 3.9   TEE short-axis view shows that aortic valve is tricuspid (*arrow*) **a**, severe AI (*arrow*) **b**, and aortic valve area is 0.64 cm² by direct planimetry **c**

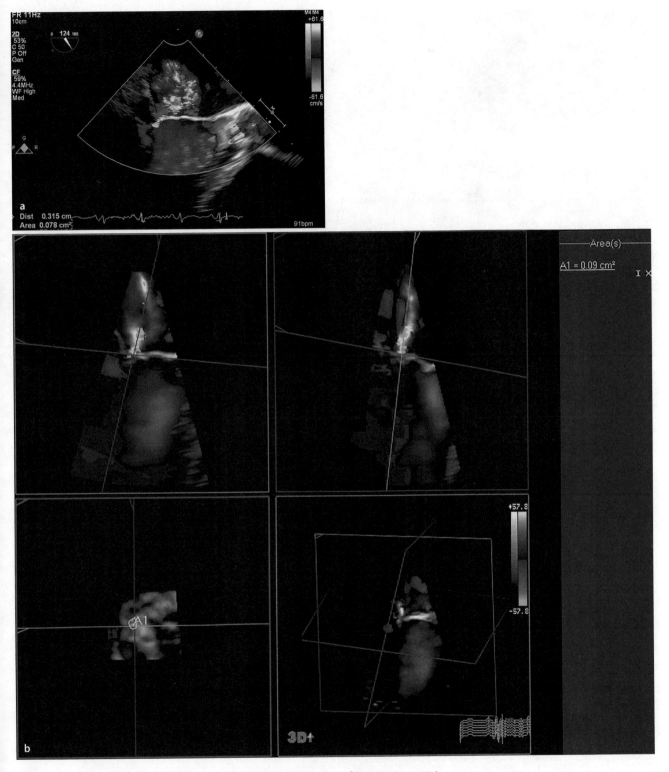

□ **Fig. 3.10** MR VC is 3.1 mm in TEE long-axis view **a** but MRVCA is 0.09 cm² by full volume 3D **b**

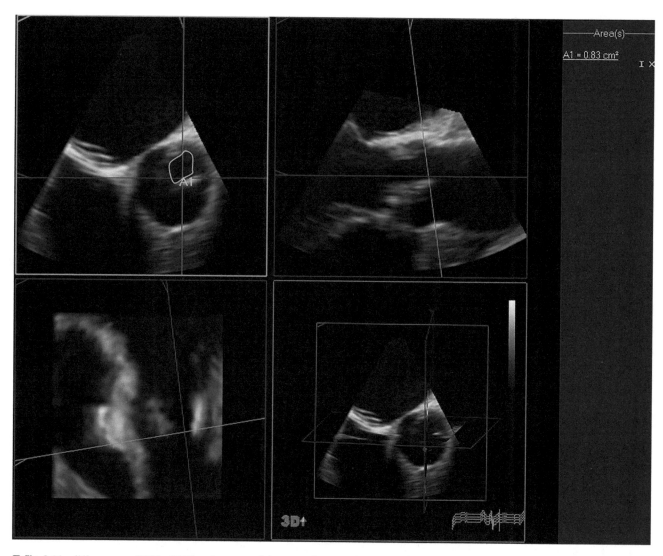

☐ Fig. 3.11   AVA measures 0.83 by 3DQ by placement of the *green* plane in right upper quadrant and left lower quadrant at tip of leaflets

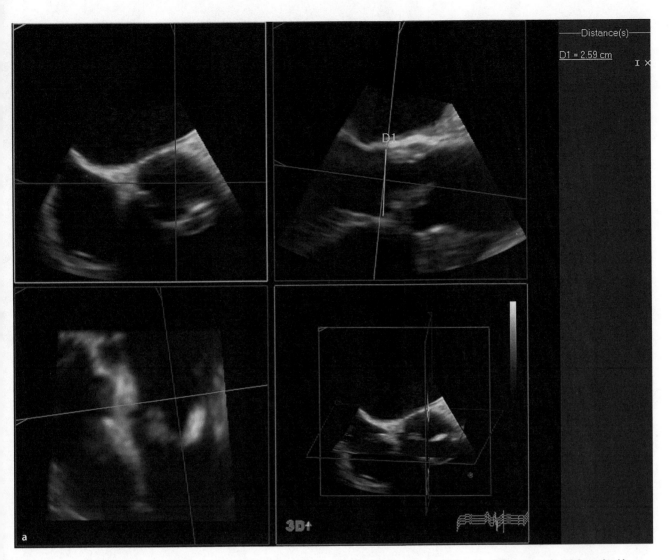

■ **Fig. 3.12** AV annulus measures 26 mm by 3DQ by double oblique method **a** and 27.4 mm and 25 mm in different axes by 3DQ method **b**

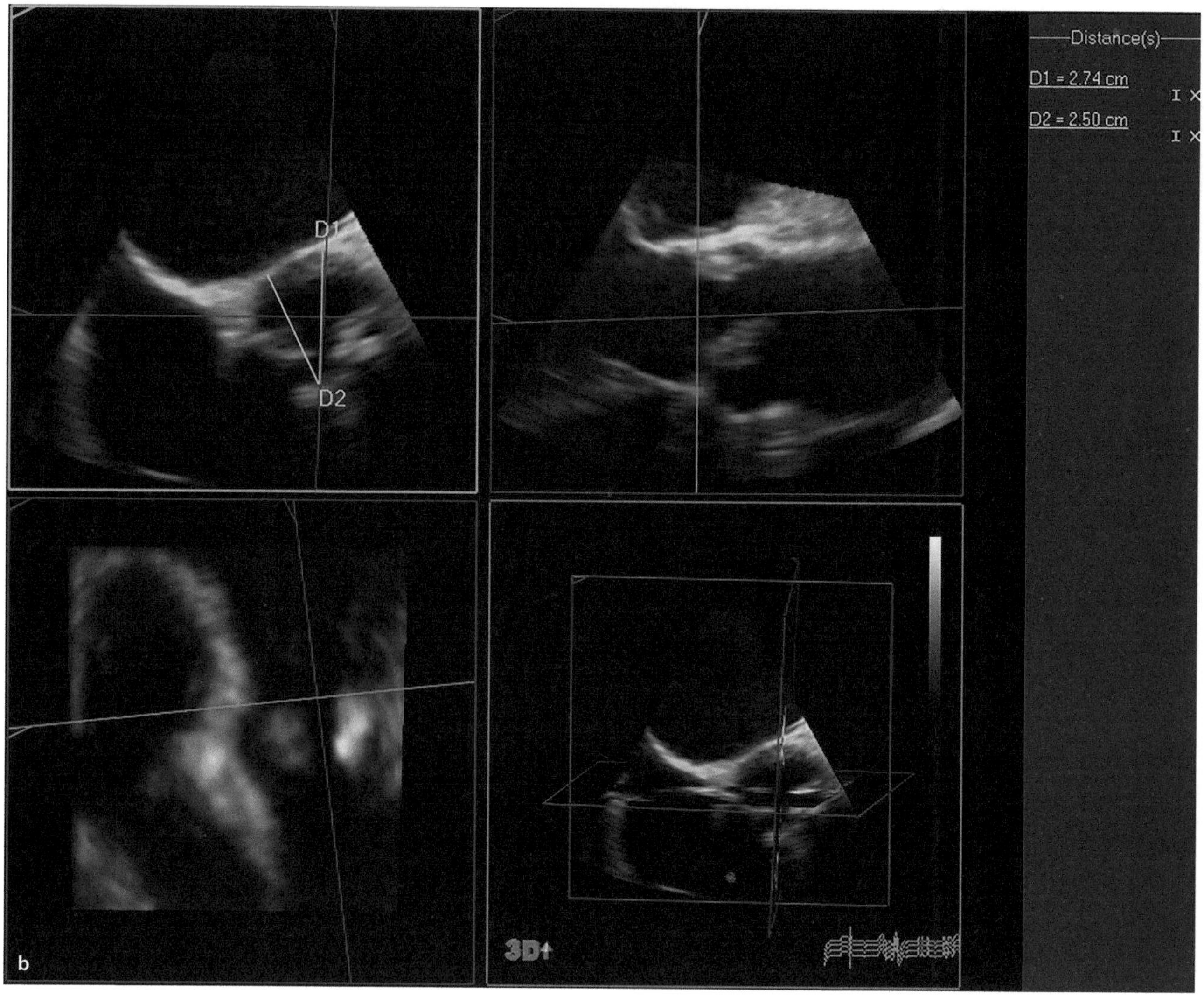

Fig. 3.12 (continued)

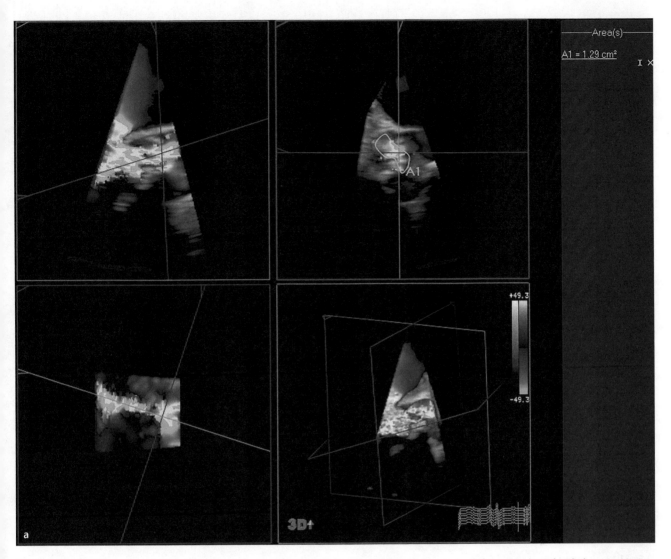

Fig. 3.13 AIVCA measures 1.29 cm² by full volume in en face view (left upper quadrant), *blue* and *red* planes are aligned with the regurgitant jet in right upper quadrants and left lower quadrants, respectively **a**, AI regurgitation anatomic surface area measures 0.63 cm² **b**

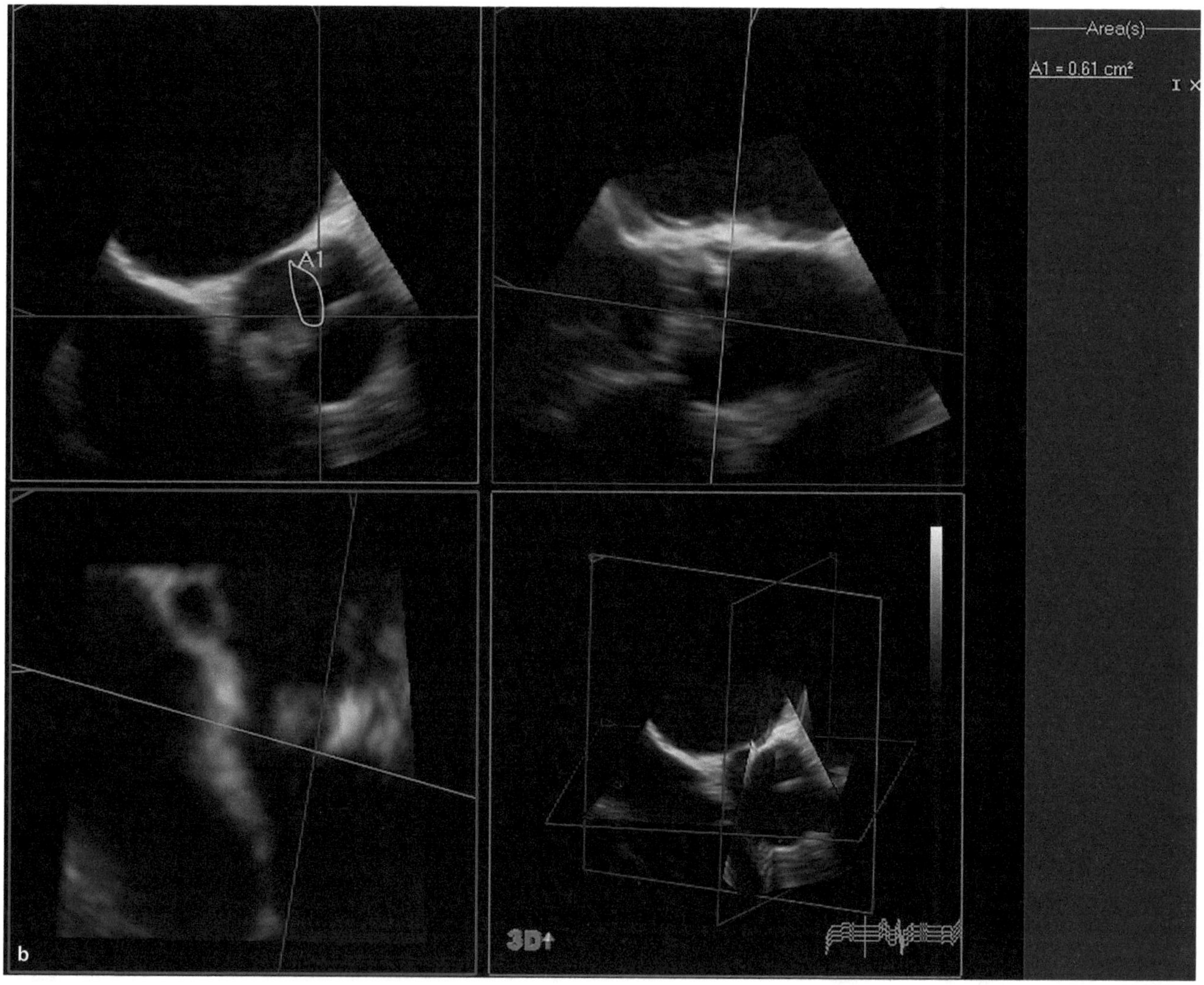

Area(s)

A1 = 0.61 cm²

□ **Fig. 3.13**   (continued)

Diagnosis   Critical AS (AVA/BSA = 0.3–0.4 cm²/m²) and severe AI, mild to moderate MR, tricuspid aortic valve.

Comment   AVR.

3.5   Case 3: Moderate Valvular AS, Bicuspid Aortic Valve, and Interrupted Aortic Arch

A 44-year-old man presented by dyspnea on exertion functional class II of 1 month exacerbation and hypertension since 15 years ago. Blood pressure of upper extremities was about 175 mmHg and in lower extremities 145 mmHg.

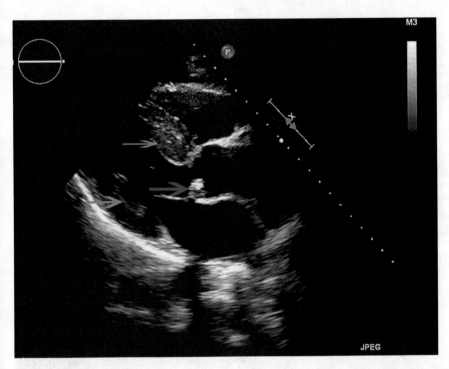

☐ Fig. 3.14 Left ventricular hypertrophy (*green arrows*) and thick aortic leaflets (*pink arrow*) are visible in parasternal long-axis view

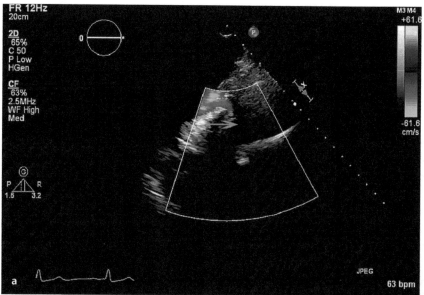

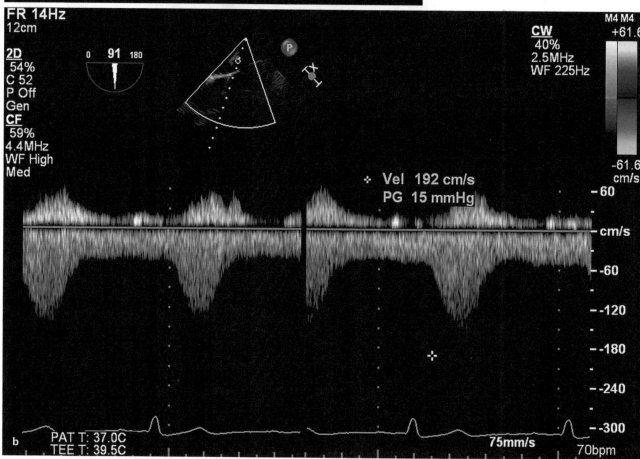

Fig. 3.15 Aortic arch is interrupted in suprasternal long-axis view and no flow is detectable in this view (*arrow*) **a** and peak gradient is 15 mmHg by continuous wave Doppler **b**

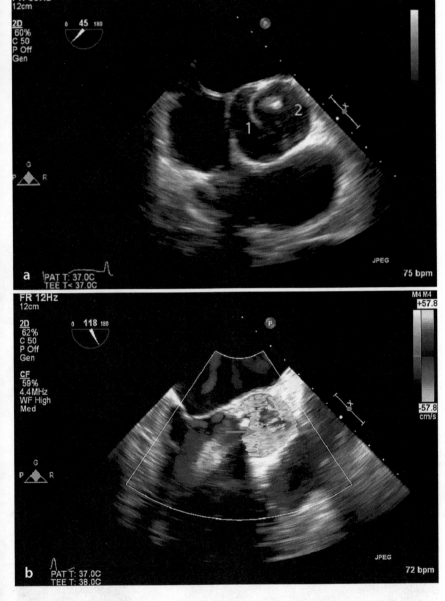

■ **Fig. 3.16**   Bicuspid aortic valve is evident in TEE short-axis view **a** and severe turbulency is evident in TEE long-axis view (*arrow*) **b**

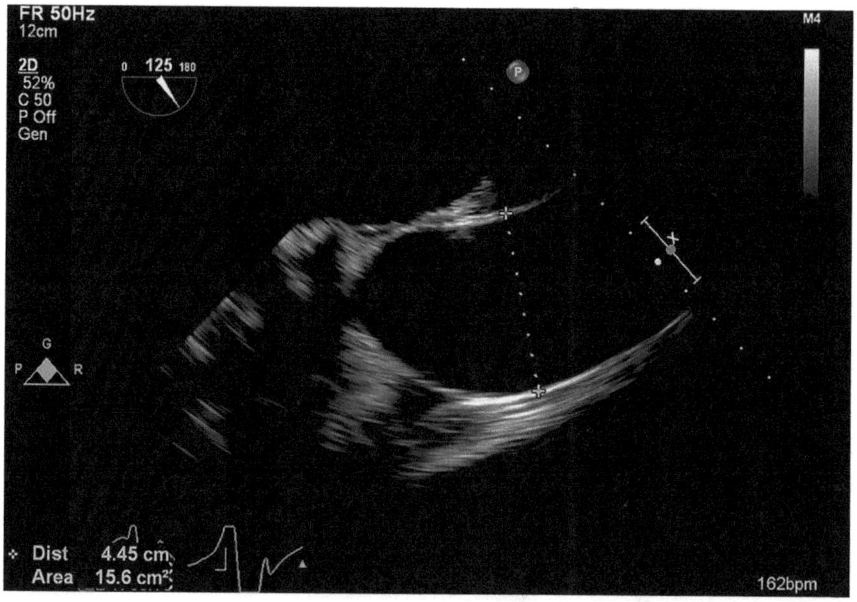

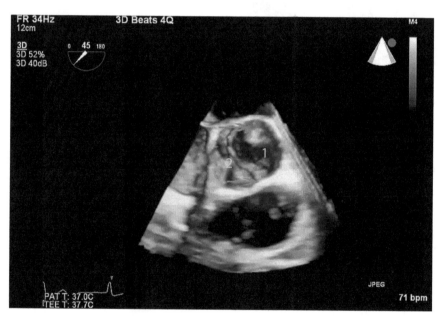

Fig. 3.17   Ascending aorta measures 45 mm in TEE long-axis view

Fig. 3.18   Calcification of aortic commissures is evident by live 3D mode of aortic valve by TEE short-axis view (*arrows*), bicuspid aortic valve is only detectable in systole

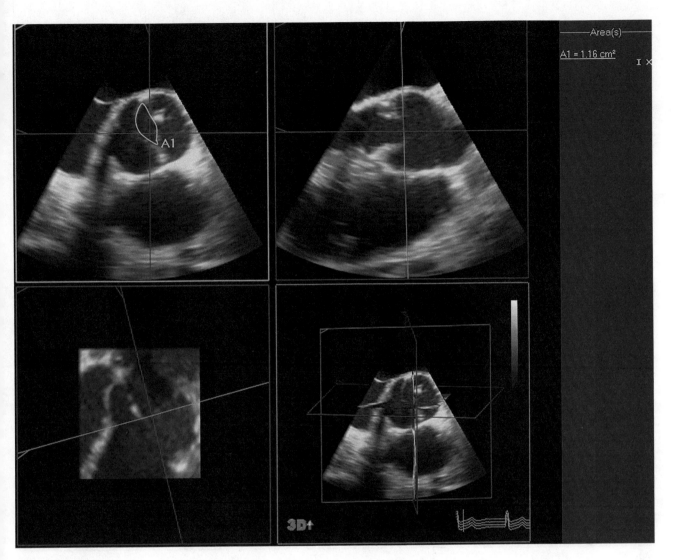

❏ **Fig. 3.19**   Aortic valve area measures 1.16 cm² by 3DQ

3

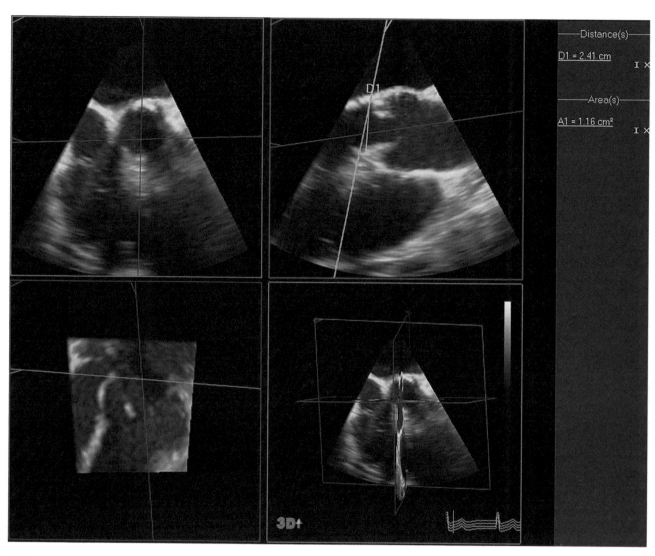

Distance(s)
D1 = 2.41 cm

Area(s)
A1 = 1.16 cm²

3D+

□ Fig. 3.20   Aortic annulus measures 24 mm by double oblique method

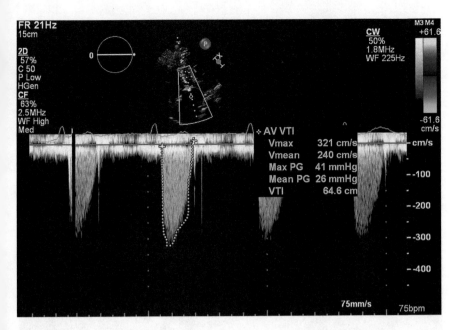

◻ **Fig. 3.21**   Peak and mean aortic valve gradient are 41 and 26 mmHg, respectively

Diagnosis   Moderate valvular AS, Bicuspid aortic valve, and interrupted aortic arch.

Comment   The patient referred for coronary angiography and evaluation for ischemia.

Lesson   In interrupted aortic arch, there may be no gradient in descending aorta and it can be misleading.

3.6   Case 4: Bicuspid Aortic Valve with Moderate Valvular Aortic Stenosis

A 55-year-old man presented by one time of dizziness.

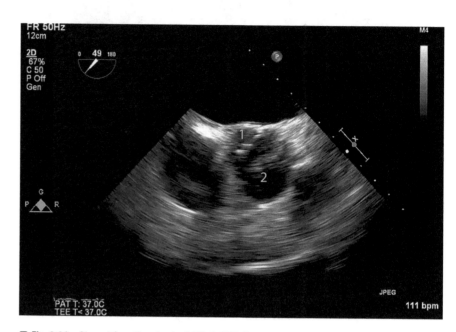

■ **Fig. 3.22**   Bicuspid aortic valve is visible in TEE short-axis view

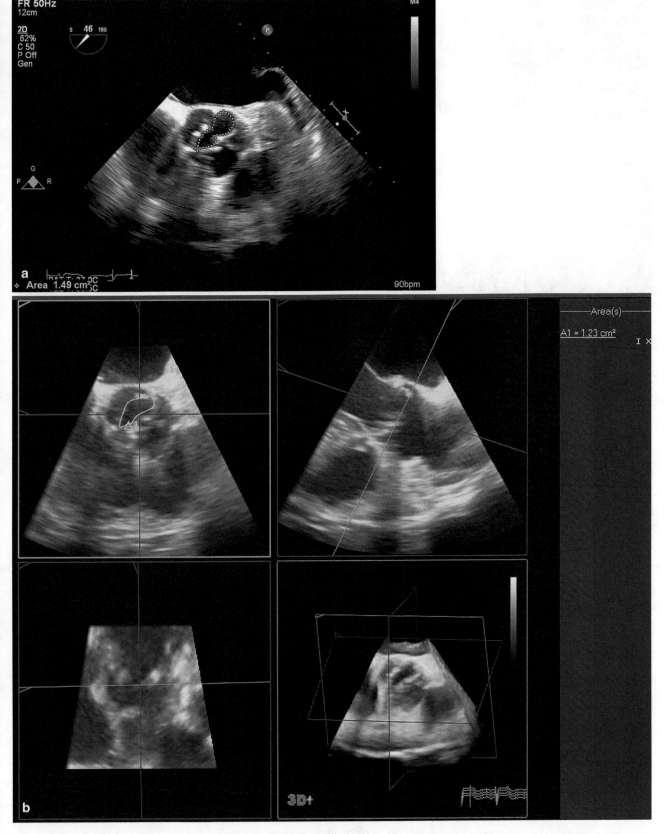

■ Fig. 3.23   Aortic valve area measures 1.5 cm² by direct planimetry by two-dimensional echocardiography in TEE short-axis view **a** and 1.2 cm² by TEE 3DQ method by 3D zoom **b**

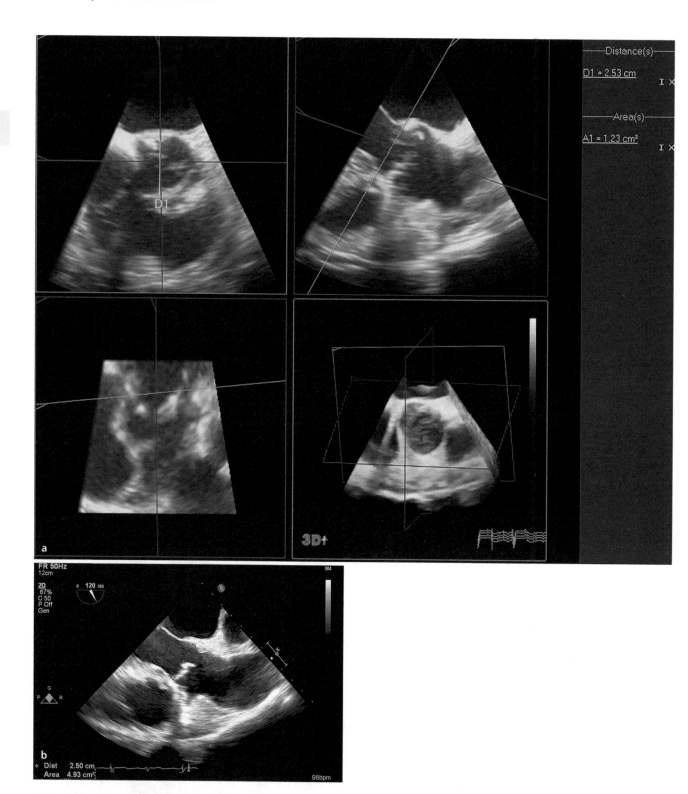

Fig. 3.24 Aortic annulus measures 25.3 mm **a** by double oblique method and 25 mm in parasternal long-axis view **b**

Diagnosis   Moderate valvular aortic stenosis, Bicuspid aortic valve, LVEF = 55%.

Comment   Follow-up.

Lesson   Aortic valve area was 1.5 cm² by TEE 2D echocardiography and 1.2 cm² by TEE 3DQ by 3D zoom, it is due to this fact that bt 2D echocardiography, the plane of measurement of aortic valve area may not be put in tip of aortic leaflets but by 3DQ, the aortic valve area is measured just at the tip of aortic leaflets.

3.7   Case 5: Bicuspid Aortic Valve, Mild AS, Mild AI

A 25-year-old man presented by dyspnea on exertion functional class II of recent exacerbation.

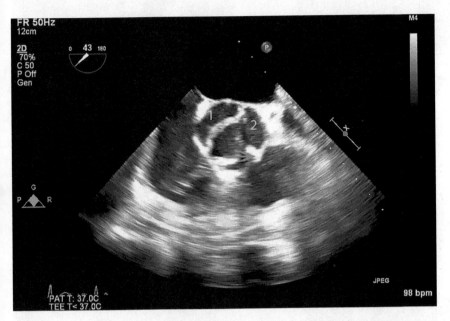

Fig. 3.25 Bicuspid aortic valve is demonstrated by TEE short-axis view with a graph (*arrow*)

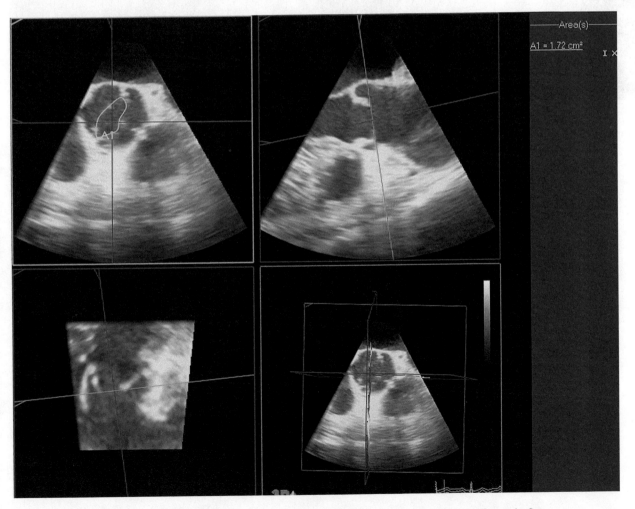

Fig. 3.26 Aortic valve area measures 1.7 cm² by direct planimetry by 3DQ, 3D zoom method at the tip of aortic leaflets

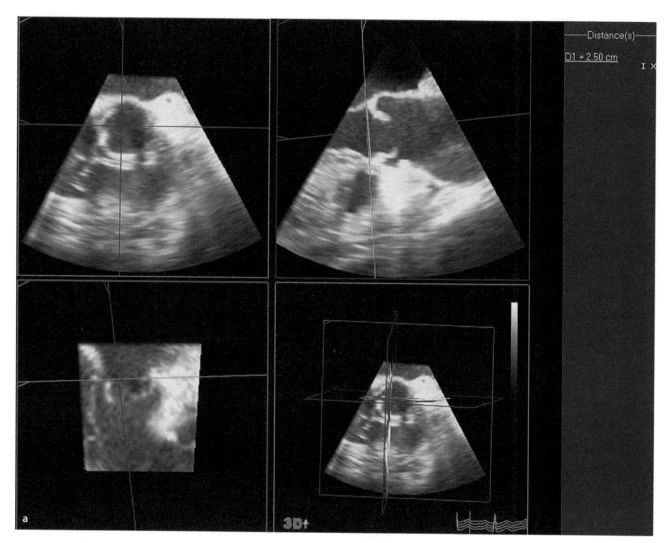

Fig. 3.27 Aortic annulus measures 25 mm by double oblique method **a**, 24 mm in its minor axis and 26.8 mm in another axis **b**, aortic annulus is 24 mm in parasternal long-axis view by 2D echocardiography **c**

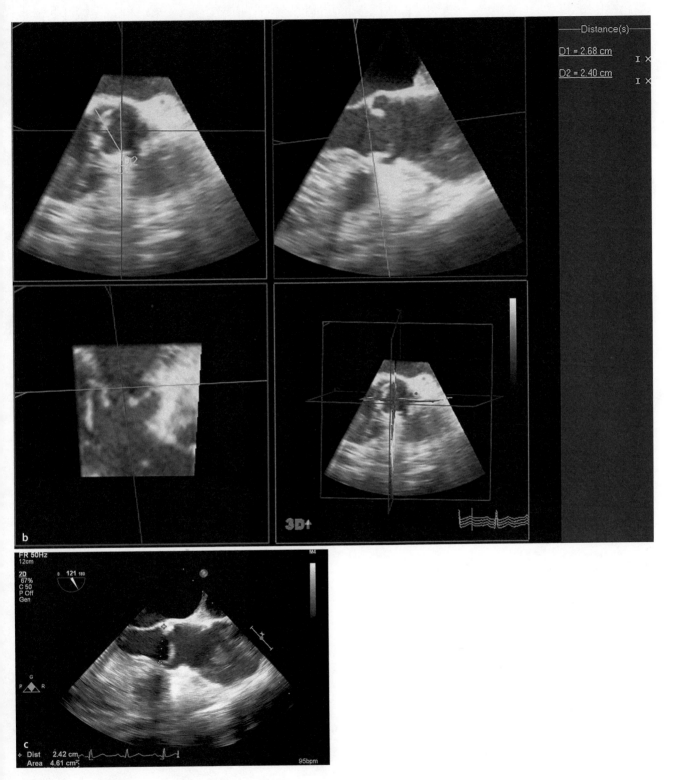

Fig. 3.27 (continued)

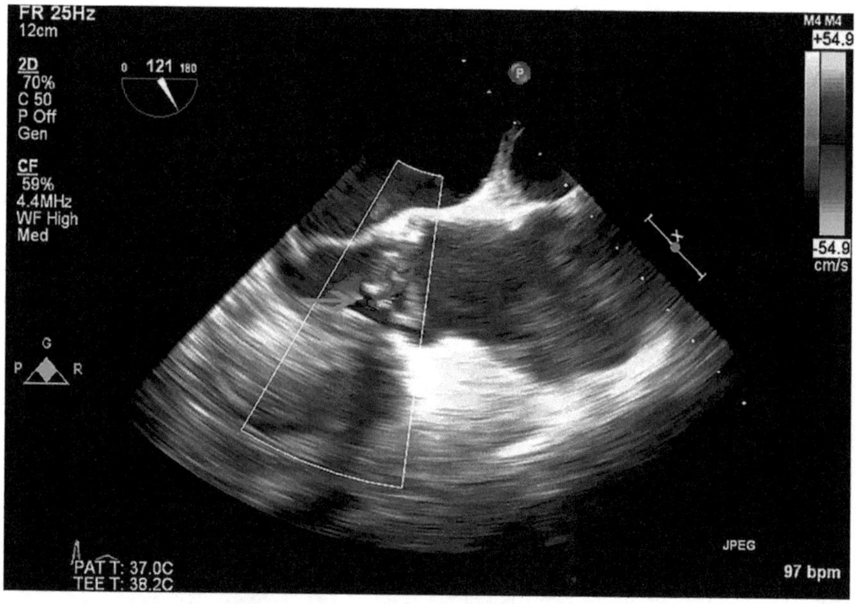

■ Fig. 3.28   Mild AI is shown in this TEE long-axis view (*arrow*)

Diagnosis   Bicuspid aortic valve, mild AS, mild AI.

Recommendation   Follow-up.

Lesson   Aortic annulus which is measured in TEE long-axis (conventional method) is the same with aortic annulus by 3DQ method in sagittal plane (in this patient 24 mm), but by double oblique method or other axis the annulus is larger (26 and 26.8 mm, respectively).

3.8   Case 6: Low Flow, Low Gradient Severe AS

A 55-year-old man referred for echocardiography before heart transplantation. He had a history of dyspnea on exertion functional class III of recent exacerbation. He underwent coronary angiography and had minimal coronary artery disease and there was 20 mmHg gradient between LV and aorta in cardiac catheterism. Transthoracic echocardiography revealed LVEDd = 60 mm, LVESd = 52 mm, septum and posterior walls measured 11 mm, and LVEF about 15–20%. Aortic valve was severely thick and calcified. He had a history of Hodgkin disease 30 years ago and underwent chemotherapy and radiotherapy.

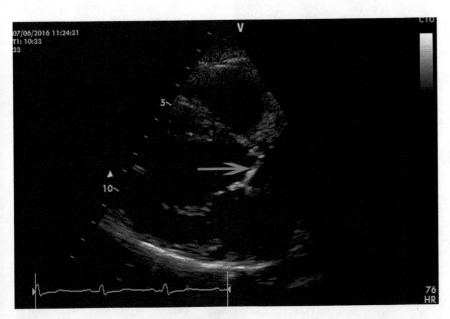

◘ **Fig. 3.29** Parasternal long-axis view shows that aortic valve is severely thick and calcified and restricted leaflet opening during systole (*arrow*)

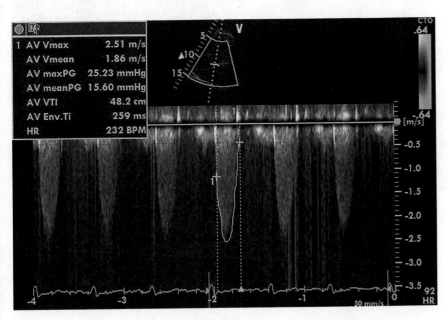

◘ **Fig. 3.30** Peak gradient across aortic valve measures 25 and mean gradient measures 15.6 mmHg, respectively

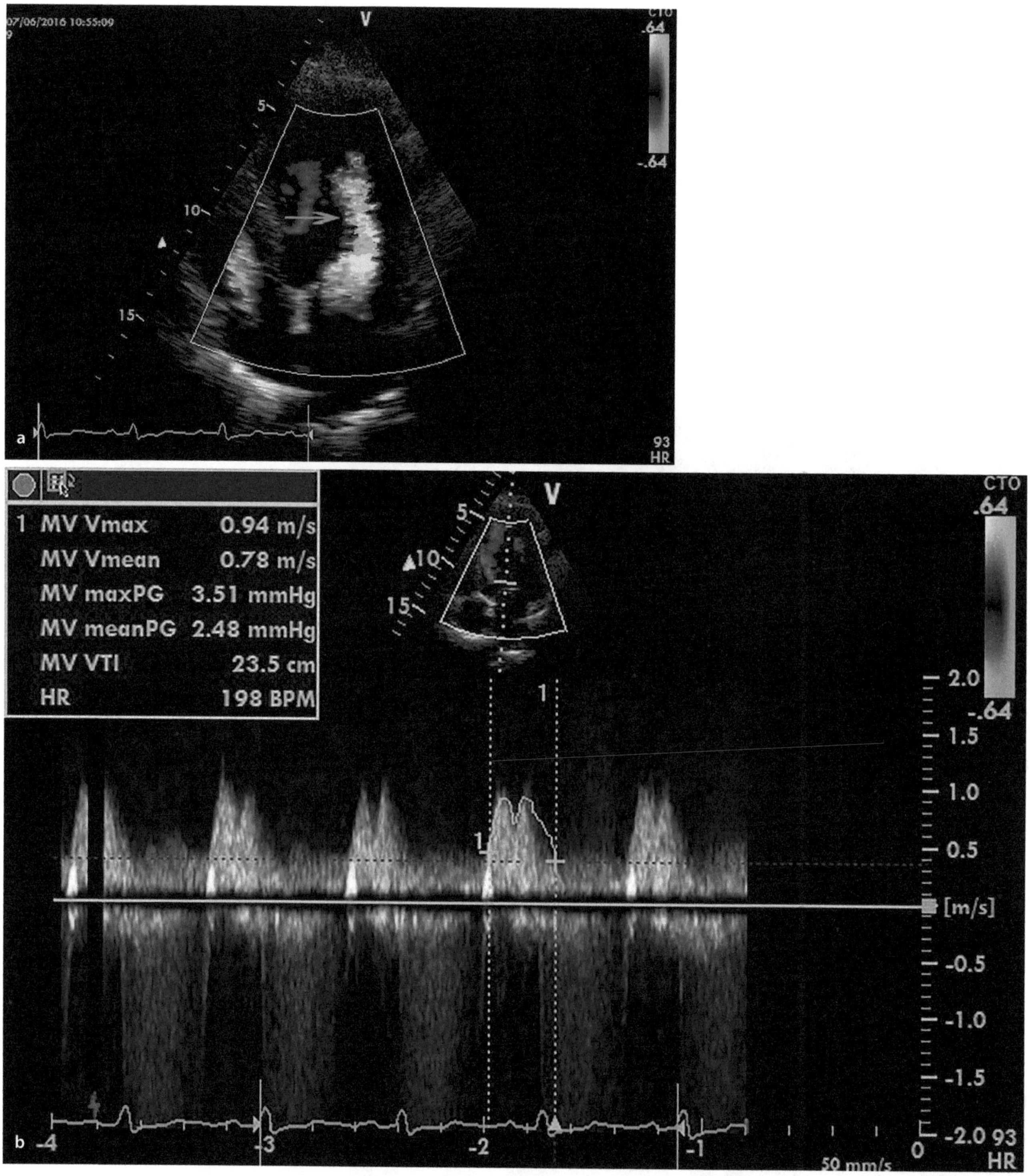
07/06/2016 10:55:09
V
CTO
.64
-.64
5
10
15
a
93
HR
1 MV Vmax 0.94 m/s
MV Vmean 0.78 m/s
MV maxPG 3.51 mmHg
MV meanPG 2.48 mmHg
MV VTI 23.5 cm
HR 198 BPM
2.0
1.5
1.0
0.5
[m/s]
-0.5
-1.0
-1.5
-2.0
b
-4
-3
-2
-1
0
50 mm/s

■ **Fig. 3.31** Apical four-chamber view shows that there is diastolic turbulency across mitral valve (*arrow*) **a**, peak and mean gradient measures 3.5 and 2.5 mmHg, respectively **b**

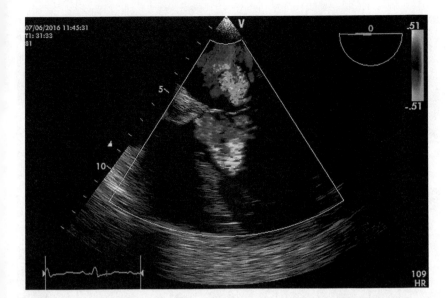

☐ **Fig. 3.32** Transesophageal echocardiography reveals moderate mitral regurgitation in 0°
view (*arrow*)

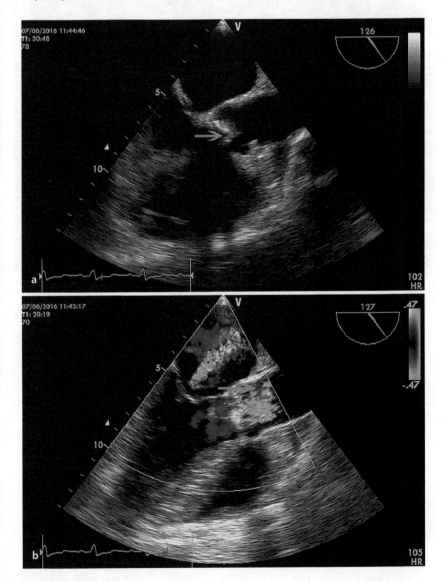

☐ **Fig. 3.33** Aortic valve is severely thick and calcified (*arrow*) **a**, systolic turbulency is seen
across aortic valve in favor of severe aortic stenosis (*arrow*) **b** in TEE long-axis view (*arrow*)

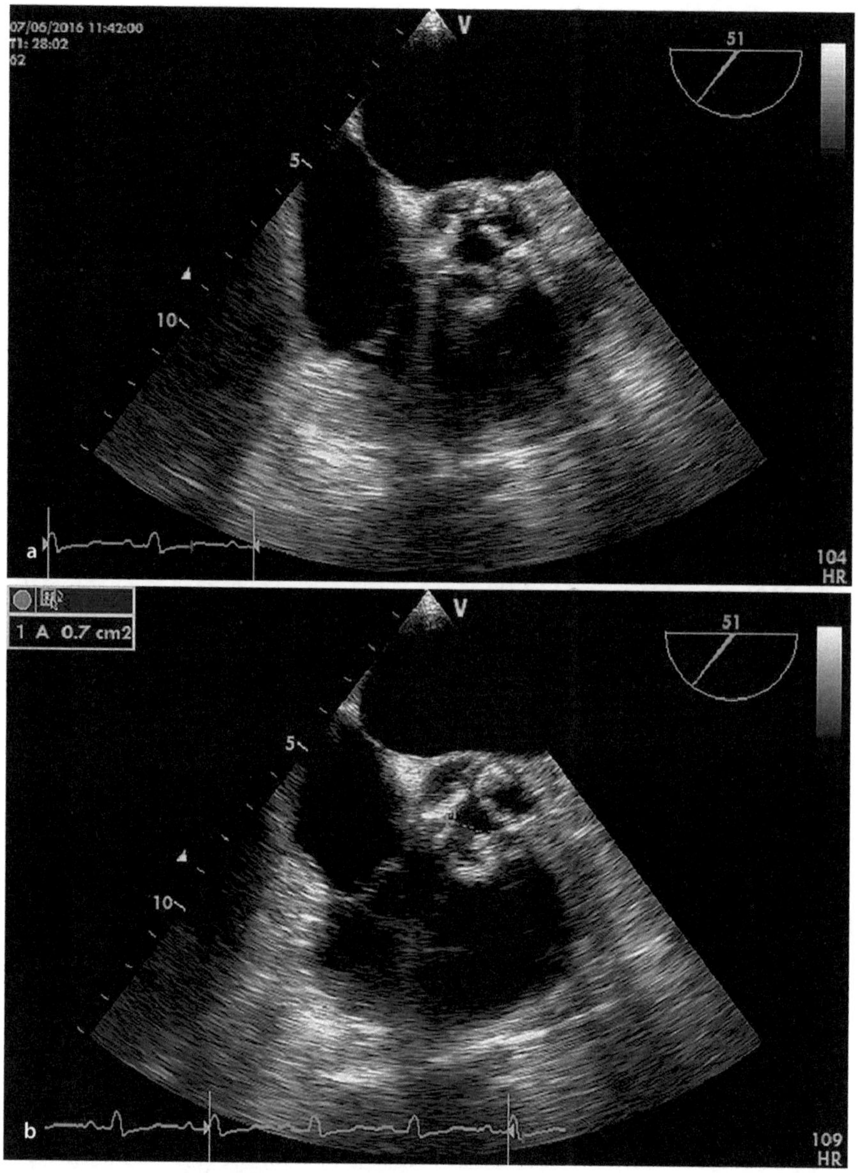

□ **Fig. 3.34** Aortic leaflets are severely thick and calcified especially in borders by TEE short-axis view (*arrow*) **a**, aortic valve area measures 0.7 cm² by direct planimetry in this view **b**

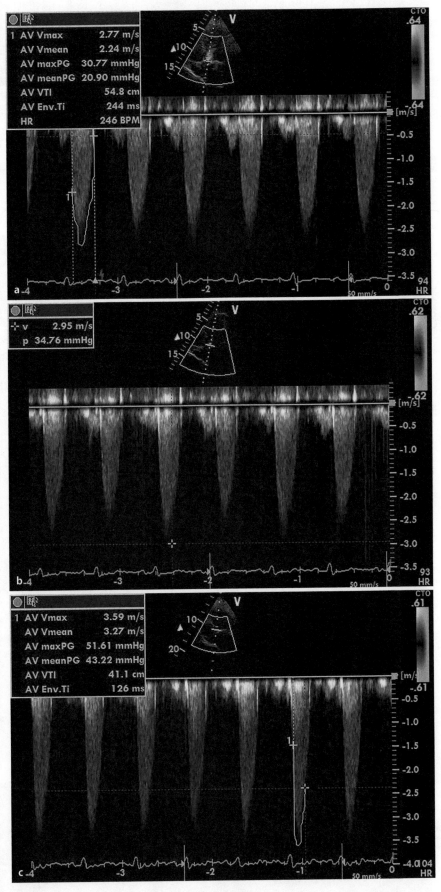

Fig. 3.35 After 10, 15, and 20 microgram dobutamine, peak gradient gradually increases to 20, 35, and 52 mmHg, respectively **a–c** and mean gradient reached to 20 and 43 mmHg **a, c**

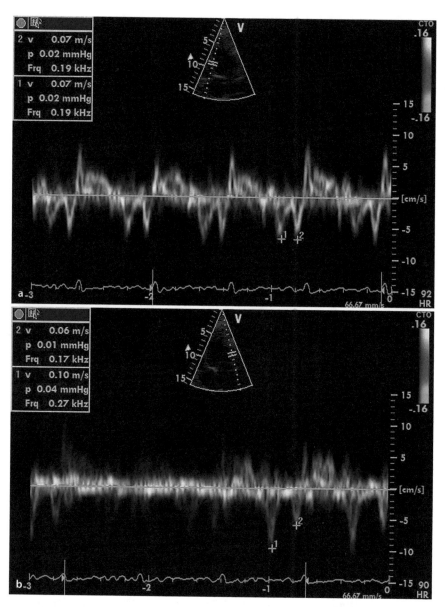

Fig. 3.36 Septal e and a wave measure 7 and 7 cm/s, respectively **a** and lateral e and **a** wave measure 10 and 6 cm/s, respectively **b**

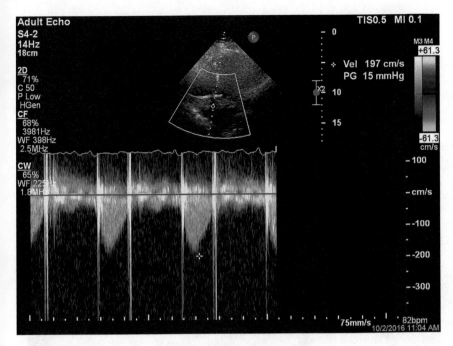

Fig. 3.37 Peak gradient across prosthetic aortic valve measures 15 mmHg

Diagnosis   Severe low flow low gradient AS, mild AI, AV annulus = 19 mm.

Comment   The patient was candidate for TAVI or AVR.
The patient underwent AVR, LVEF achieved to 50%.

Lesson

1. Septal and lateral e wave of cut off of 8 cm/s demonstrated 93% sensitivity and 88% specificity for the diagnosis of restrictive cardiomyopathy [6]. In this patient, septal e wave measures 10 cm/s and is not in favor of restrictive cardiomyopathy.

2. Low flow, low gradient AS occurs in LVEF <50%, AVA <1 cm^2, and mean gradient less than 40 mmHg. Low dose dobutamine stress echocardiography is indicated in these cases.

3. About 30% of patients with aortic valve area <1 cm^2 do not have mean and peak aortic gradient in the range of severe AS. Most of them are true valvular AS with decreased contractility and some of them are pseudo-AS which there is AS with reduced LV contractility due to another cause. Dobutamine stress echocardiography is performed for accurate diagnosis. If stroke volume increased to more than 20% with no change in aortic valve area, it is true valvular AS and if AVA increases >0.2 cm^2 but mild increase in gradients and less than 20% increase in stroke volume, it is pseudo-AS [7].

3.9   Case 7: Paradoxical Low Gradient Severe AS

A 92-year-old man presented by multiple episodes of syncopal attacks.

Physical examination revealed ejection systolic murmur at aortic area. ECG was normal, LVEF = 55%.

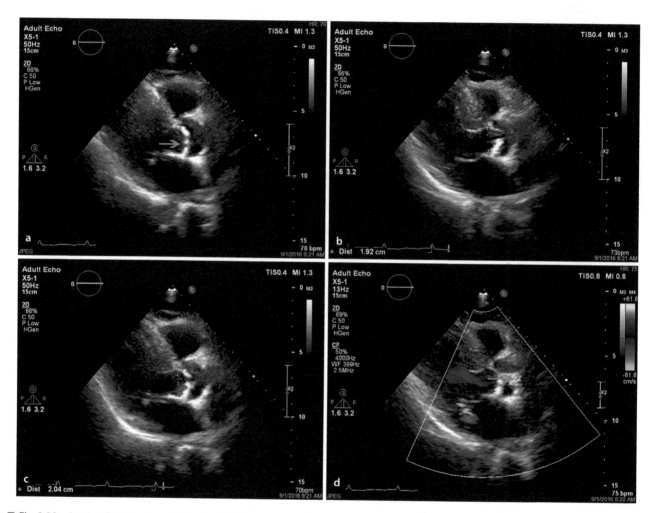

🔲 **Fig. 3.38**   Aortic valve is severely thick and calcified in parasternal long-axis view (*arrow*) **a**, aortic annulus measures between 19 and 20.4 mm in this view **b**, **c**, systolic turbulency across aortic valve is seen in this view (*arrow*) **d**

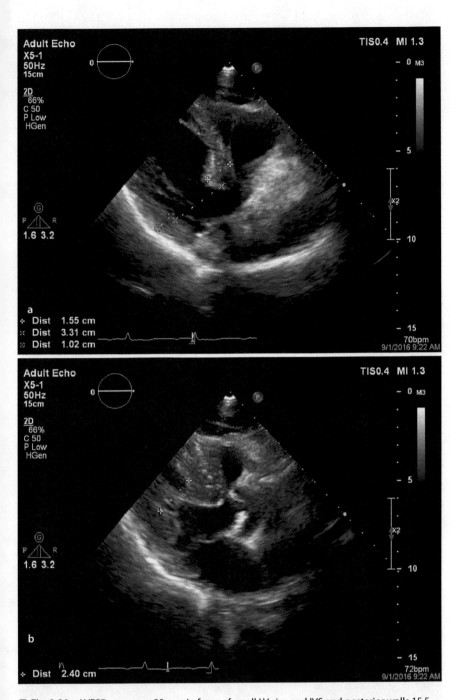

Fig. 3.39 LVESD measures 33 mm in favor of small LV size and IVS and posterior walls 15.5 and 10 mm, respectively **a**, LVESD measures 24 mm **b** in parasternal long-axis view

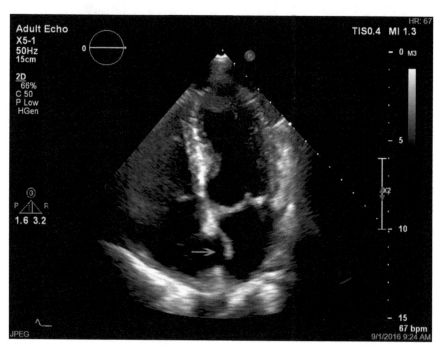

◨ **Fig. 3.40**   Thick and calcified aortic leaflets are visualized in this parasternal short-axis view (*arrow*)

◨ **Fig. 3.41**   IAS was aneurysmal in apical four-chamber view (*arrow*)

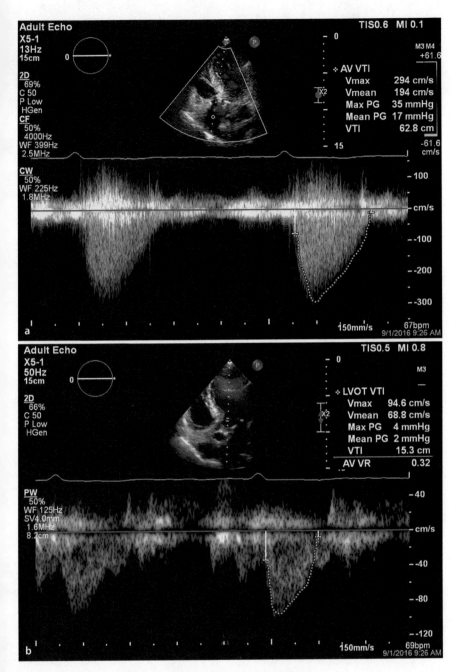

Fig. 3.42 Peak and mean gradients across aortic valve measure 35 and 17 mmHg, respectively, and aortic VTI measures 63 cm **a**, LVOT VTI = 15 cm **b**

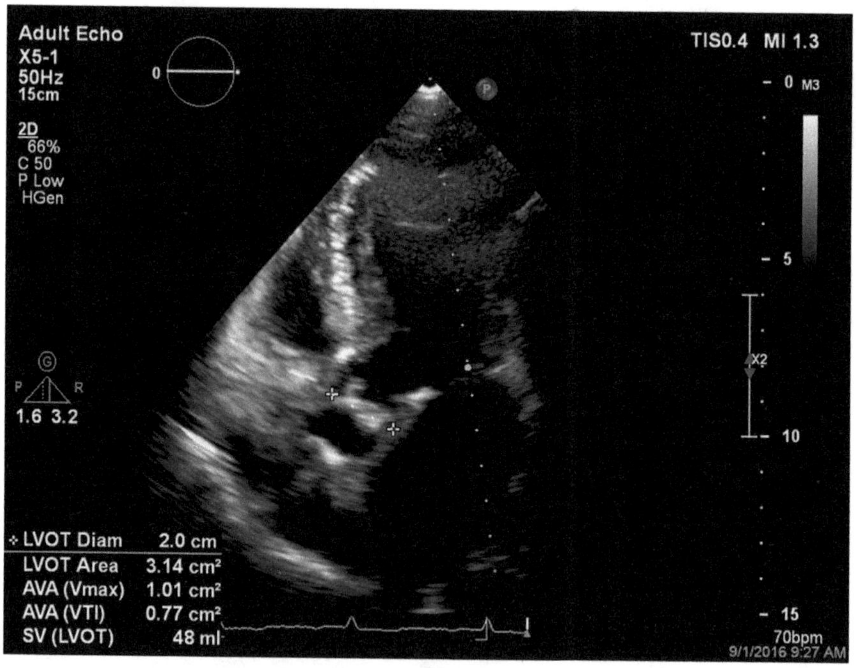

Fig. 3.43 Aortic valve area measures 0.77 cm² and LV stroke volume is 48 cm³

Diagnosis   Severe paradoxical AS.

Comment   TEE and considering TAVI for this patient.

Lesson   In this patient, AVA is <0.8 cm² but mean aortic gradient is 17 mmHg, LVEF is normal, stroke volume index = 48/1.7 = 28 cm³/m².

In paradoxical AS, stroke volume index is less than 35 cm³/m² [1]. Paradoxical AS occurs typically in elderly with small LV cavity and hypertrophied LV.

3.10   Case 8: Severe AS Post-CABG

A 70-year-old man presented by dyspnea and chest pain of 2 month duration. He had a history of CABG 8 years ago. Physical examination revealed ejection systolic murmur at aortic area. LVEF = 45–50% and anterior and lateral wall were hypokinetic.

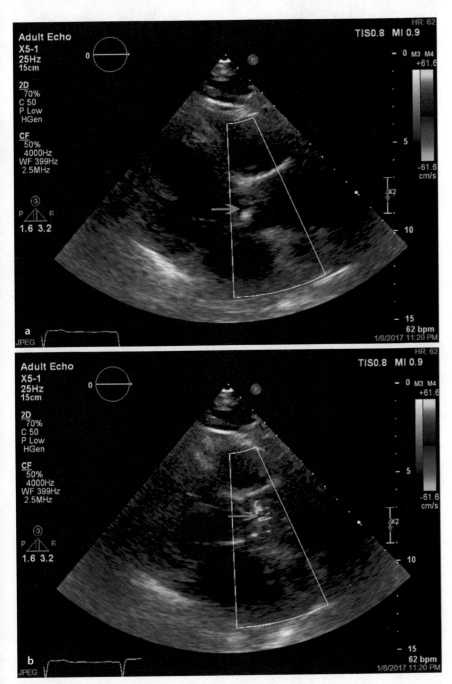

☐ **Fig. 3.44**   Aortic valve is thick and calcified in parasternal long-axis view (*arrow*) **a**, there is systolic turbulency (*arrow*) in ascending aorta in favor of aortic stenosis **b**

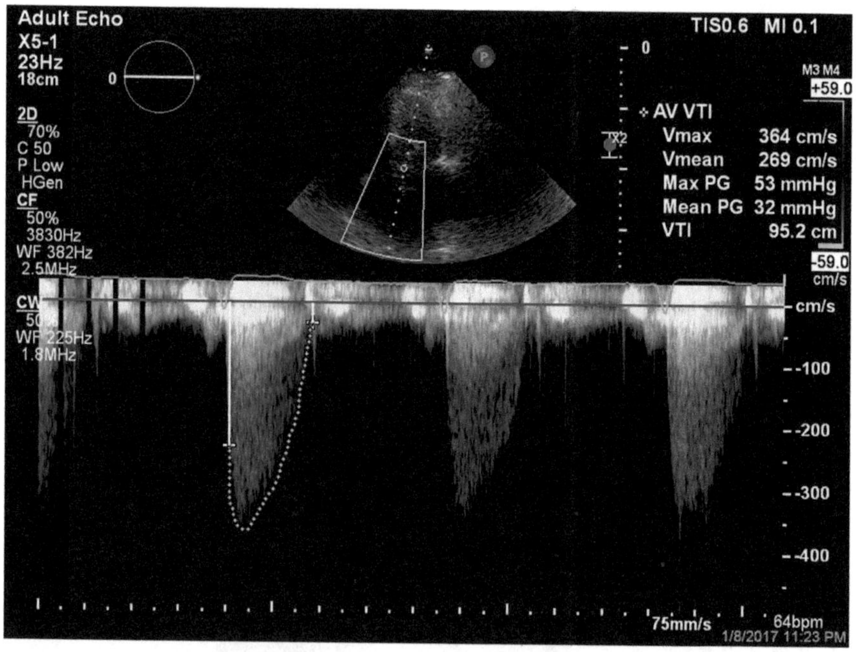

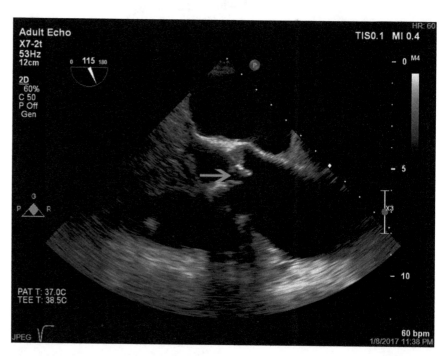

Fig. 3.45 Peak and mean gradient were 53 and 32 mmHg, respectively

Fig. 3.46 Restricted opening of aortic leaflets are demonstrated in TEE long-axis view (*arrow*)

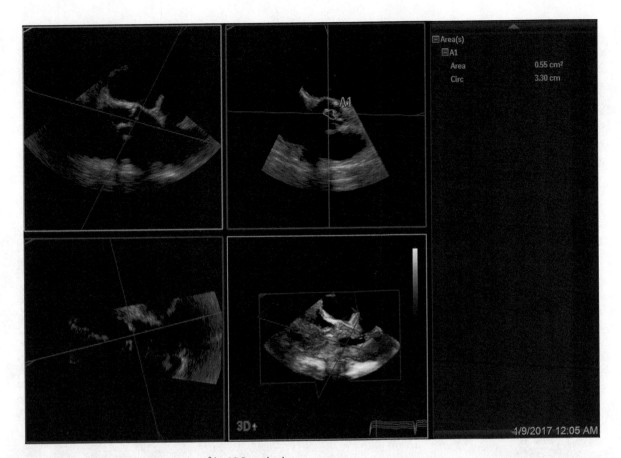

Fig. 3.47 Aortic valve area measures 0.55 cm² by 3DQ method

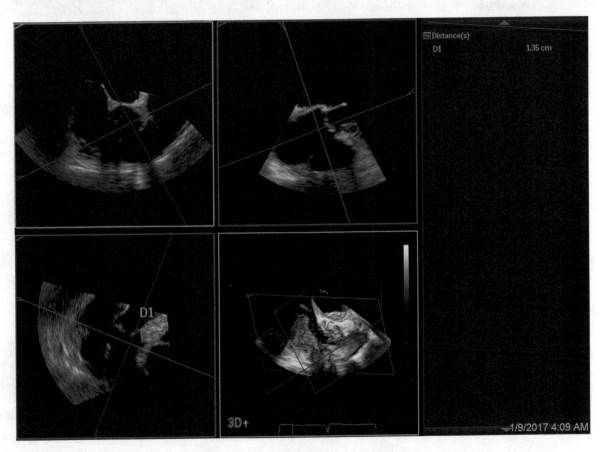

Fig. 3.48 Distance of left main from aortic leaflets is 13.5 mm in *blue* plane

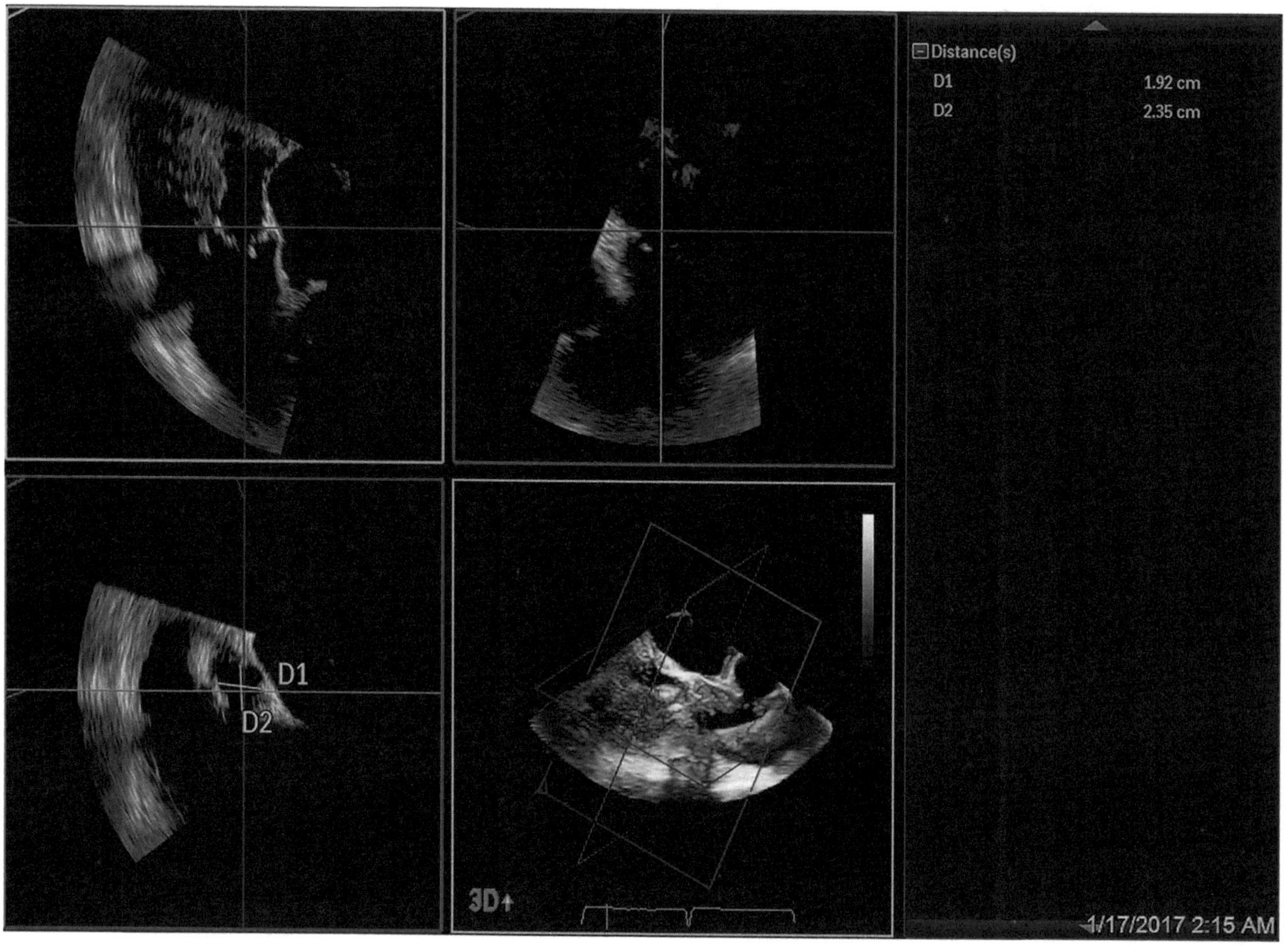

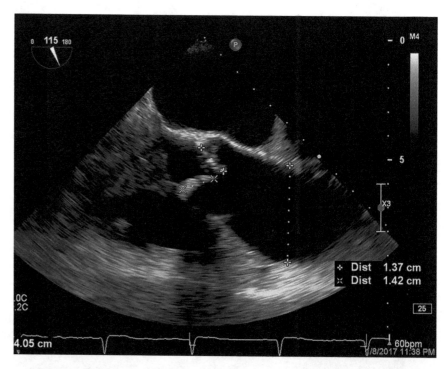

Fig. 3.49 Aortic annulus measures 19.2*23.5 mm by 3DQ

Fig. 3.50 Left coronary cusp measures 13.7 mm and right coronary cusp measures 14.2 mm in TEE long-axis view

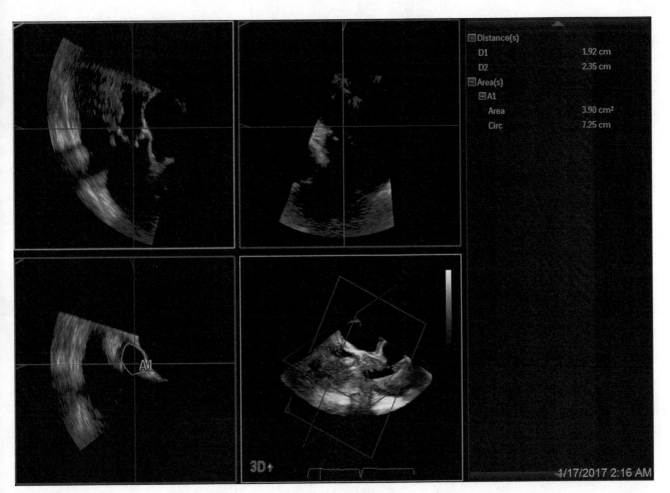

Fig. 3.51 Aortic annulus area measures 7.25 cm, annulus will be calculated as follows: 7.25/3.14 = 2.3 cm or 23 mm, aortic annulus area = 3.9 cm², annulus = 22 mm

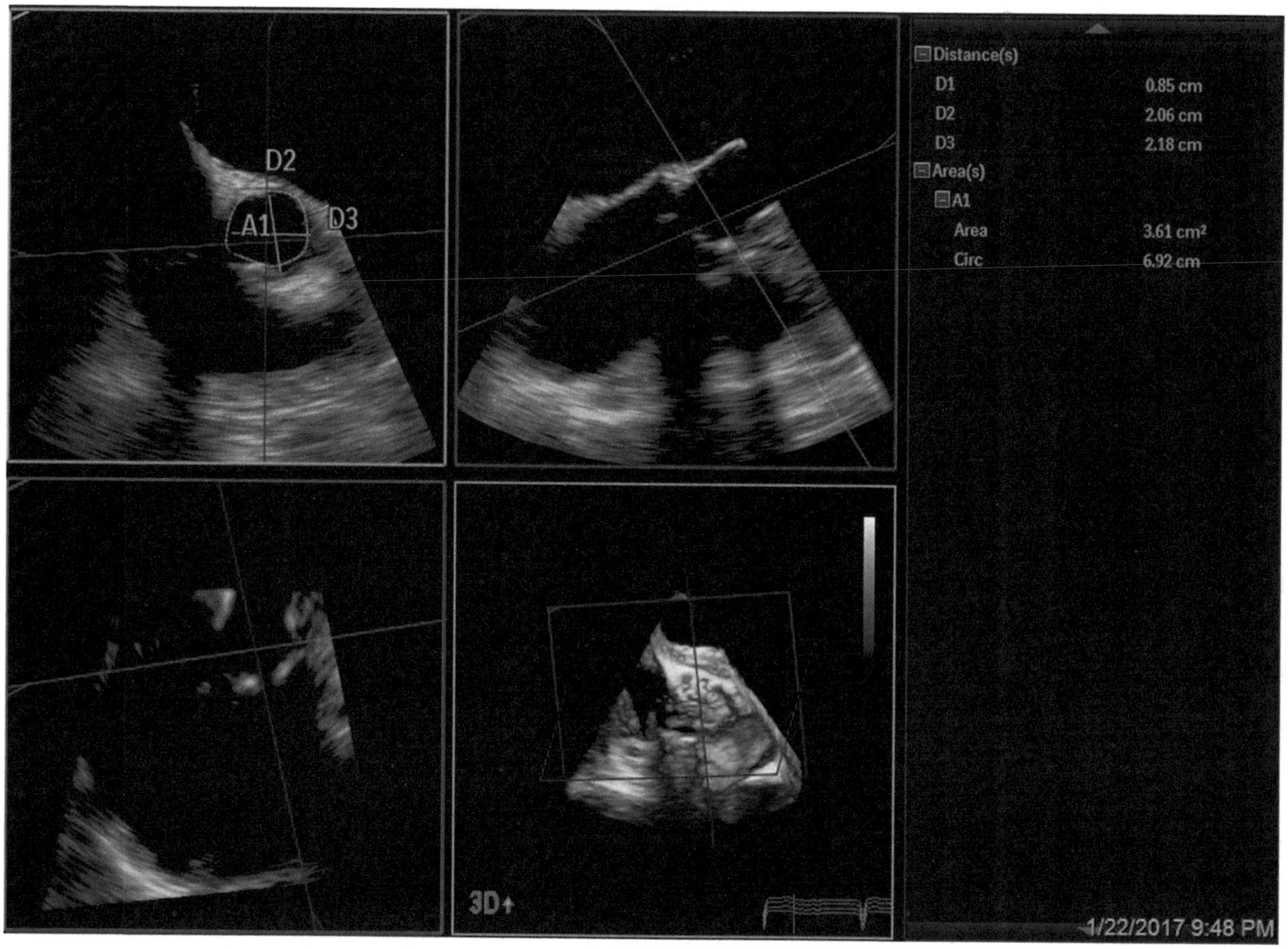

Fig. 3.52   8.5 mm below aortic valve, LVOT measures 20.6*21.8 mm, area = 3.6 cm² (LVOT = 21 mm) and perimeter = 6.9 cm (LVOT = 19 mm)

Diagnosis   Severe AS, aortic valve area measures 0.8 cm² by CE.

Comment   TAVI.
It seems that Edward Sapien = 23 mm or core valve 26 mm.

3.11   Case 9: Bicuspid Aortic Valve with Severe AS and Severe AI

A 70-year-old woman presented by dyspnea on exertion functional class III of recent exacerbation. Physical examination revealed ejection type systolic murmur at aortic area. ECG was normal and coronary angiography was normal.

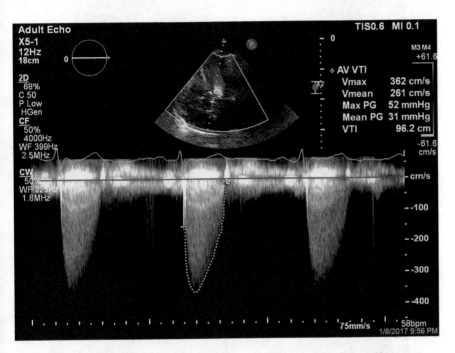

◼ **Fig. 3.53** Peak and mean gradients across aortic valve measure 52 and 31 mmHg, respectively

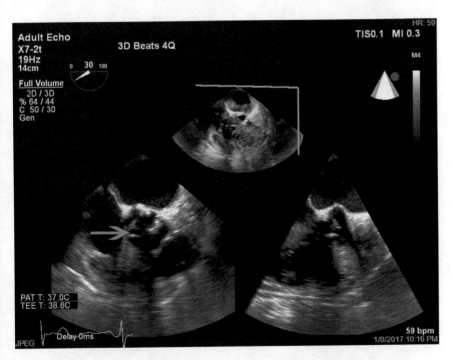

◼ **Fig. 3.54** Bicuspid aortic valve is visualized by TEE full volume (*arrow*)

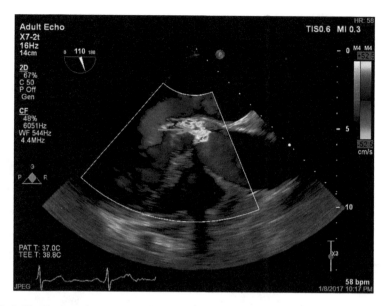

◘ **Fig. 3.55**   Moderately severe AI is shown in TEE long-axis view (*arrow*)

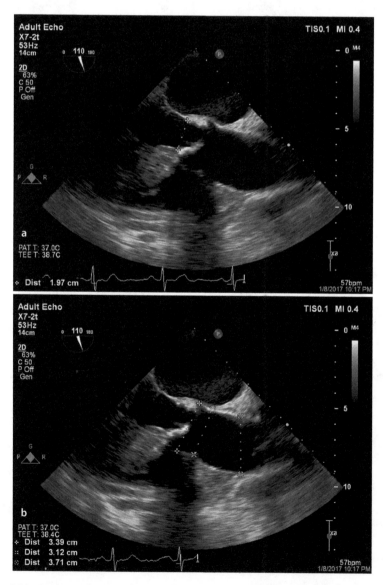

◘ **Fig. 3.56**   Aortic annulus measures 20 and sinus of valsalva, sinotubular junction, and ascending aorta measure 37, 31, and 34 mm, respectively **a, b**

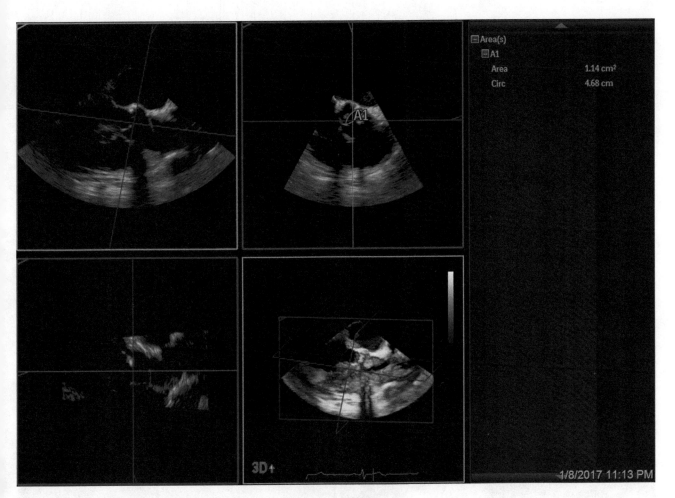

◘ **Fig. 3.57** Aortic valve area measures 1.14 cm² by direct planimetry by TEE 3DQ method

Diagnosis Aortic valve area measures 0.55 cm² by continuity equation method, severe AS, and moderately severe AI in a symptomatic patient with BAV.

Comment AVR.

3.12   Case 10: TAVI Procedure

A 82-year-old man who underwent CABG 12 years ago referred for dyspnea on exertion FC III. TTE showed LVEF = 35%, and severe valvular aortic stenosis, PG = 76, and MG about 40 mmHg.

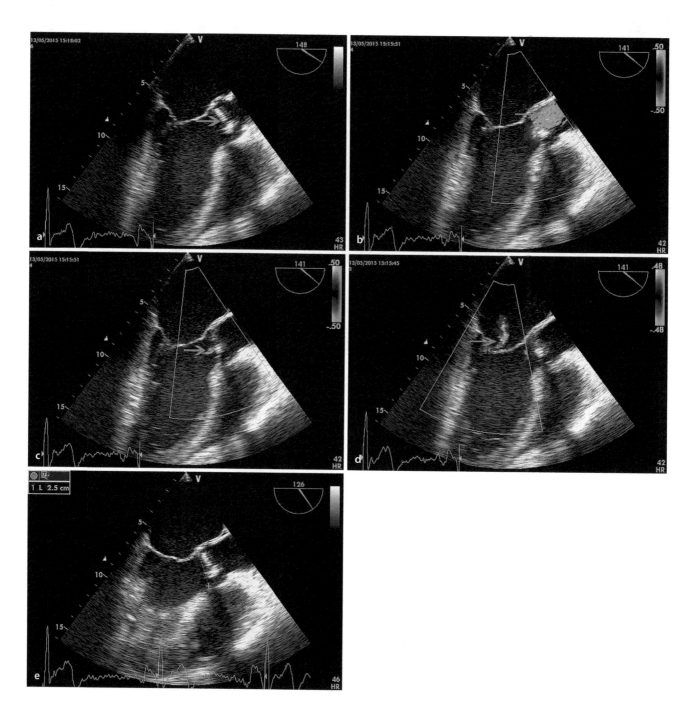

☐ **Fig. 3.58**   Aortic valve is severely thick and calcified in TEE long-axis view **a**, severe turbulency in ascending aorta in favor of severe AS (*arrow*) **b**, mild AI (*arrow*) **c**, and mild MR (*arrow*) **d** are visible in this view, aortic annulus measures 25 mm **e**

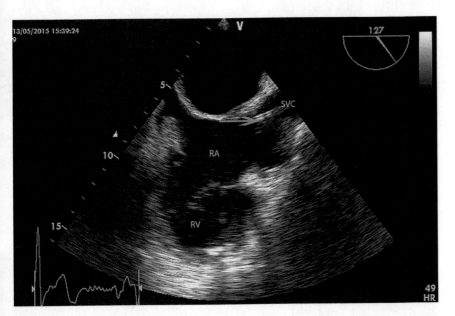

Fig. 3.59 Temporary pacemaker is visible in RA and RV via SVC. *SVC* superior vena cava, *RA* right atrium

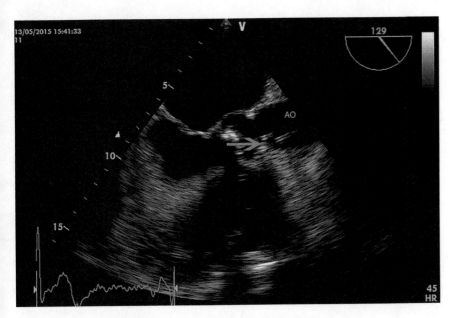

Fig. 3.60 The guide wire is placed in ascending aorta (*arrow*). *AO* aorta

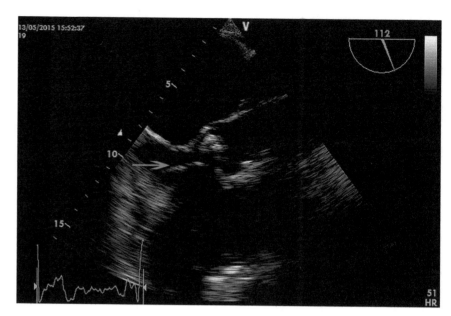

◘ **Fig. 3.61**   The guide wire is passed through aortic valve difficult and is placed in LV (*arrow*)

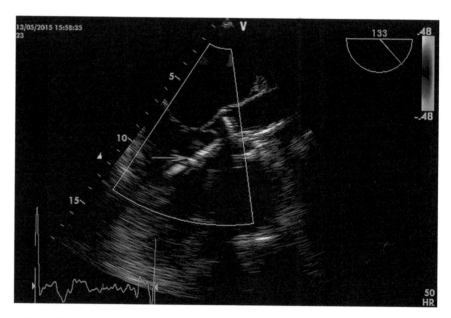

◘ **Fig. 3.62**   The balloon number 25 is passed over the guide wire in LV (*arrow*)

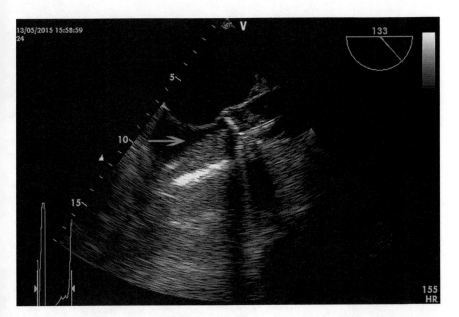

Fig. 3.63 Rapid atrial pacing is done during balloon inflation (*arrow*) for 3 s, systolic blood pressure reached to 40 mmHg during rapid atrial pacing

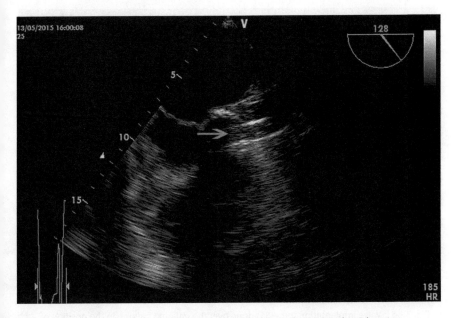

Fig. 3.64 Second time of balloon inflation (*arrow*) is done during rapid atrial pacing

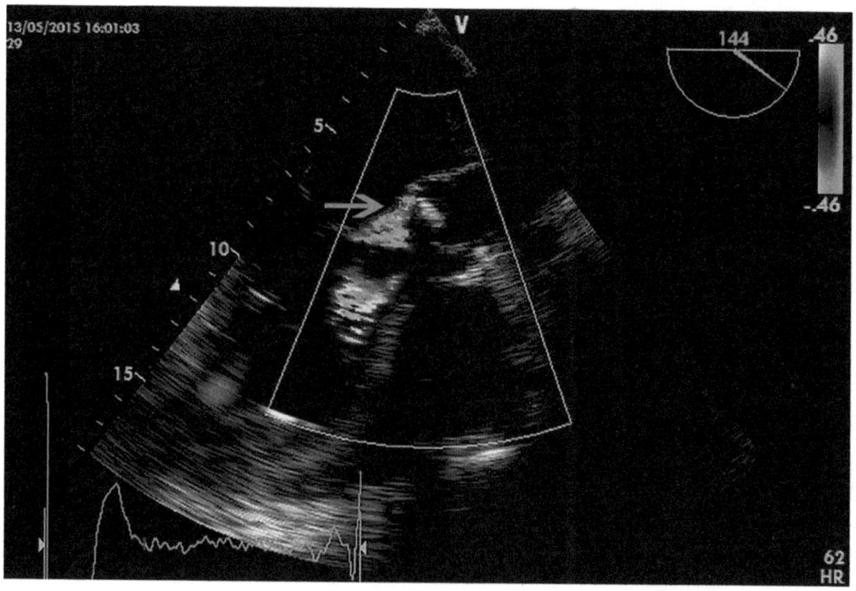

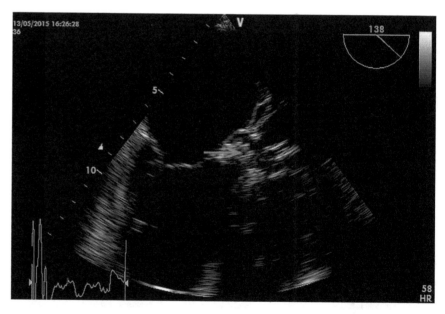

Fig. 3.65 Moderate AI is visible after second balloon dilation (*arrow*)

Fig. 3.66 Valve implantation (*arrow*) is done over the inflating balloon in the position of aortic valve during rapid pacing

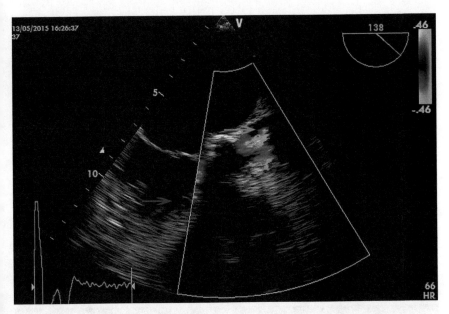

Fig. 3.67 Turbulency across aortic valve is nearly disappeared after valve implantation (*arrow*) and guide wire is still within LV (*pink arrow*)

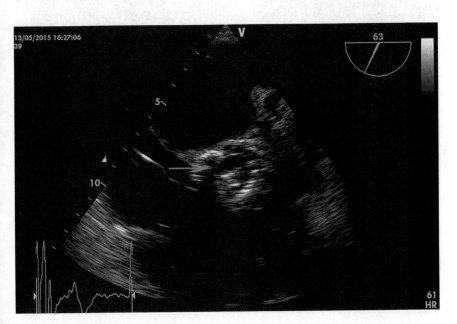

Fig. 3.68 Good function of implanted aortic valve is seen in TEE short-axis view

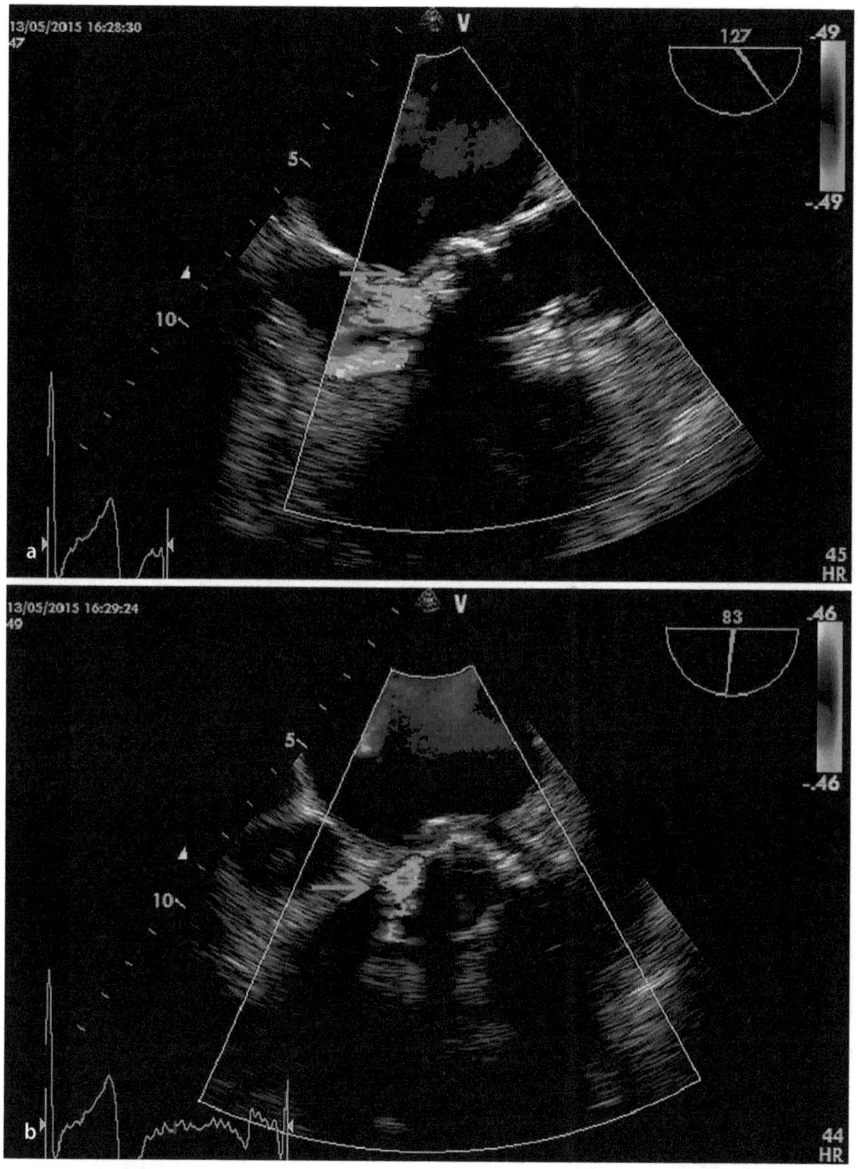

■ **Fig. 3.69**   Moderate paravalvular leak is visible in TEE long **a** and short-axis **b** views, paravalvular leak is mainly from NCC side and mild from LCC side (*pink arrow*) **b**

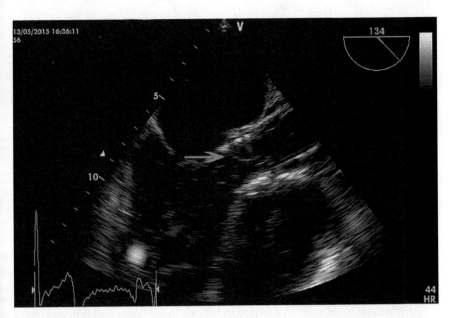

Fig. 3.70 Other time of balloon inflation (*arrow*) was performed for reducing paravalvular leak

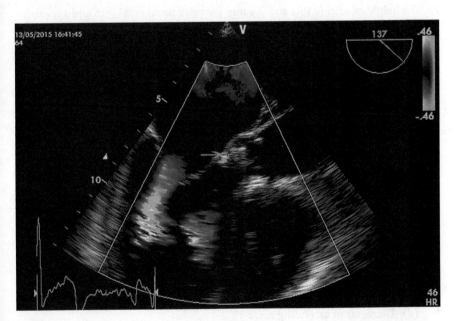

Fig. 3.71 Mild paravalvular leak is visible between AV and MV after last balloon inflation (*arrow*)

Diagnosis   Successful TAVI procedure with Edward Sapien valve number 26.

Lesson

1. For aortic annulus 18–21, Edward Sapien valve number 23 mm and for aortic annulus = 23–25 mm, Edward Sapien valve number 26 mm is selected.
2. It is previously mentioned that the Edward Sapien valve is selected larger than aortic annulus measured at parasternal long-axis to prevent paravalvular leak, but with precise annulus sizing with CT scan and 3D TEE, it has been demonstrated that the annulus measured at parasternal long-axis is annulus size in sagittal plane and annulus size in coronal plane is larger.
3. Aortic annulus diameter with TEE is 1.36 mm larger than TTE.
4. During TAVI, aortic leaflets are pushed toward aortic wall and there is the danger of occlusion of coronary arteries by aortic leaflets. Coronary ostia to annulus diameter should be measured before TAVI and aortic right and left coronary leaflet length should be measured in long-axis view.
5. The position of Edward Sapien aortic valve for TAVI is subcoronary [2]
6. The Edwards SAPIEN prosthesis consists of a balloon expandable, cylindrical frame composed of stainless steel to which is attached a trifoliate, equine pericardium heart valve. A fabric skirt is sewn to the frame and functions to mitigate paravalvular aortic regurgitation. The anchoring of the prosthesis and function of the valve are both intra-annular. This valve is currently available in two sizes: 23 for aortic annulus 18–22 mm and 26 mm for aortic annulus 21–25 mm.
7. The height of skirt is 10.1 and 7.4 mm for valve number 23 mm and 11.4 and 8.67 mm for valve 26 mm [8].
8. The average height of right coronary leaflet measures 14.1 mm and left coronary leaflet measures 14.2 mm [8], these measurements were done with necropsy [9].
9. The mean distance between RCA and aortic annulus is 13.2 ± 2.64 mm and between left main and aortic annulus is 12.6 ± 2.61 mm in a study on post-mortem hearts. These figures are 17.2 ± 3.3 for RCA and 14.4 ± 2.9 mm for left main artery in a study by multislice computed tomography [8]. As the result, height of left and right coronary cusps (about 14 mm) are greater than the distance between left main and RCA from annulus (13.2 and 12.6 mm) in normal hearts.
10. The ventricular end of aortic prosthesis is positioned 2–6 mm below the aortic valve leaflets, if left bundle branch passes 2–3 mm below this point, the possible risk of crush of conductive tissue exits [8].
11. The echocardiographic measurements before TAVI include:
    (a) Diameter of aortic annulus which will be described later in detail
    (b) Diameter of sinus of valsalva at mid sinusal level
    (c) Diameter of sinutubular junction
    (d) Diameter of ascending aorta
    (e) Diameter of LVOT
    (f) Diameter of IVS
    (g) Width and height of sinus of valsalva
    (h) Distance of left main and RCA from aortic annulus [8].
12. Heavy bulk calcification of aortic valve leaflets are associated by the risk of paravalvular leak because of the gap between external prosthesis surface and calcified aortic leaflets.
13. Calcification of landing zone of prosthesis may cause asymmetry of deployment and compression on coronary ostia.

14. Large calcification of edge of aortic leaflets may cause coronary ostial obstruction.
15. Large calcification of sinotubular junction may affect balloon expansion and cause left ventricular displacement of valve during implantation.
16. The minimal distance between coronary ostia and aortic annulus should be more than 10–11 mm for both commercial available valves.
17. Core valve is used for sinus of valsalva >27 mm and height >10 mm.
18. Now Edward Sapien valves are available for aortic annulus 16–27 mm, prosthesis 20–29 mm and core valve valves are available for aortic annulus 17–29 mm, prosthesis 23–31 mm [10].
19. Sinotubular junction should be smaller than 40–43 mm for core valve.
20. The position of core valve in LVOT is 5–10 mm below aortic annulus and for Edward Sapien is 2–4 mm below aortic annulus.
21. Core valves consist of three portions: Outflow portion which is positioned in aortic root, midportion which contains host leaflets and coronary ostia, and inflow portion which is positioned in left ventricular outflow tract and contains patient native aortic leaflets and skirt of pericardium prevents paravalvular leak.
22. Core valve has about 50 mm length with 12 mm skirt, the prosthesis size is determined by external size of left ventricular end, the midportion diameter of valve number 26 and 29 measure 22 and 24 mm and aortic end diameter 40 and 43 mm and height 53 and 55 mm, respectively. The valve size 26 is designed for annulus = 20–23 mm and valve 29 mm is designed for aortic annulus 24–27 mm. The diameter of ascending aorta should not be more than 45 mm [2].
23. Bicuspid aortic valve is a relative contraindication for TAVI, although it has been reported in expert hands [10].
24. Core valve is designed for arterial access, and has a supravalvular position [10].
25. Up to 40% of LBBB is reported after core valve implantation due to this fact that core valve is positioned about 5–10 mm in LVOT [8].
26. If severe calcification of aortic valve presents, the smaller valve should be selected [10].
27. In general, it is said that there is oversizing for both core valve and Edward Sapien valves [10], but indeed this may be due to the fact that aortic annulus is oval shape and the diameter that conventionally measured is annulus in parasternal long-axis view which is the smallest aortic diameter (sagittal plane) while the annulus in coronal plane is larger.

3.13   Case 11: Visualization of Four Pulmonary Veins and Measurement of Aortic Annulus for TAVI

A 45-year-old woman presented by dyspnea on exertion functional class II. Transthoracic echocardiography showed severe MS, moderately sever MR, severe TR, no LA, and LAA clot. She was candidate for cardiac surgery (MVR + TV annuloplasty) and the question was about aortic valve, AVA was 1.7 by continuity equation and mild to moderate AI, Does AVR is needed?

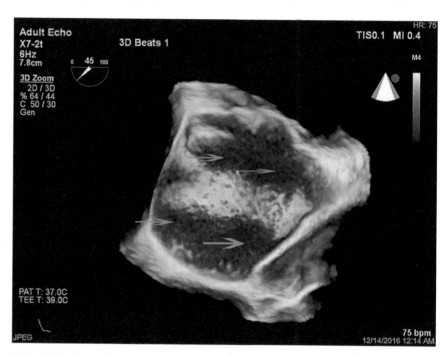

Fig. 3.72 Four pulmonary veins are visualized in this 45° view by 3D zoom of interatrial septum from LA side (*arrows*)

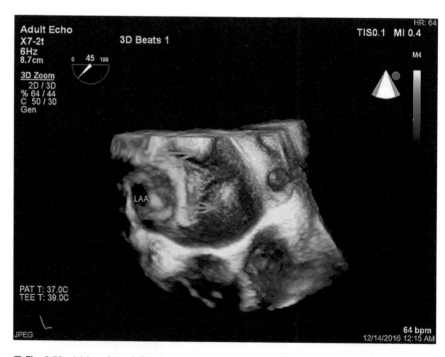

Fig. 3.73 LAA and two left pulmonary veins are visualized in this 45° view by 3D zoom, there is no clot in LAA

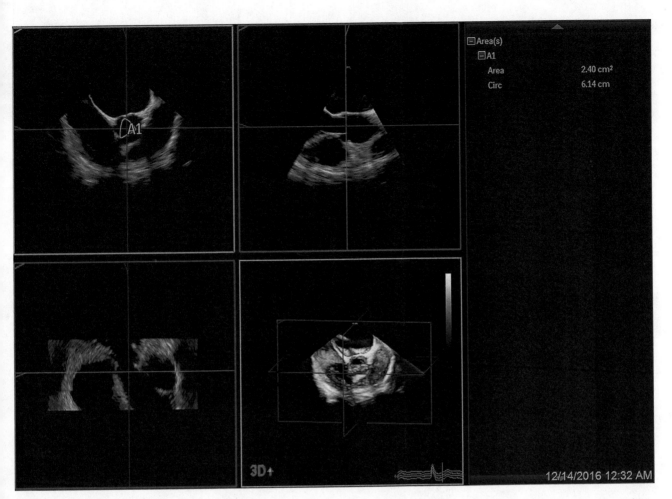

Fig. 3.74 Aortic valve area measures 2.4 cm² by direct planimetry by full volume of aortic valve, it is of notice that *blue* plane is positioned at tip of aortic leaflets and then measurement is done in *green* plane

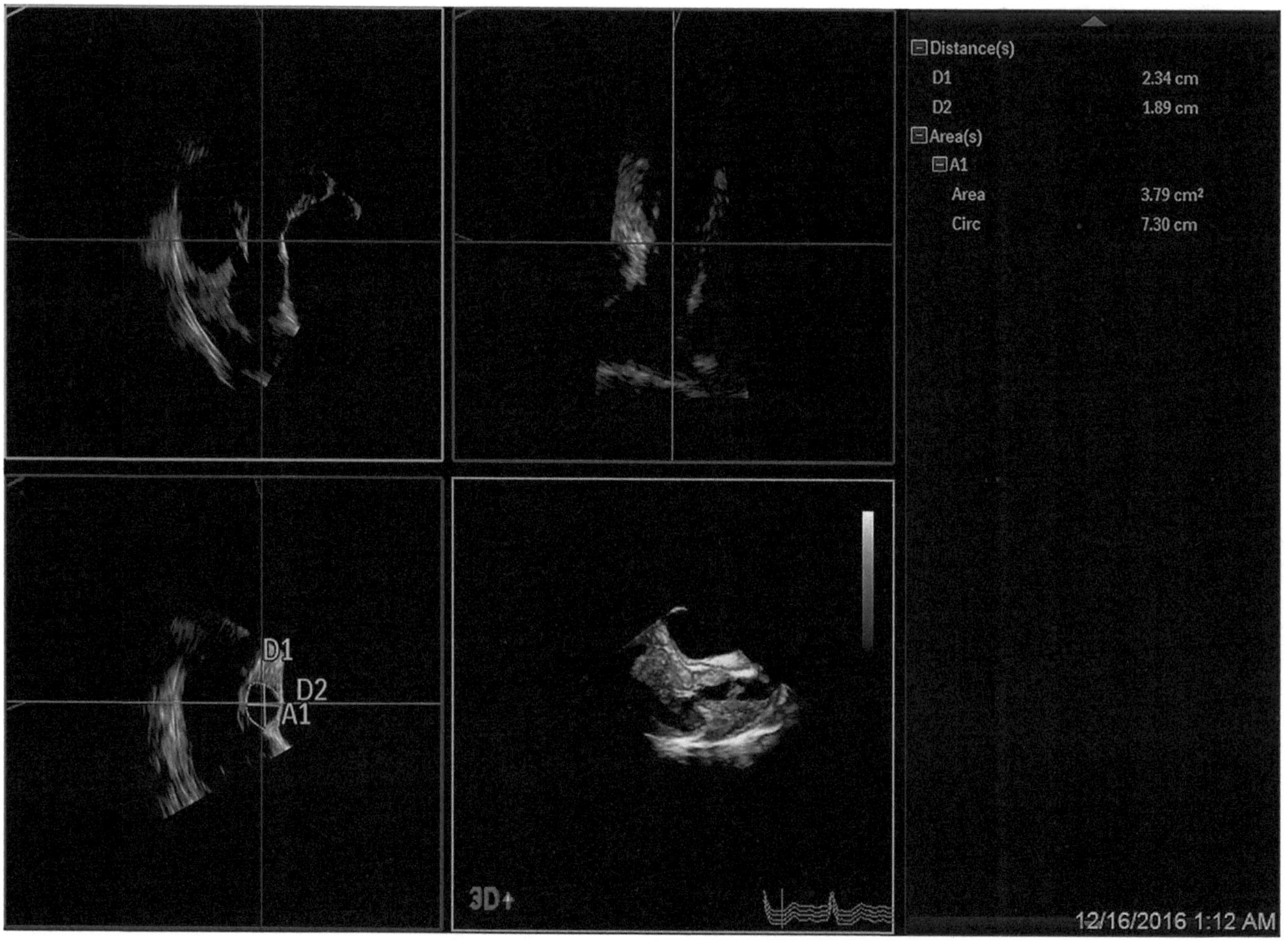

Distance(s)	
D1	2.34 cm
D2	1.89 cm
Area(s)	
A1	
Area	3.79 cm²
Circ	7.30 cm

□ Fig. 3.75 Full volume of aortic valve is captured in long-axis of aortic valve, then three planes are locked and *blue* plane is turned 90° counterclockwise, *blue* plane is positioned in hinge point of aortic leaflets and in left lower quadrant view (*blue* plane), aortic annulus is measured in two orthogonal views (sagittal and coronal views) (23 and 19 mm, respectively) and area and perimeter of aortic valve are measured (3.8 cm² and 7.3 cm, respectively)

Aortic annulus area = 3.8 cm²,

Diameter of annulus is calculated as follows: aortic annulus area = 3.8 cm²/0.785 = 4.84,

D2 = 4.84,

D = 2.20 cm,

Aortic annulus area = 7.3 cm,

Diameter of aortic annulus is calculated as follows: 7.3/3.14 = 2.32 cm.

So aortic annulus is measured 23 and 19 mm in coronal and sagittal views directly, 22 mm by calculating via area and 23.2 mm when calculated via perimeter. This method of aortic annulus sizing is previously described by Khalique et al. [11].

3.14   Case 12: Type A Aortic Dissection

A 34-year-old man with history of sudden onset chest pain with radiation to both his arms after an emotional stress. In physical examination, there was a diastolic murmur grade III/VI in aortic area and equal pulses in both upper extremities.

Transesophageal echocardiography was performed for more evaluation of aortic dissection and extension of dissectional flap.

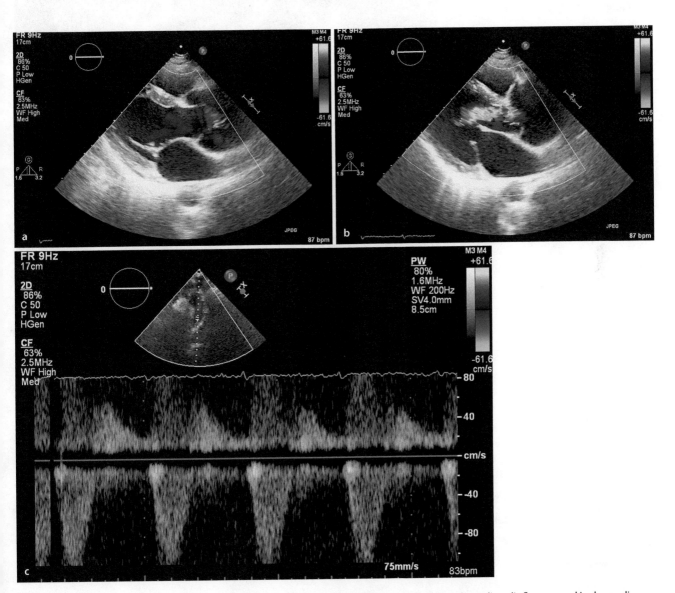

◻ **Fig. 3.76**   Parasternal long-axis view shows dilated aortic root **a**, severe aortic regurgitation, **b** and pan diastolic flow reversal in descending aorta **c**

3

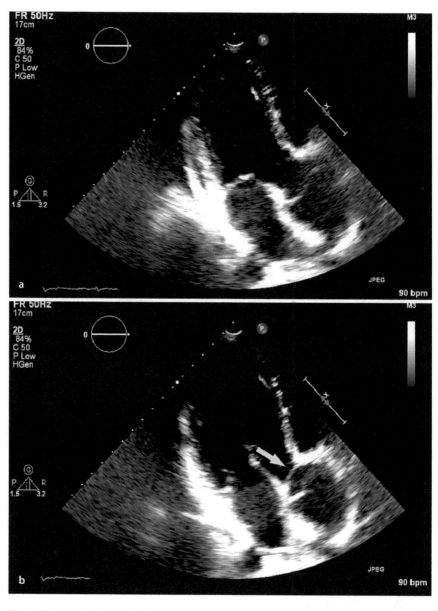

Fig. 3.77 Apical three chamber view depicts a hyper echogenic linear density in sinus of valsalva that it protrudes to left ventricular out flow tract during diastolic time (*arrow*) in favor of aortic dissection (**a, b** systolic and diastolic time)

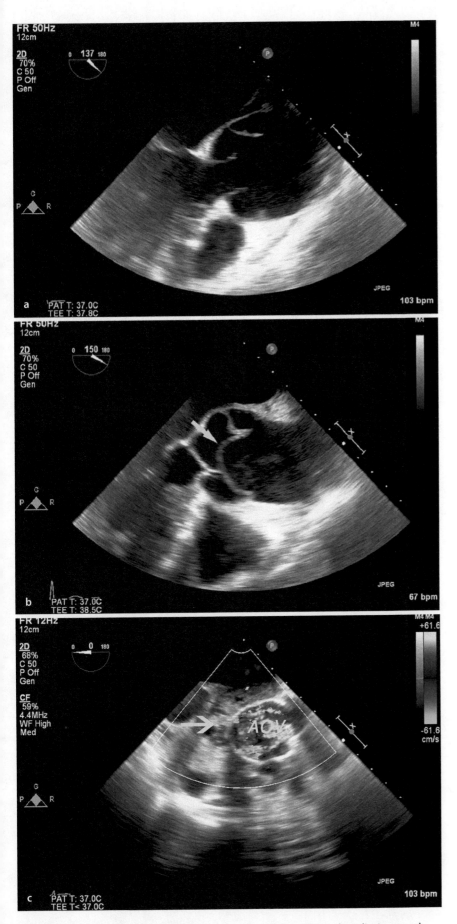

Fig. 3.78 Mid esophageal long-axis view shows flap of dissection in diastolic time **a** and systolic time **b** with severe AI in TEE short-axis view (*arrow*) **c**

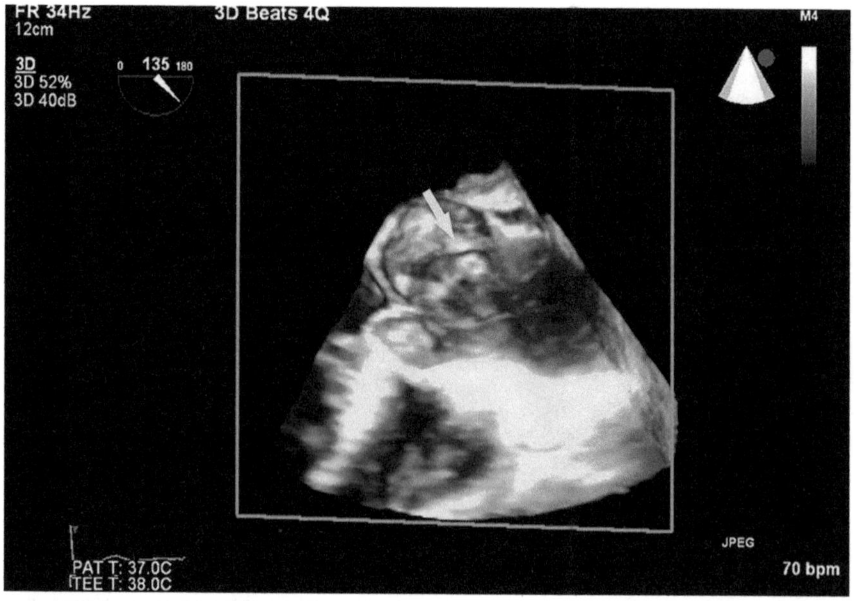

Fig. 3.79   3D full volume view of aorta in 120° shows large area of intimal-media detachment (*arrow*) in ascending aorta with flap protrusion toward left ventricular out flow tract. For optimal resolution post-image processing should be consider and increase smoothness up to 4 number

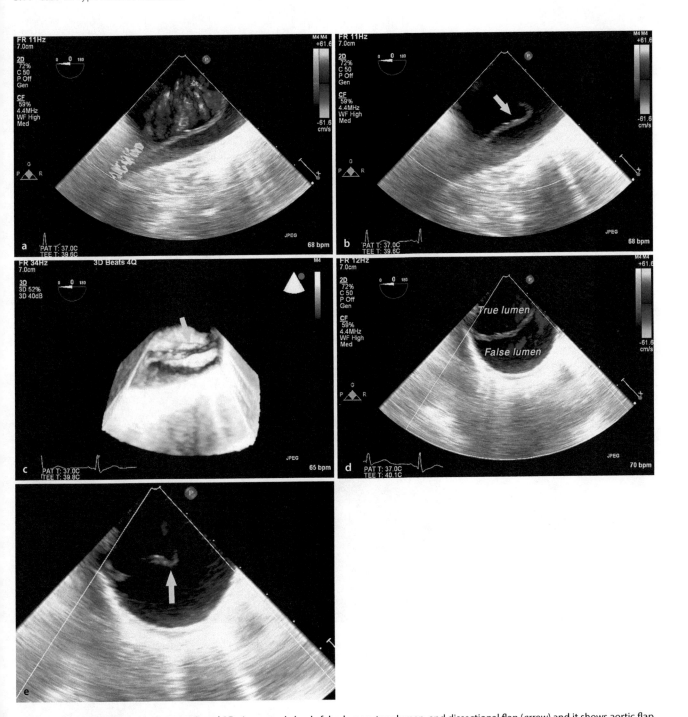

□ **Fig. 3.80** Upper esophageal aortic 2D and 3D view reveal clearly false lumen, true lumen, and dissectional flap (*arrow*) and it shows aortic flap extension to arch **a–c** and descending aorta **d, e**

Diagnosis   Patient with diagnosis of type A of aortic dissection and severe aortic regurgitation was sent to operation room and Bentall operation for patient was done.

Two weeks after operation the patient presented with chest pain and was sent for reevaluation of aorta.

Transthoracic echo shows prosthetic aortic valve with acceptable gradients but evaluation of aortic valve mobility was not possible due to metallic valve shadow.

Transesophageal echocardiography was performed for more evaluation of aortic prosthetic valve and Bentall operation complications.

The patient was evaluated for infective endocarditis and close follow-up for increased peri-aortic thickness was done, after 2 weeks peri-aortic thickness decreased in size slowly and resolved.

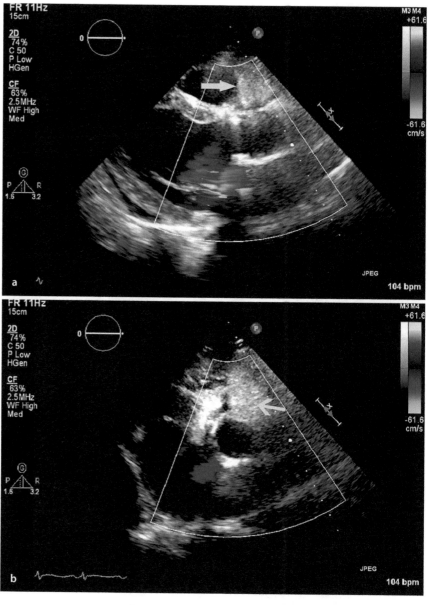

☐ **Fig. 3.81** Parasternal long-axis view shows a hyper echogenic density above of aorta (**a**, *arrow*) and parasternal short-axis view shows peri-aortic thickness (**b**, *arrows*)

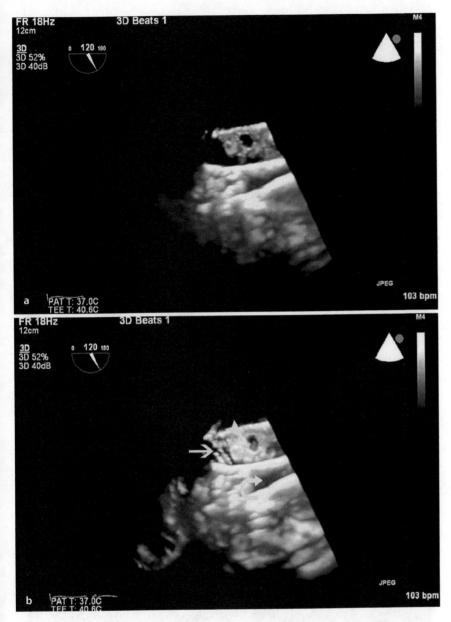

Fig. 3.82 3D zoom parasternal demonstrates good mobility of prosthetic valve (**a, b,** *arrow*) and re-implantation site of left main to composite graft is visible clearly (*head arrow*) and it depicts a free space around of composite graft (*crew arrow*). *AOV* aortic valve

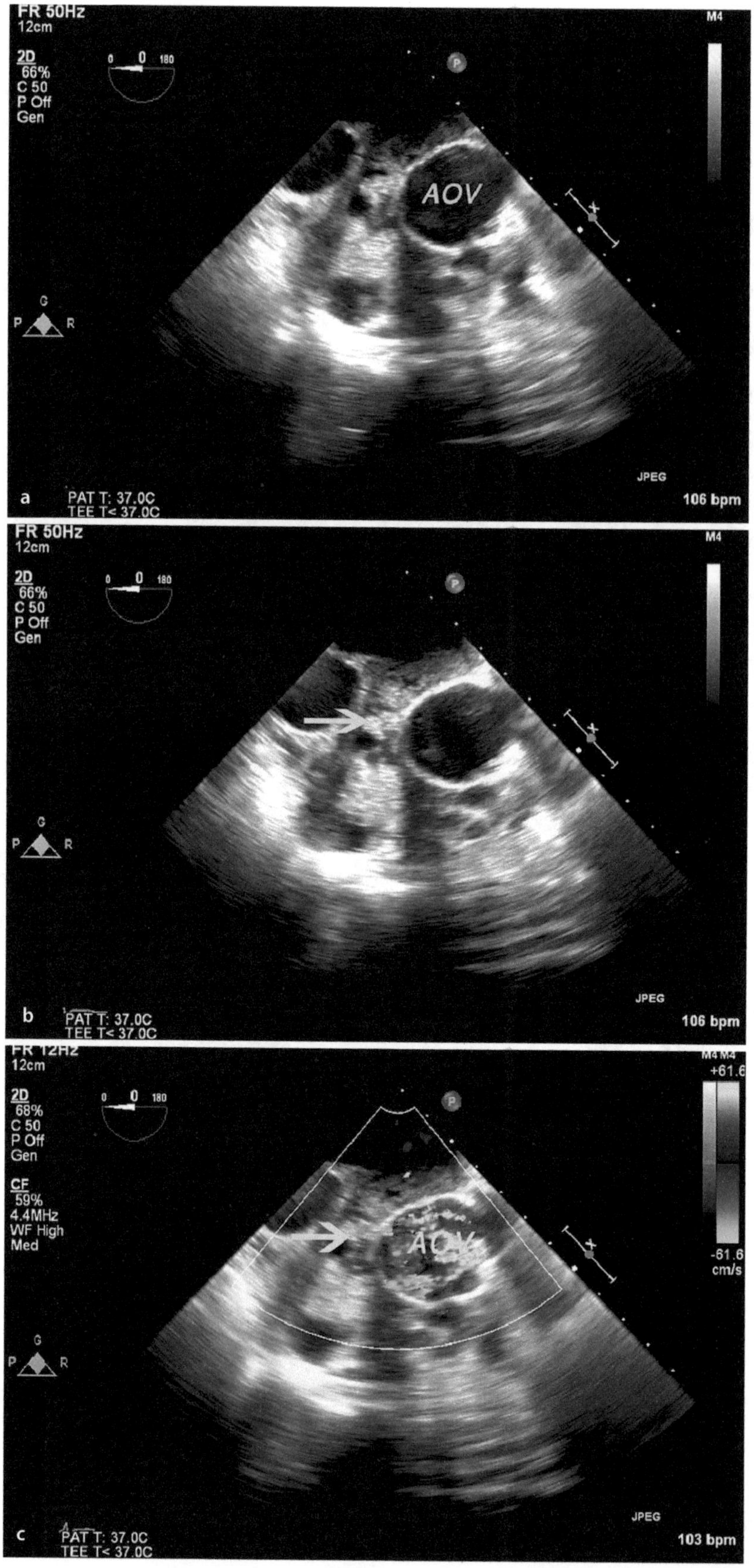

Fig. 3.83   Mid esophageal short-axis view shows that peri-aortic thickness is full of hyper echogenic material without any flow in it and no evidence of abscess formation, these are highly suggestive for hematoma (**a**–**c**, *arrows*) and with low probability insertion of Teflon felt during operation

Diagnosis   Hematoma around of composite graft.

What is the cause of early and late mortality after Bentall operation?

Early mortality and morbidity post-operation are defined as complications during first month after operation, and late complications occur after first month. Early mortality and morbidity include low cardiac output, arrhythmia, pulmonary problems, sepsis, cerebrovascular attack, and bleeding and late complications are congestive heart failure, type B dissection, CVA, myocardial infarction, and sudden death.

What are the points for follow-up after Bentall operation?

Patient with Bentall operation should be followed for persistent intimal flap, progression of disease, pseudo aneurysm formation, recurrent dissection.

Type A aortic dissection involves ascending aorta and type B involves descending aorta. In acute type A aortic dissection, emergent surgery is the treatment of choice and acute type B aortic dissection needs endovascular intervention if complicated. Complication includes: limb or visceral ischemia, abdominal pain due to expansion, and retrograde involvement of ascending aorta [12].

References

1. Nishimura RA, Otto CM, Bonow RO, Carabello BA, Erwin 3rd JP, Guyton RA, et al. 2014 AHA/ACC guideline for the Management of Patients with Valvular Heart Disease: executive summary: a report of the American College of Cardiology/American Heart Association task force on practice guidelines. Circulation. 2014;129(23):2440–92.

2. Zamorano JL, Badano LP, Bruce C, Chan KL, Goncalves A, Hahn RT, et al. EAE/ASE recommendations for the use of echocardiography in new transcatheter interventions for valvular heart disease. J Am Soc Echocardiogr. 2011;24(9):937–65.

3. Joint Task Force on the Management of Valvular Heart Disease of the European Society of Cardiac, European Association for Cardio-Thoracic Surgery, Vahanian A, Alfieri O, Andreotti F, Antunes MJ, et al. Guidelines on the management of valvular heart disease (version 2012). Eur Heart J. 2012;33(19):2451–96.

4. Fang L, Hsiung MC, Miller AP, Nanda NC, Yin WH, Young MS, et al. Assessment of aortic regurgitation by live three-dimensional transthoracic echocardiographic measurements of vena contracta area: usefulness and validation. Echocardiography. 2005;22(9):775–81.

5. Chin CH, Chen CH, Lo HS. The correlation between three-dimensional vena contracta area and aortic regurgitation index in patients with aortic regurgitation. Echocardiography. 2010;27(2):161–6.

6. Butz T, Piper C, Langer C, Wiemer M, Kottmann T, Meissner A, et al. Diagnostic superiority of a combined assessment of the systolic and early diastolic mitral annular velocities by tissue Doppler imaging for the differentiation of restrictive cardiomyopathy from constrictive pericarditis. Clin Res Cardiol. 2010;99(4):207–15.

7. Awtry E, Davidoff R. Low-flow/low-gradient aortic stenosis. Circulation. 2011;124(23):e739–41.

8. Piazza N, de Jaegere P, Schultz C, Becker AE, Serruys PW, Anderson RH. Anatomy of the aortic valvar complex and its implications for transcatheter implantation of the aortic valve. Circ Cardiovasc Interv. 2008;1(1):74–81.

9. Vollebergh FE, Becker AE. Minor congenital variations of cusp size in tricuspid aortic valves. Possible link with isolated aortic stenosis. Br Heart J. 1977;39(9):1006–11.

10. Zamorano JL, Goncalves A, Lang R. Imaging to select and guide transcatheter aortic valve implantation. Eur Heart J. 2014;35(24):1578–87.

11. Khalique OK, Kodali SK, Paradis JM, Nazif TM, Williams MR, Einstein AJ, et al. Aortic annular sizing using a novel 3-dimensional echocardiographic method: use and comparison with cardiac computed tomography. Circ Cardiovasc Imaging. 2014;7(1):155–63.

12. Braverman AC. Disease of the aorta. In: Mann DL, Zipes DP, Libby P, Bonnow RO, Branwald E, editors. Braunwald's heart disease. 2. Philadelphia, PA: Elsevier Saunders; 2015. p. 1277–311.

Tricuspid Valve Disease

Videos can be found in the electronic supplementary material in the online version of the chapter.
On http://springerlink.com enter the DOI number given on the bottom of the chapter opening page.
Scroll down to the Supplementary material tab and click on the respective videos link.

© Springer International Publishing AG 2017
H. Sadeghian, Z. Savand-Roomi, *3D Echocardiography of Structural Heart Disease*,
DOI 10.1007/978-3-319-54039-9_4

4.1   Tricuspid Stenosis, Tricuspid Regurgitation

There are two categories of tricuspid valve involvement:
1. Congenital, like Ebstein disease
2. Acquired

Most acquired tricuspid valve disease occurred due to rheumatismal disease. There may be direct involvement of tricuspid valve by rheumatismal disease, or involvement of mitral and aortic valve causes elevated pulmonary arterial pressure and results in tricuspid regurgitation. About 80% of cases of TR are secondary TR due to RV volume or pressure overload [1].

Low-pressure TR occurs with involvement of TV due to disease like carcinoid.

Severe TR is defined as significant TR in the presence of RA and RV dilation. Severe TR should be repaired in the time of CABG or other left-sided valve surgery (class I recommendation) [1, 2].

Moderate primary TR should be repaired in the time of left-sided valve surgery (class IIa recommendation) [2]; mild or moderate functional TR should be repaired at the time of left-sided valve surgery if TV annulus is significantly dilated (TV annulus > 40 mm) (class IIa recommendation) [1, 2]. TV annulus has a saddle shape and with dilation; the anteroposterior [1] and lateral to septal diameter is increased [3].

Severe TS is defined as TVA ≤ 1 cm^2 by planimetry or PHT [1].

4.2   Case 1: Severe TS, Severe TR, Severe MS, Mild MR

A 52-year-old woman presented with lower extremities edema and dyspnea on exertion functional class II of recent duration. She was a known case of rheumatismal involvement of bone and joints from 20 years ago but unaware of heart involvement until now.

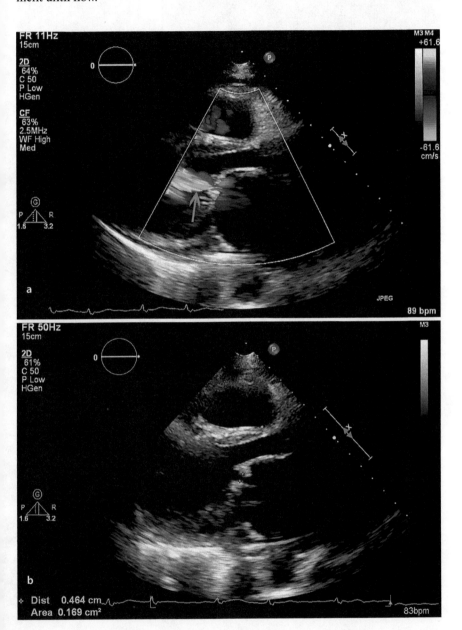

◼ **Fig. 4.1** Parasternal long-axis view shows diastolic turbulency across mitral valve in favor of significant mitral stenosis (*arrow*) **a**, mitral valve opening is 4.6 mm in this view **b**

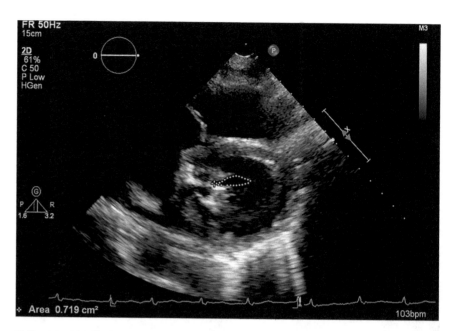

Fig. 4.2 Mitral valve area measures 0.7 cm² by planimetry in parasternal short-axis view by 2D echocardiography

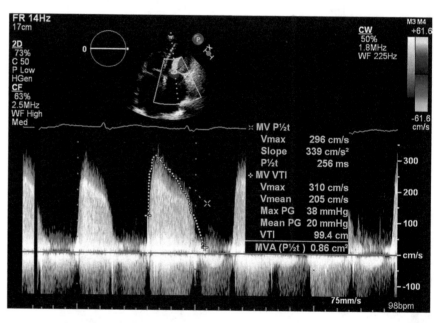

Fig. 4.3 Peak and mean gradients across mitral valve are 38 and 20 mmHg, respectively, and mitral valve area measures 0.86 cm² by PHT

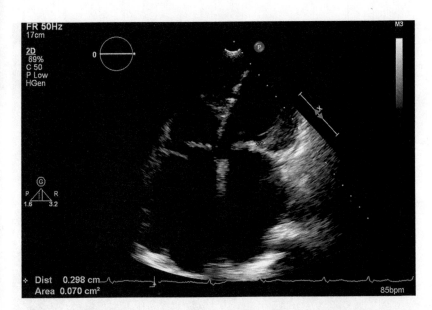

◘ **Fig. 4.4** Length of chorda of posterior mitral leaflet is 3 mm in apical four-chamber view

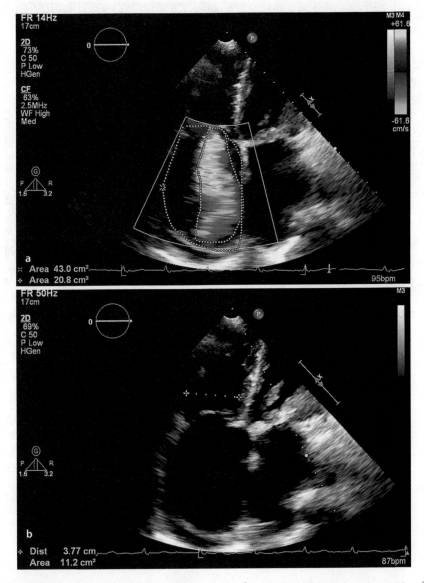

◘ **Fig. 4.5** Surface of tricuspid regurgitation is 21 cm² and surface of the right atrium is 43 cm²
a, the right ventricle is mildly dilated and 37 mm in apical four-chamber view **b**

4

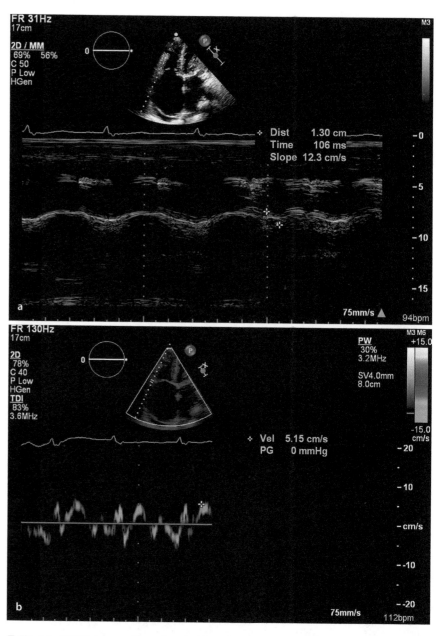

■ **Fig. 4.6** TAPSE measure 13 mm in apical four-chamber view **a** and RV sm measures 5 cm/s **b**

4.2 · Case 1: Severe TS, Severe TR, Severe MS, Mild MR

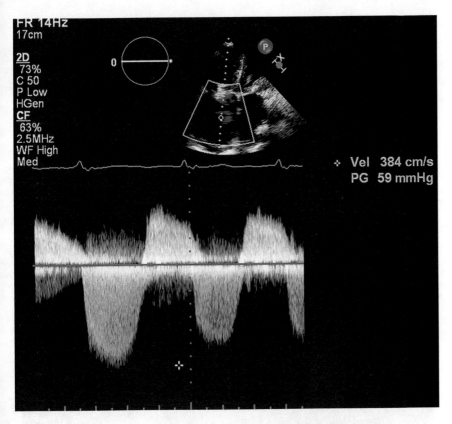

Fig. 4.7 Tricuspid regurgitation gradient is 59 mmHg in apical four-chamber view

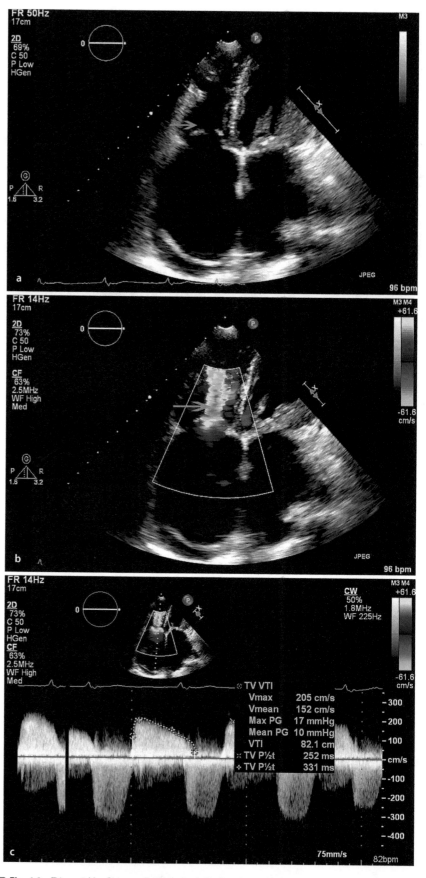

Fig. 4.8 Tricuspid leaflets are thick and calcified and restricted motion (*arrow*) **a**, there is diastolic turbulency across tricuspid valve in apical four-chamber view **b**. Peak and mean gradients across tricuspid valve measure 14.5 and 9 mmHg, respectively **c**, PHT of tricuspid is 290 mmHg and TVA calculated as follows: TVA = 190/PHT = 190/290 = 0.65 cm²

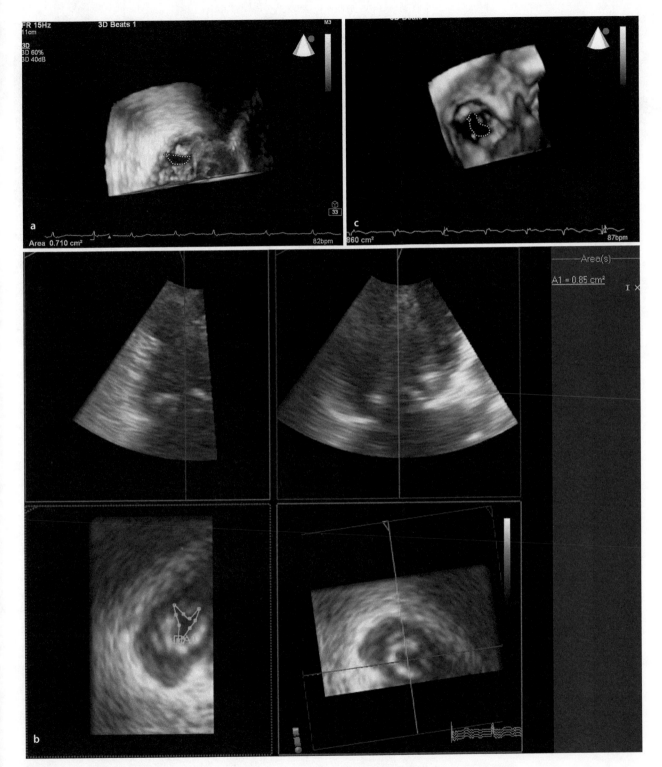

☐ **Fig. 4.9** Four-dimensional reconstruction of tricuspid valve by 3D zoom shows TVA is equal to 0.71 cm² by direct planimetery, this view is from ventricular side and septal leaflet put in 6 o'cklock position **a** [4] and measurement of TV area by 3DQ is done in apical 4 chamber transthoracic view and TVA measures 0.85 cm² **b**, TVA measures 0.86 cm² by direct plannimetery 3D zoom from RA side **c** [4] and TVA measures 0.7 cm² by direct plannimetery on 2D echocardiography transgastric view 16° **d**

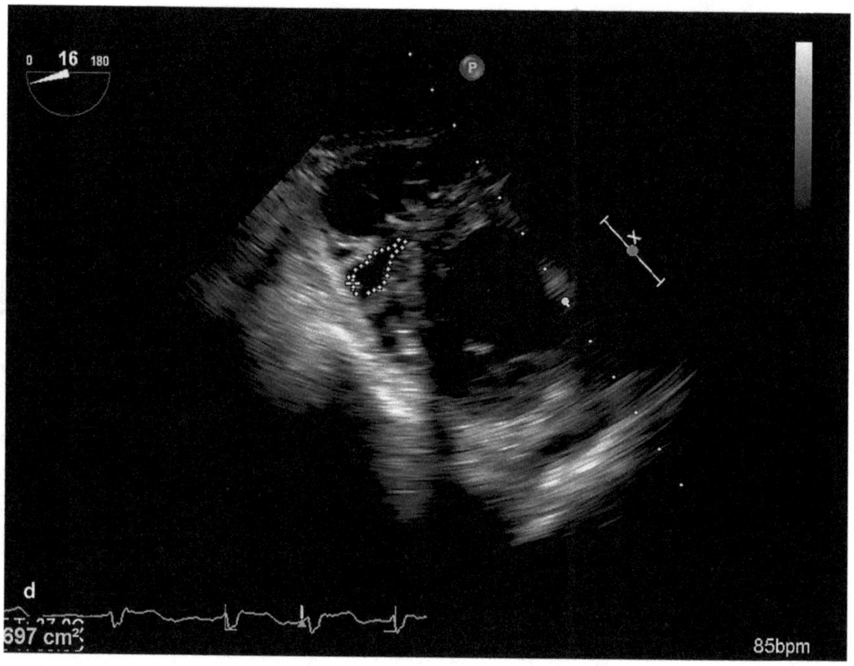

Fig. 4.9 (continued)

Diagnosis   Severe mitral stenosis, mild mitral regurgitation, severe tricuspid stenosis, severe tricuspid regurgitation, moderate RV systolic dysfunction.

Comment   MVR and TVR.

4.3   Case 2: Severe TS Post-MVR

A 52-year-old woman is under follow-up after MVR in our center.

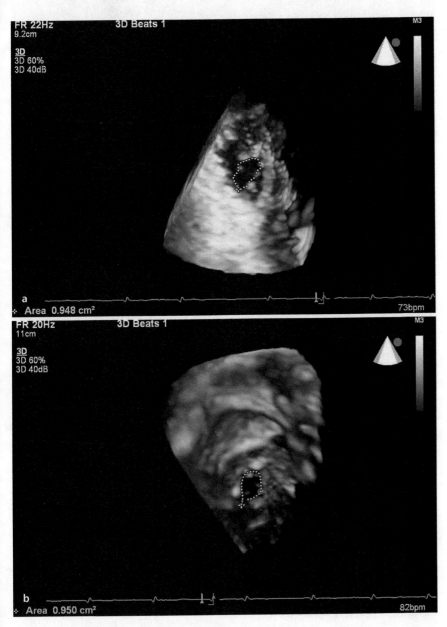

■ **Fig. 4.10** TVA is 0.95 cm² by direct planimetry by 3D echo from both RV and RA sides **a, b** [4]

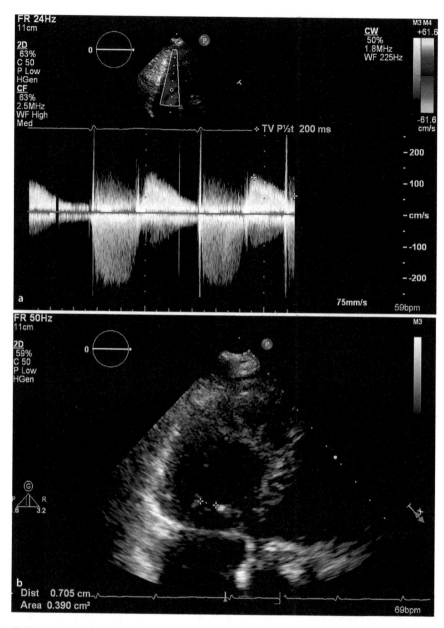

■ Fig. 4.11   TV PHT is 200 ms and TV leaflets' opening is 0.7 cm [4]

Diagnosis   Severe TS post-MVR.

Comment   If symptomatic, try for valvuloplasty of tricuspid valve if the TR is not severe.

4.4   Case 3: Severe TS and Moderate TR and Severe MS

A 43-year-old woman referred for cardiac surgery. She was a known case of mitral stenosis and underwent PTMC 8 months ago.

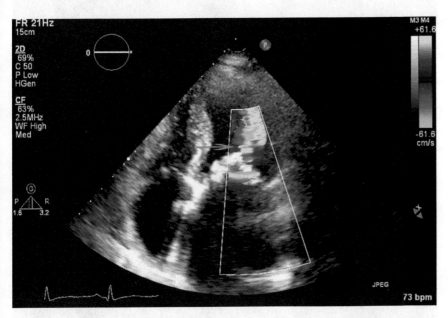

◻ **Fig. 4.12** Thickness of both mitral leaflets has a score of 4, calcification is of grade 4, mobility of AMVL has a score of 3 and PMVL has a score of 4, and length of chorda of PMVL measures 3 mm, so PMVL is nearly attached to the left ventricular free wall, and subvalvular apparatus of AMVL and PMVL has a score of 3 and 4, respectively. Total score of AMVL and PMVL are 14 and 16, respectively, so the patient was not a good candidate for PTMC from the beginning

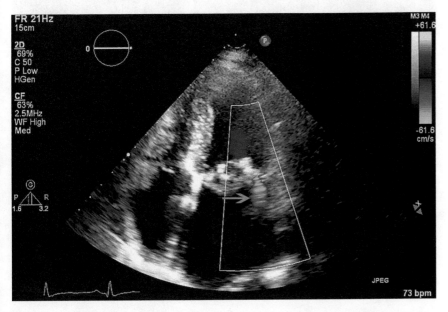

◻ **Fig. 4.13** There is a perforation in base of PMVL (*arrow*), and mitral regurgitation originates from this site of perforation (*arrow*)

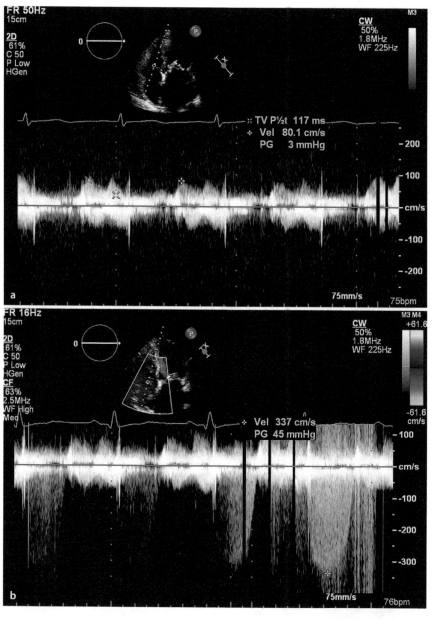

☐ Fig. 4.14 Peak and mean gradients across tricuspid valve are 7 and 3 mmHg, respectively, and TV PHT is 117 ms, so TVA with PHT is 190/117 = 1.62 cm² **a**. TRG is 45 mmHg **b**, TVA with direct planimetry and view from ventricular side with 3D zoom is 1.4 cm² **c**, and from the right atrial view 1.3 cm² **d**, TVA measures 1.15 cm² by 3DQ method **e**

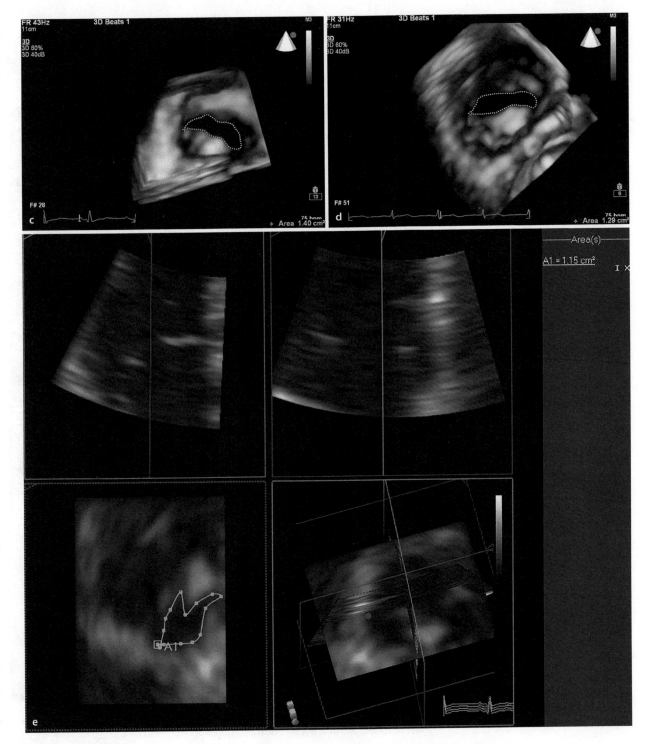

■ **Fig. 4.14** (continued)

Diagnosis Severe TS and moderate TR and severe MS with score 14–16.

Comment The patient referred for MVR and TVR.

Lesson

1. TVA measurement with direct planimetry with 3D zoom is a reliable method.
2. OMVC is an acceptable method when score is not high.
3. In the presence of TR, TV repair is possible but in the presence of severe TR and TS, TVR is recommended.

4.5   Case 4: Severe TS and Severe TR, Severe MS, Mild MR

A 46-year-old woman presented with dyspnea on exertion functional class III of recent exacerbation.

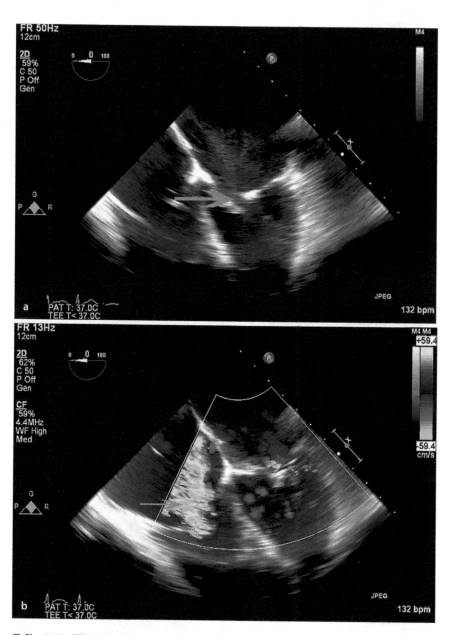

■ **Fig. 4.15** TEE 0° view shows severe spontaneous contrast in LA due to severe MS (*arrow*) **a**; severe TR (*arrow*) and mild MR are evident by TEE color Doppler study **b**

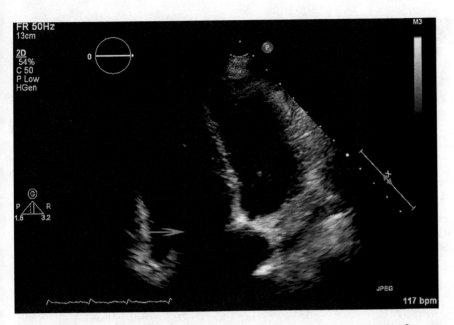

■ **Fig. 4.16**   RV is moderately dilated in TTE apical four-chamber view and restricted leaflet motion of TV is evident in this view (*arrow*)

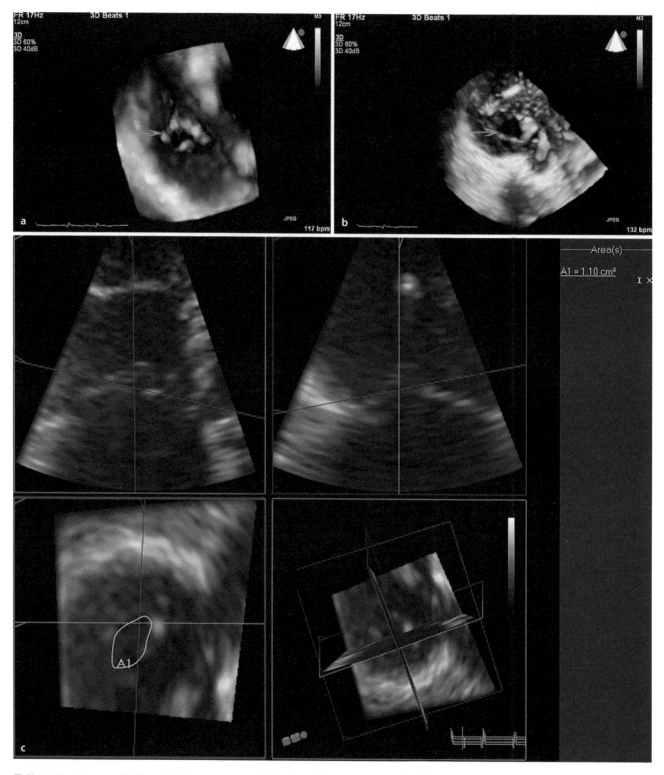

Fig. 4.17   3D zoom of TV from RA side (*arrow*) **a** and RV side (*arrow*) **b** is demonstrated in this figure; TVA measures 1.1 by 3DQ method **c**

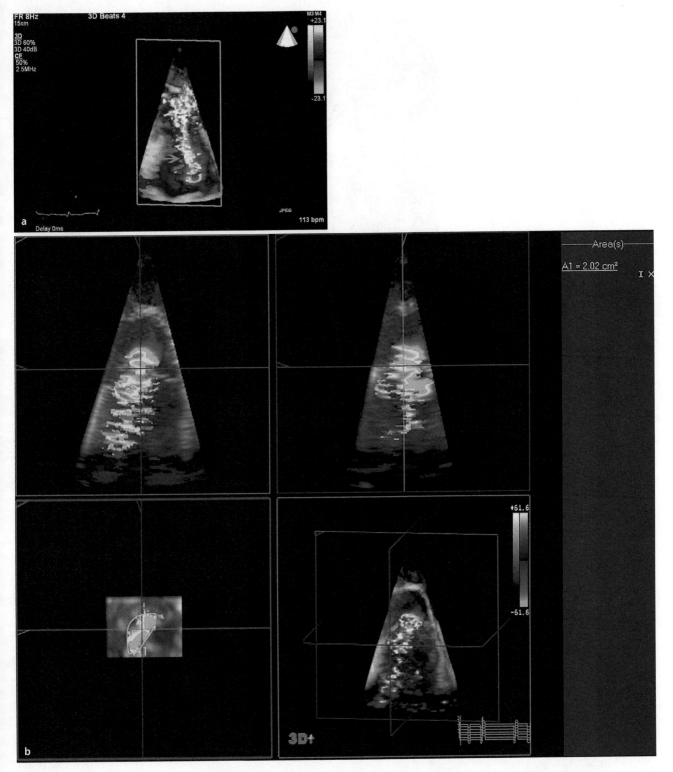

Fig. 4.18 Full volume of severe TR is evident in this view (*arrow*) **a**; TR vena contracta area measures 2 cm² in favor of severe TR **b** [5]

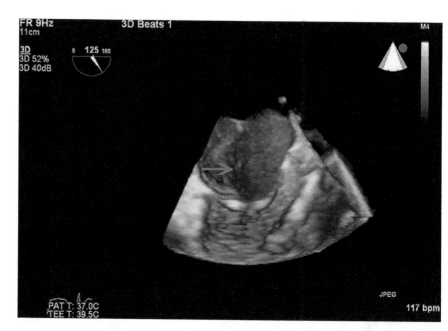

◧ **Fig. 4.19**   3D zoom in 120° reveals severe MS and severe spontaneous contrast in LA (*arrow*)

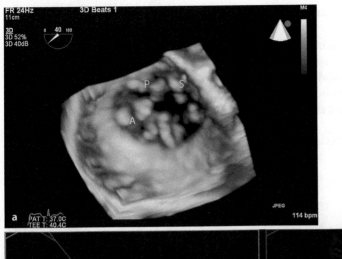

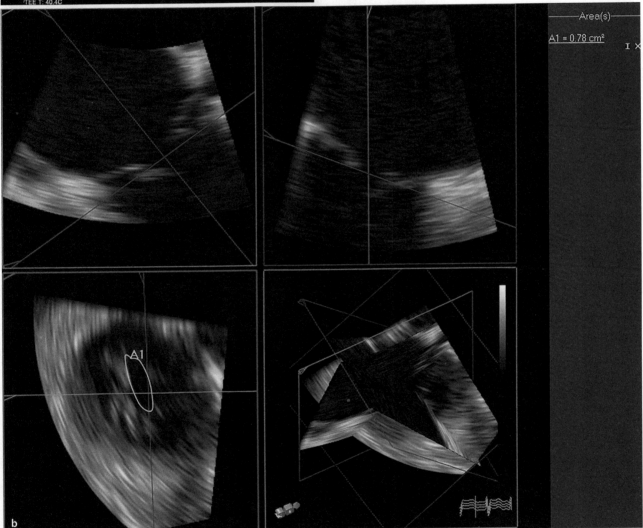

Fig. 4.20   3D zoom of TV by TEE 40° reveals three leaflets of TV **a**; TVA measures 0.8 cm² by 3DQ method **b**. *S* septal, *A* anterior, *P* posterior leaflets of TV

Diagnosis   Severe MS, mild MR, severe spontaneous contrast in LA and LAA, severe TS, and severe TR.

Comment   MVR or OMVC + TV repair or TVR.

4.6   Case 5: Carcinoid Disease with Severe TR and Severe PI

A 46-year-old woman with history of flashing and abdominal pain and palpitation and diarrhea with 2-month duration and her sonography revealed a mass in the liver; she was candidate for liver surgery with diagnosis of hydatid cyst and was referred to our echocardiography laboratory for pre-operation evaluation. In the physical examination, a harsh systolic murmur grade III/VI was heard in the left sternal border.

Transthoracic echocardiography reveals normal left ventricular size and function.

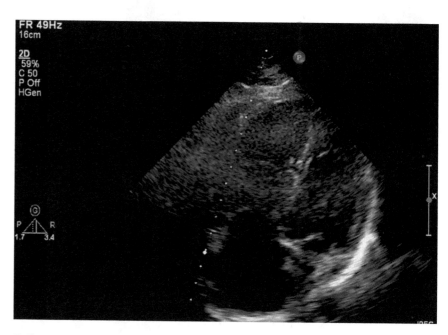

◘ **Fig. 4.21**   Apical four-chamber view shows moderate right ventricular dilation

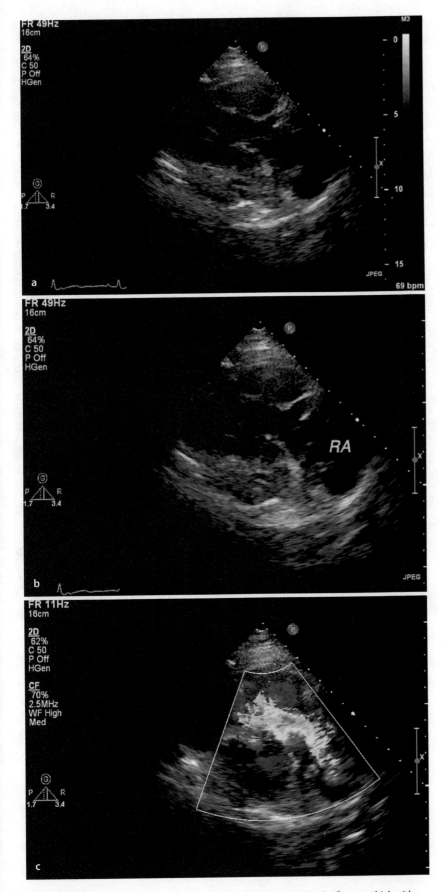

◘ **Fig. 4.22** Right ventricular inflow tract view depicts tricuspid valve leaflets are thick with restricted motion during systolic **a** and diastolic time **b** leading to severe tricuspid regurgitation **c**

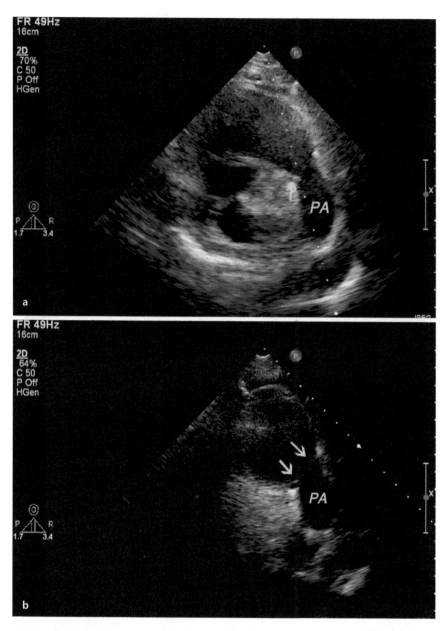

■ Fig. 4.23   Short-axis great vessel view reveals thick pulmonary valve (*arrows*, **a**, **b**)

Transesophageal echocardiography was done for further evaluation of tricuspid valve.

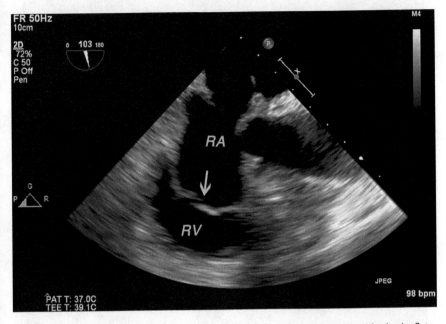

◻ **Fig. 4.24** Mid-esophageal 103° view of tricuspid valve confirms thick tricuspid valve leaflets (*arrow*)

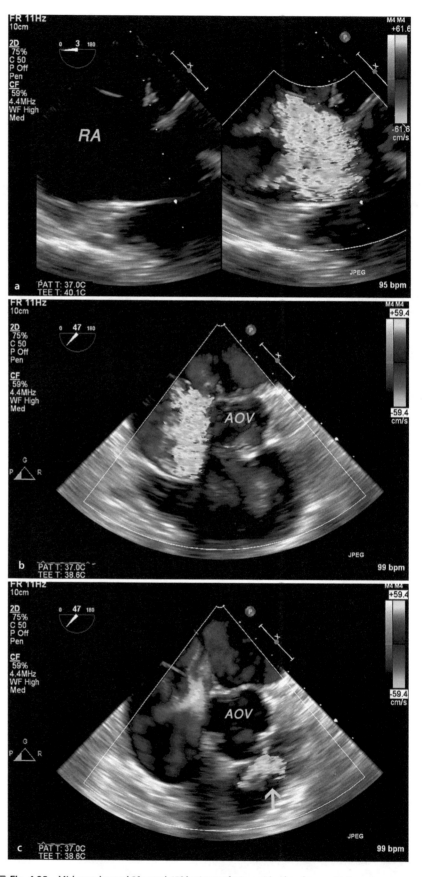

◻ Fig. 4.25 Mid-esophageal 3° **a** and 47° **b** views of tricuspid valve demonstrate severe tricuspid regurgitation during systolic time (*arrow*), and pulmonary regurgitation is filled more than 50% of the right ventricular outflow tract (**c**, *arrow*) in favor of severe pulmonary insufficiency during diastolic time

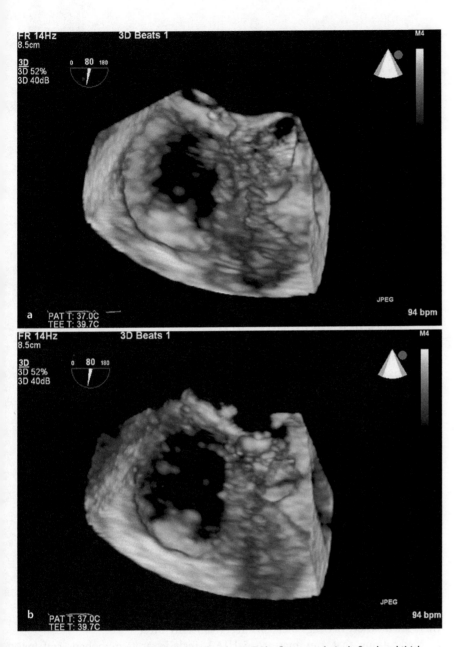

Fig. 4.26 3D zoom view of tricuspid valve shows TV leaflets are relatively fixed and thick during systolic **a** and diastolic time **b**

Diagnosis With respect to the deformity of tricuspid valve leaflets, carcinoid tumor was a possible diagnosis for the patient. So she was sent for detection of 5-HIAA (5-hydroxyindoleacetic acid) in 24 h urine sample which was about ten times more than normal range. The patient was sent for endoscopy, it was normal, and three-phasic abdominal CT scan reveals liver mass with the source of carcinoid and it is not a hydatid cyst. The patient was sent for resection of tumor, and 1 month after resection, level of 5-HIAA decreased to normal level.

4.6.1 What is a Carcinoid Tumor?

Carcinoid tumor is a rare disease, arising in 1.2–2.1 per 100,000 people in general population per year. They are most commonly found in the GI tract and bronchus. Primary midgut carcinoid tumor metastasizes to the liver or regional lymph node.

The most common manifestations of the carcinoid syndrome are vasomotor changes, gastrointestinal hypermobility, bronchospasm, and hypotension. These symptoms are caused by the release of vasoactive substances, including serotonin (5-hydroxytryptamine), histamine, bradykinin, and prostaglandins.

4.6.2 What is a Carcinoid Heart?

It eventually occurs in 50% of patients with carcinoid syndrome and may be an initial presentation of carcinoid disease in as many as 20% of patients.

Carcinoid heart is a heart with its tricuspid and pulmonic valve affected by serotonin. Serotonin makes them thick and rigid. Carcinoid heart is characterized by pathognomonic plaque-like deposits of a fibrous tissue. These deposits occur most commonly on the endothelium of valve cusps, leaflets, papillary muscle and cords, and occasionally on the intimae of the pulmonary arteries or aorta.

4.6.3 What is the Cause of Involvement of the Right-Sided Valve in a Carcinoid Heart?

Serotonin is extracted to 5-HIAA in the lung, so the level of serotonin in pulmonary veins is very low and it could not affect the left-sided valves.

4.6.4 How is 5-HIAA Used?

The 5-HIAA urine is used to help diagnose and monitor carcinoid tumors. Carcinoid tumor secretes serotonin a lot, and 5-HIAA is the primary metabolite of serotonin that is extracted in the urine. Concentration of 5-HIAA may be significantly increased when a person has carcinoid tumor that produces serotonin.

A significantly increased level of 5-HIAA in 24 h urine sample is suggestive but not diagnostic of a carcinoid tumor. In order to diagnose the condition, the tumor itself must be located and a sample of it examined (biopsy).

4.6.5 Is There Anything Else that Affects 5-HIAA Level?

There are a variety of drugs that can affect the 5-HIAA test.

Medications that can increase 5-HIAA include acetaminophen, caffeine, ephedrine, diazepam, nicotine, glyceryl guaiacolate (an ingredient found in some cough medications), and phenobarbital.

Medications that can decrease 5-HIAA include aspirin, ethyl alcohol, imipramine, levodopa, MAO inhibitors, heparin, isoniazid, methyldopa, and tricyclic antidepressants.

4.7 Case 6: Severe TR Due to Quadricuspid Tricuspid Valve

An old man with a history of long-standing systolic murmur in the left sternal border. He presented with severe dyspnea and ascites and lower extremities edema. He had a history of CABG 2 years previously.

Transthoracic echocardiography showed severe left ventricular dilation and dysfunction and regional wall motion abnormality in the left anterior descending artery (LAD) territory and severe right ventricular dilation and dysfunction with abnormal septal motion in favor of volume overload.

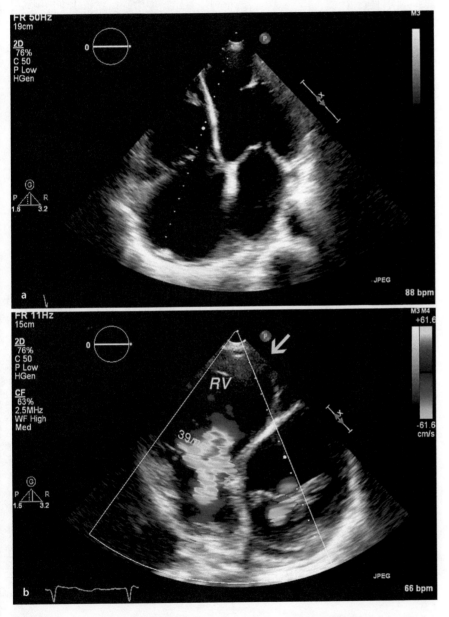

◘ **Fig. 4.27** Apical four-chamber view shows dilated right ventricle **a**, and off-axis four-chamber view **b** depicts severe right ventricular dilation, and its apex is more apical than the left ventricle (*arrow*), and it shows also severe tricuspid regurgitation with annular dilation mechanism; TV annulus is measured 39 mm (25 mm/m²). *RV* right ventricle

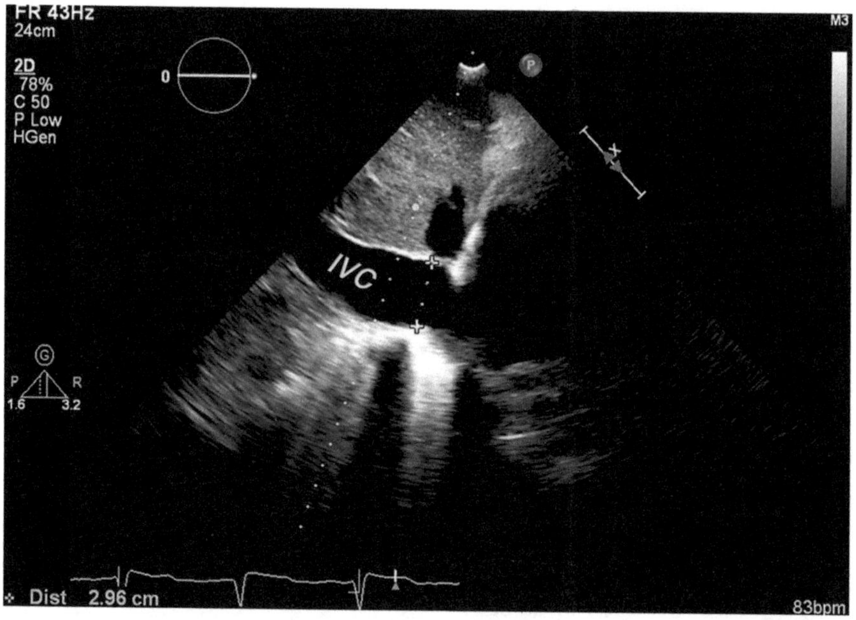

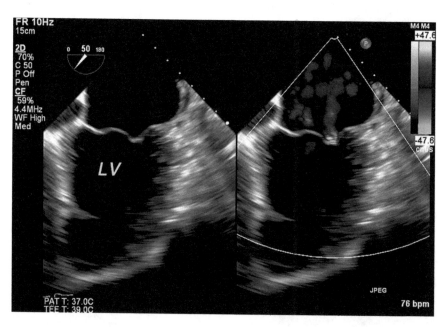

Fig. 4.28   Subcostal view shows dilation of inferior vena cava (IVC) with reduced collapse

Transesophageal echocardiography was performed for more evaluation of tricuspid valve.

Fig. 4.29   Mid-esophageal two-chamber view shows mild mitral regurgitation

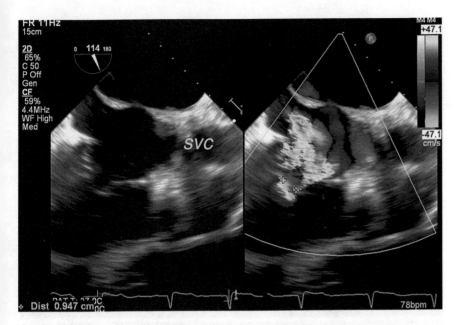

☐ Fig. 4.30 Mid-esophageal bicaval view demonstrates tricuspid regurgitation, and vena contracta is about 9.4 mm in size indicative for severe tricuspid regurgitation

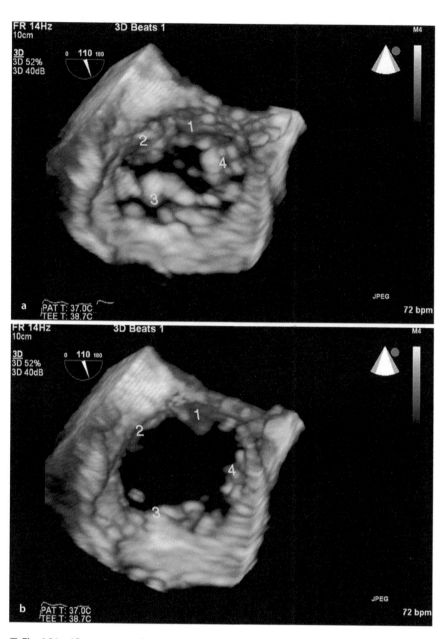

■ **Fig. 4.31**   3D zoom view of tricuspid valve from the right atrium side **a** and **b**, systolic and diastolic time, respectively) demonstrates quadricuspid tricuspid valve with severe annular dilation and restriction tricuspid valve leaflets that cause large non-coaptation area and severe tricuspid regurgitation subsequently

Diagnosis   Advance ischemic cardiomyopathy and a quadricuspid tricuspid valve with severe tricuspid regurgitation and severe right ventricular dysfunction.

Recommendation   With respect to severe right and left ventricular dysfunction, operation for patient was not possible so medical therapy and follow-up were recommended.

4.7.1 What is the Congenital Anomaly of Tricuspid Valve?

The most common anomaly is Ebstein anomaly, tricuspid atresia, congenital tricuspid stenosis, and congenital cleft of the anterior leaflet.

Ebstein anomaly occurs in approximately 1% of congenital disease and is associated with maternal lithium use during the first trimester of pregnancy.

4.7.2 Tricuspid Atresia

This is the third most common cause of cyanotic congenital heart defects.

4.7.3 Congenital Tricuspid Stenosis

The tricuspid valve may have incompletely developed leaflets, shortened or malformed chordae, small annuli, abnormal size and number of papillary muscles, or any combination of these defects. It is rare and is usually associated with other anomalies, such as severe pulmonary stenosis or atresia and secondary hypoplasia of the right ventricle.

4.7.4 Congenital Cleft of the Anterior Leaflet

Congenital cleft of the anterior leaflet of tricuspid valve is rare and usually associated with perimembranous ventricular septal defects.

4.7.5 What is the Variation in Number of Cusps in the Tricuspid Valve?

A cadaveric study by Mishra et al. showed normal tricuspid valve with three cusps was found only in 51% of hearts, bicuspid tricuspid valve was detected in 1%, and quadricuspid tricuspid valve was seen in 31% of cadavers, and a number of accessory cusps ranged from one to four [6].

4.8   Case 7: Severe TS and Severe TR Due to Rheumatismal Involvement

A 60-year-old man with a history of lower extremities edema for a 2-month duration, and he had a history of MVR (mitral valve replacement) for 10 years. Physical examination showed metallic sound in mitral area and a pansystolic murmur grade III/VI and a faint diastolic murmur at the left sternal border.

Transthoracic echocardiography showed normal left ventricular size and function.

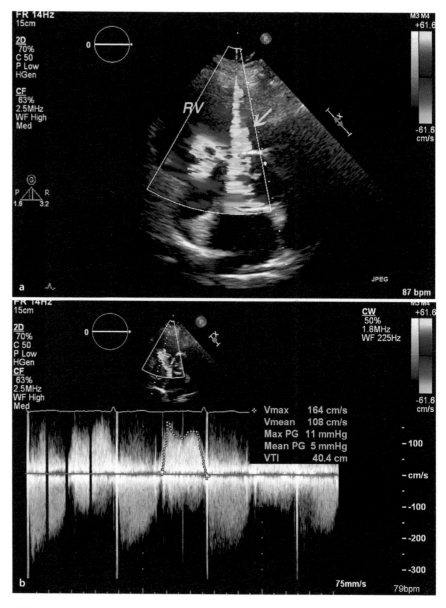

■ **Fig. 4.32**   Apical four-chamber view shows severe tricuspid regurgitation and a lot of acoustic shadow (*arrow*) due to mitral prosthetic valve **a**, and color Doppler study across tricuspid valve depicts peak and mean gradients of tricuspid valve about 11 mmHg and 5 mmHg, respectively, that they are significantly increased and in favor of tricuspid stenosis **b**. *RV* right ventricle

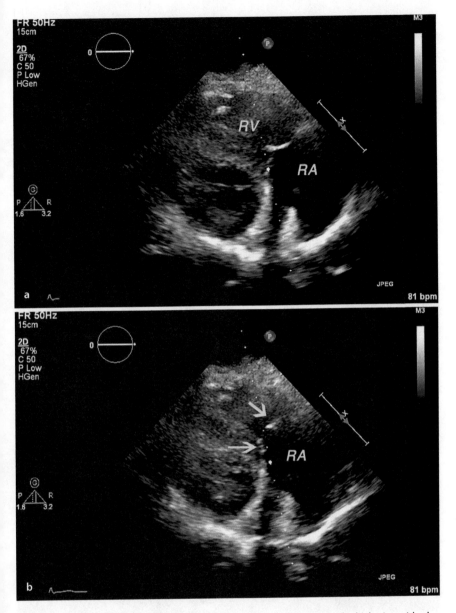

□ **Fig. 4.33** Parasternal right ventricular inflow tract view reveals precisely thick tricuspid valve **a** and doming of tricuspid leaflets in diastolic time (*arrows*, **b**). *RA* right atrium, *RV* right ventricle

Transesophageal echocardiography was performed for more evaluation of mitral prosthetic valve and tricuspid valve.

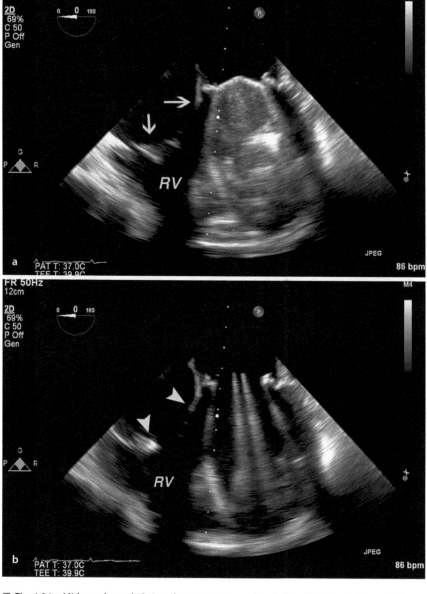

Fig. 4.34 Mid-esophageal 0° view demonstrates good mobility of leaflets during systolic **a** and diastolic time **b** in favor of good function of prosthetic mitral valve, and it also reveals restricted tricuspid leaflet during systolic time (*arrows*) and their doming during diastolic time (*head arrow*). *RV* right ventricle

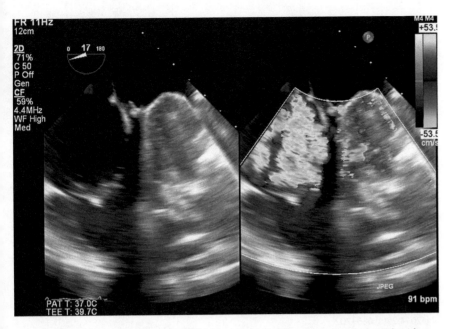

Fig. 4.35 Mid-esophageal 17° view shows severe tricuspid regurgitation in the right side and doming of leaflets in the left side

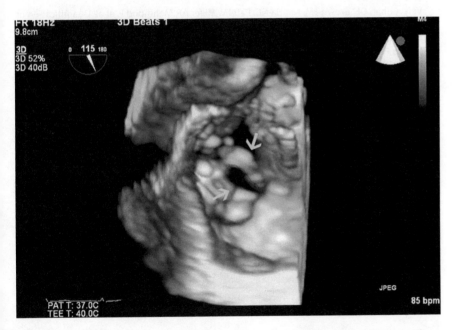

Fig. 4.36 3D zoom view of tricuspid valve from the right atrial side shows thick tricuspid leaflet and tricuspid stenosis from en face view (*arrow*); tricuspid valve area is measured about 1 cm² by 3DQ (doesn't show)

Diagnosis   Severe rheumatismal tricuspid stenosis and tricuspid regurgitation and good function of prosthetic mitral valve.

Recommendation   Patient was referred for tricuspid valve replacement, and the surgeon did minimal invasive operation for the patient with very good result.

4.8.1 When Do You Send Patient for Right-Sided Valve Surgery Along with a Good Left-Sided Prosthetic Valve Function?

Severe TR alone is not an indication for redo surgery after left-sided valve surgery; it should be associated with progressive RV dilation or dysfunction or symptomatic patient for consideration of redo surgery and TVR or TV repair.

References

1. Nishimura RA, Otto CM, Bonow RO, Carabello BA, Erwin 3rd JP, Guyton RA, et al. 2014 AHA/ACC guideline for the Management of Patients with valvular heart disease: executive summary: a report of the American College of Cardiology/American Heart Association task force on practice guidelines. Circulation. 2014;129(23):2440–92.
2. Joint Task Force on the Management of Valvular Heart Disease of the European Society of Cardiology, European Association for Cardio-Thoracic Surgery, Vahanian A, Alfieri O, Andreotti F, Antunes MJ, et al. Guidelines on the management of valvular heart disease (version 2012). Eur Heart J. 2012;33(19):2451–96.
3. Shiota T. Role of modern 3D echocardiography in valvular heart disease. Korean J Intern Med. 2014;29(6):685–702.
4. Anwar AM, Geleijnse ML, Soliman OI, McGhie JS, Nemes A, ten Cate FJ. Evaluation of rheumatic tricuspid valve stenosis by real-time three-dimensional echocardiography. Heart. 2007;93(3):363–4.
5. Velayudhan DE, Brown TM, Nanda NC, Patel V, Miller AP, Mehmood F, et al. Quantification of tricuspid regurgitation by live three-dimensional transthoracic echocardiographic measurements of vena contracta area. Echocardiography. 2006;23(9):793–800.
6. Mishra PP, Mishra A, Pouranam V. Variations in the number and morphology of cusps of the tricuspid valve: a cadaveric study. Int J Biomed Res. 2016;7(01):039–43.

Pulmonary Valve Disease

Videos can be found in the electronic supplementary material in the online version of the chapter. On http://springerlink.com enter the DOI number given on the bottom of the chapter opening page. Scroll down to the Supplementary material tab and click on the respective videos link.

© Springer International Publishing AG 2017
H. Sadeghian, Z. Savand-Roomi, *3D Echocardiography of Structural Heart Disease*,
DOI 10.1007/978-3-319-54039-9_5

5.1   Pulmonary Stenosis, Pulmonary Regurgitation

Pulmonary stenosis is often a congenital heart disease; involvement of pulmonary valve due to acquired disease like carcinoid is rare.

Most congenital pulmonary stenoses do not progress over time, some regress, and some progress with time. Mild to moderate valvular PS are usually asymptomatic; mild valvular PS is usually not progressive [1].

Pulmonary valve is a tricuspid valve; there are some forms of bicuspid pulmonary valve which produces pulmonary stenosis.

Rheumatic involvement of pulmonary valve is rare, but elevated pulmonary arterial pressure due to left-sided valve disease due to rheumatism and functional pulmonary regurgitation is common.

There are also subvalvular and supravalvular pulmonary stenosis.

Subvalvular pulmonary stenosis is often a compensatory mechanism for preventing pulmonary hypertension. It occurs frequently in association with VSD or as a component of tetralogy of Fallot [1].

Supravalvular pulmonary stenosis is often associated with tetralogy of Fallot [1]. In fetal life, when there is severe branch stenosis of the pulmonary artery, the blood flow is toward the pulmonary artery from the aorta via the ductus arteriosus. This flow can produce migration of cells from the aorta toward the pulmonary branches and produce branch pulmonary stenosis after birth especially in the left pulmonary artery which is in the direction of ductus arteriosus.

Pulmonary regurgitation is often an acquired disease. Mild pulmonary regurgitation presents in up to 60% of normal population. Elevated pulmonary arterial pressure is one of the most common causes of pulmonary regurgitation due to pulmonary artery and annulus dilation.

Besides, other causes of pulmonary regurgitation include interventions on pulmonary valve. Pulmonary regurgitation post valvuloplasty of the pulmonary valve due to pulmonary stenosis or pulmonary regurgitation post-surgery of tetralogy of Fallot is common.

Pulmonary stenosis with PG > 64 mmHg is considered as severe PS, and pulmonary peak gradient >36 mmHg is considered as moderate PS [1, 2].

Valvular PS can be referred for balloon valvuloplasty in the absence of significant pulmonary regurgitation. If valvuloplasty is not possible, the patient should be referred for surgery with PG > 80 mmHg [1].

Severe PR post-surgery TF in symptomatic patients should be treated with PVR; if the patient is asymptomatic in the presence of one of the following criteria, he/she should be referred for PVR (IIa):

1. Progressive RV dilation
2. Progressive RV dysfunction
3. Reduced exercise capacity
4. Sustained VT [1]

Tissue valves have a life span of 10–15 years. Normalization of RV size becomes unlikely with RVEDV index = 160 cm^3/m^2 [1].

5.2 Case 1: Severe Valvular and Subvalvular Pulmonary Stenosis, Bicuspid Pulmonary Valve

A 29-year-old woman was referred for consultation before her second pregnancy; her first pregnancy was without complication. She had dyspnea on exertion functional class II, physical examination revealed ejection systolic murmur at pulmonic area, and ECG showed right axis deviation and tall R in precordial leads.

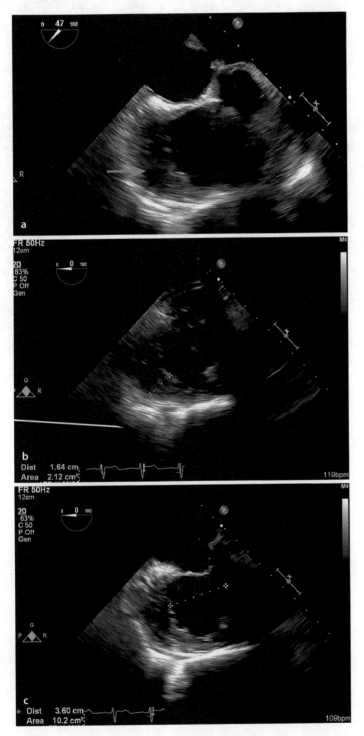

Fig. 5.1 Hypertrophy of right ventricular free wall is evident in TEE short-axis view (*arrow*) **a**, right ventricular free wall measures up to 16 mm **b**, right ventricle is dilated up to 36 mm in TEE 0° view **c**

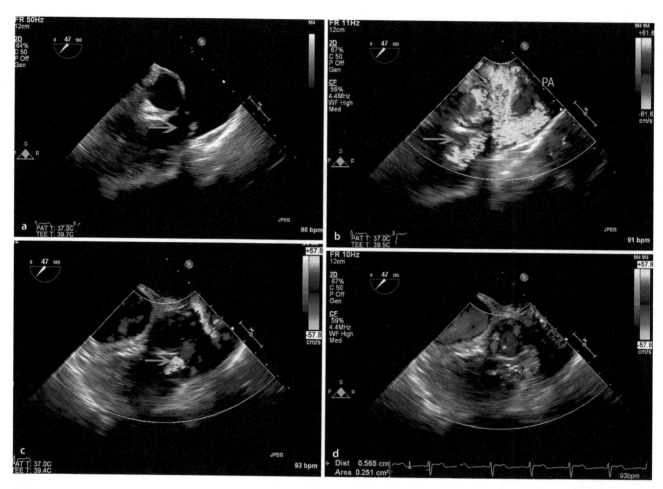

Fig. 5.2   Pulmonary valve is thick and dome in TEE short-axis view (*arrow*) **a**, systolic turbulency begins in RVOT (*arrow*) **b** in favor of valvular and subvalvular PS, there is also pulmonary regurgitation (*arrow*) **c**, vena contracta of pulmonary insufficiency is 5.6 mm **d**

5.2 · Case 1: Severe Valvular and Subvalvular Pulmonary Stenosis, Bicuspid Pulmonary Valve

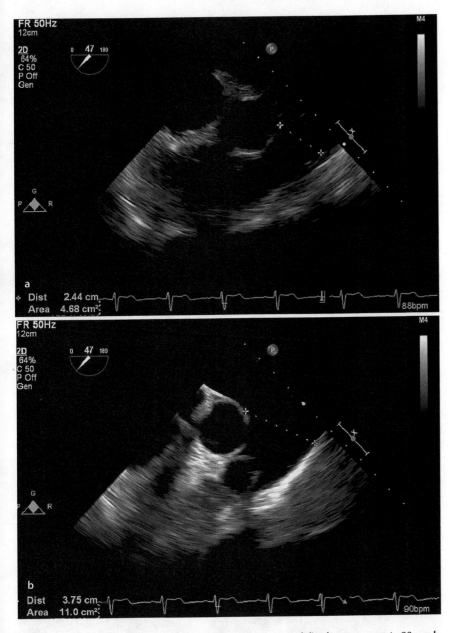

☐ Fig. 5.3 Proximal of pulmonary artery measures 24 mm **a** and distal measures up to 38 mm **b**

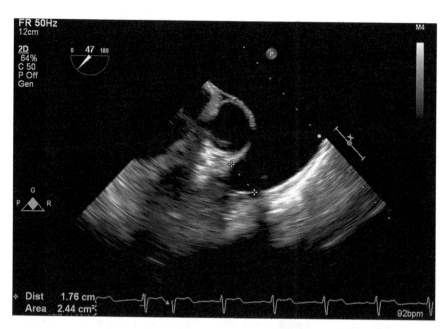

Fig. 5.4 Pulmonary annulus measures 17.6 mm in TEE short-axis view

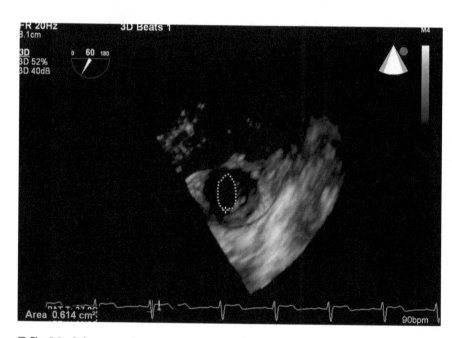

Fig. 5.5 Pulmonary valve area measures 0.6 cm² by direct planimetry in TEE short-axis view by narrow sector live 3D modality and seems bicuspid

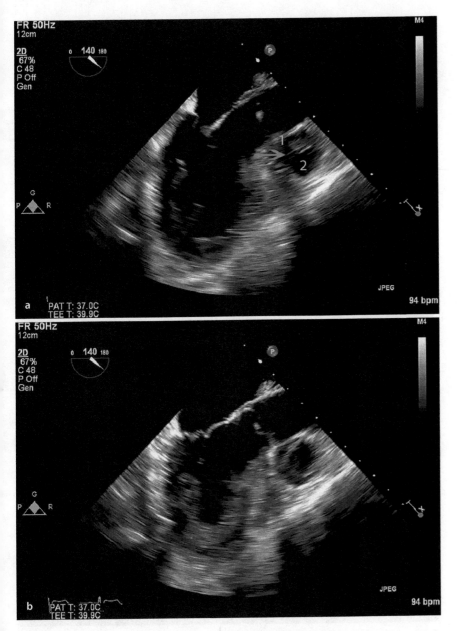

□ **Fig. 5.6** Bicuspid pulmonary valve is also evident in TEE 140° view in diastole **a** and systole **b** (*arrows*)

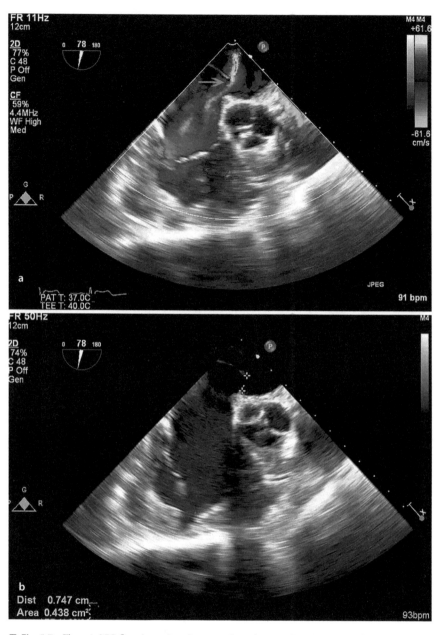

Fig. 5.7 There is PFO flow (*arrow*) **a**, distance of two layers measures 7.8 mm **b**

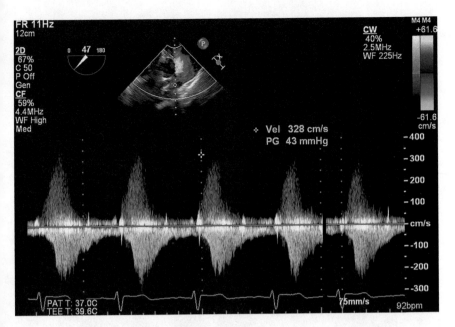

◘ **Fig. 5.8** There is 43 mmHg gradient in RVOT

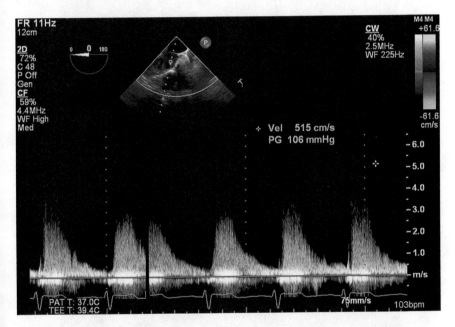

◘ **Fig. 5.9** TEE 0° view near arch shows that there is 106 mmHg gradient in pulmonary artery

Diagnosis Bicuspid pulmonary valve with 106 mmHg gradient, severe valvular and subvalvular PS, and PFO.

Comment Valvuloplasty of pulmonary valve or surgery.

Lesson
1. When there is a flow above and below of baseline by continuous wave Doppler study, it means that the cursor is not aligned, and real gradient must be higher.
2. In severe PS, there is a risk for RV suicide.

5.3   Case 2: Moderate Valvular Pulmonary Stenosis with Partially Aneurysmal IAS and PFO and Small Fenestration Within It

A 33-year-old man presented with dyspnea on exertion functional class I. Physical examination revealed systolic ejection murmur at pulmonic area, and ECG showed right-axis deviation and tall R in V1 and V2.

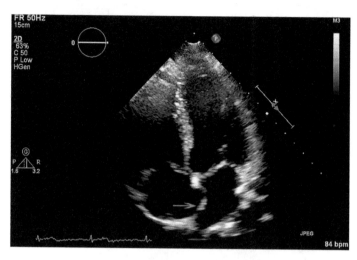

◘ Fig. 5.10   Partially aneurysmal IAS is evident in apical four-chamber view (*arrow*)

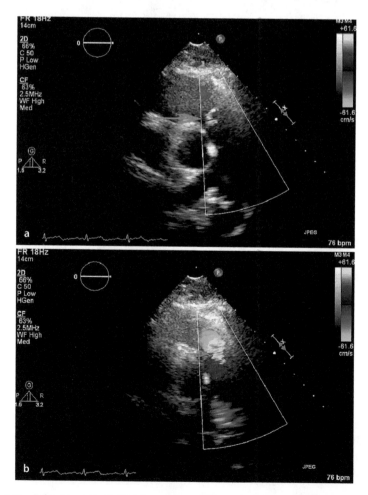

◘ Fig. 5.11   Pulmonary valve is thick in parasternal short-axis view (*arrow*) **a**, there is systolic turbulency across it (*arrow*) **b** in favor of valvular pulmonary stenosis

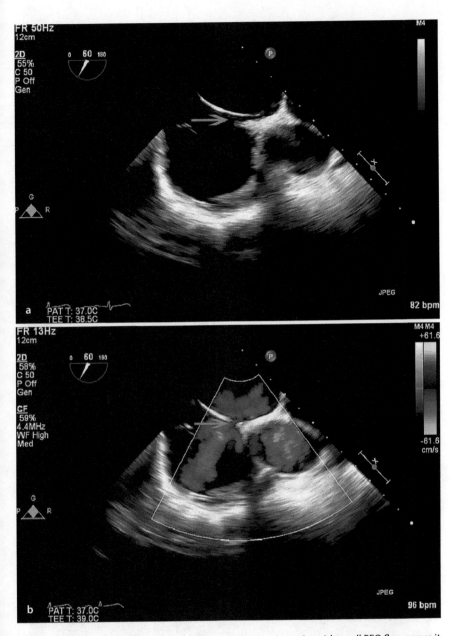

◘ Fig. 5.12 Bilayered IAS is shown in TEE short-axis view (*arrow*) **a** with small PFO flow across it (*arrow*) **b**

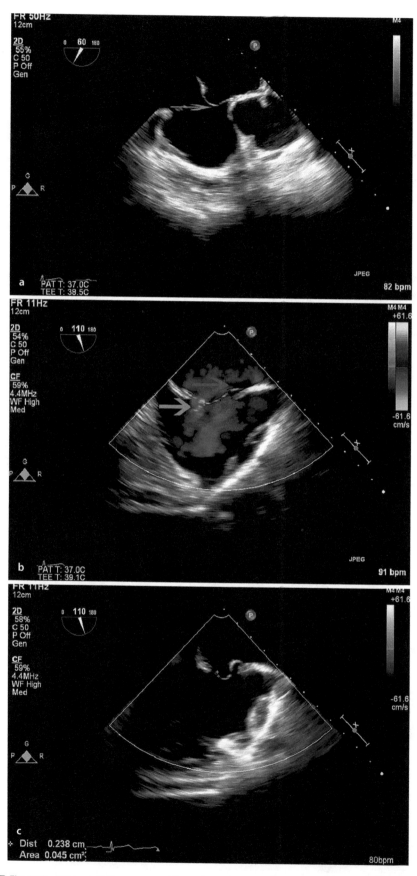

Fig. 5.13 IAS is partially aneurysmal (*arrow*) **a** with a small fenestration in its center with a left-to-right shunt flow across it (*green arrow*) **b**, and it measures about 0.2.3 mm by 2D echocardiography **c** (*pink arrow* shows PFO in **b**)

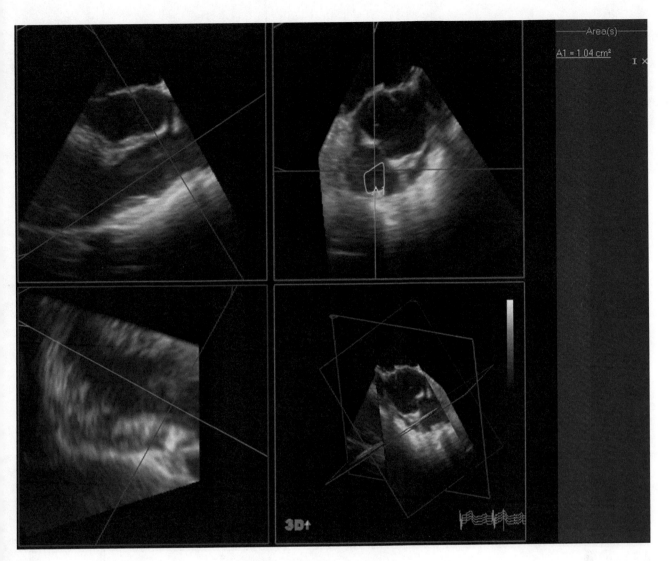

Fig. 5.14 Pulmonic valve area measures 1.04 cm² by full-volume TEE in short-axis view

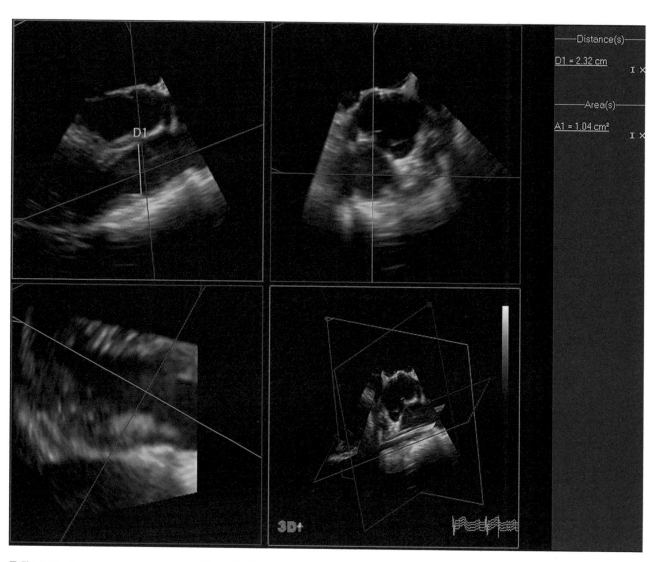

Fig. 5.15 Pulmonary annulus measures 23 mm by 3DQ

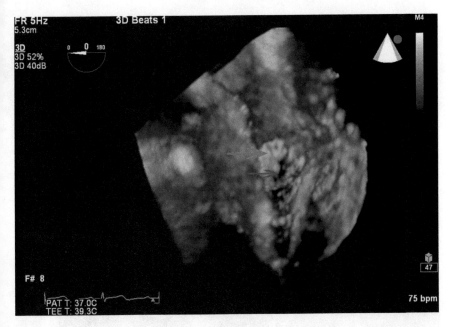

☐ **Fig. 5.16** 3D zoom of interatrial septum from the right atrial side shows the bulging of IAS (*green arrow*) and fenestration within it (*pink arrow*)

Diagnosis   Moderate valvular pulmonary stenosis (PG = 47 mmHg) with partially aneurysmal IAS with PFO and small fenestration of IAS.

Comment   Valvuloplasty of pulmonary valve if the patient is symptomatic.

5.4   Case 3: Moderate Valvular Pulmonary Stenosis with Right Ventricular Systolic Dysfunction

A 55-year-old man presented with leg edema; physical examination revealed ejection systolic murmur at pulmonic area. ECG showed tall R in V1–V3.

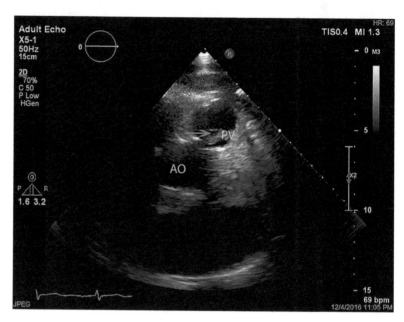

◘ Fig. 5.17   Parasternal short-axis view shows thickening of pulmonary valve (*arrow*). *AO* aortic valve, *PV* pulmonary valve

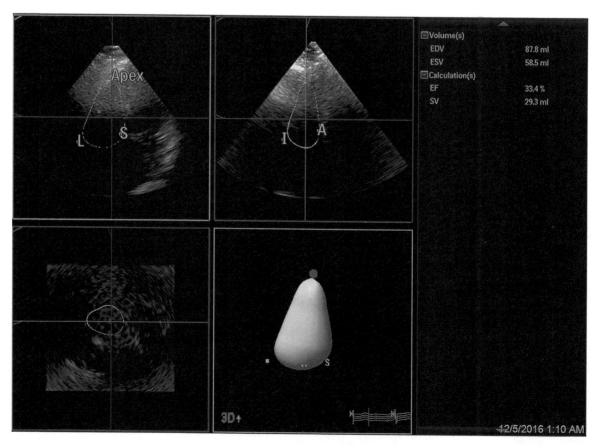

◘ Fig. 5.18   Right ventricular end-diastolic volume, end-systolic volume, and ejection fraction measure 88 cm³, 59 cm³, and 33%, respectively, by full-volume 3D

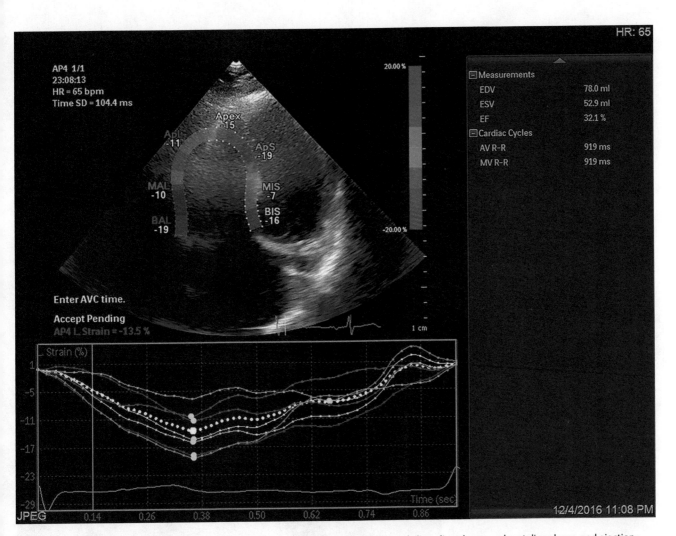

Fig. 5.19 Longitudinal right ventricular strain measures −13.5%, right ventricular end-diastolic volume, end-systolic volume, and ejection fraction measure 78 cm³, 52 cm³, and 32%, respectively, by 2D echocardiography

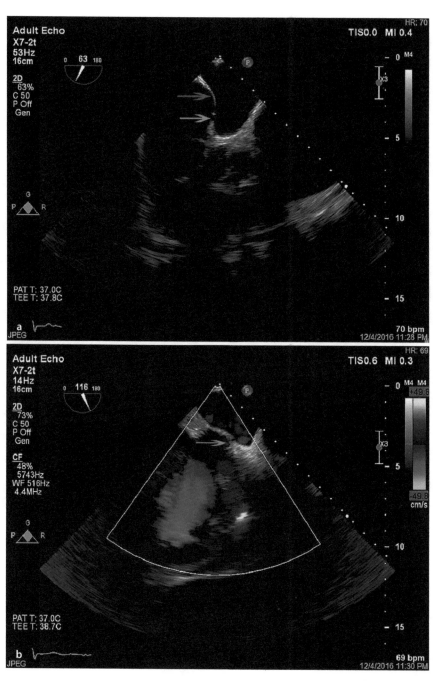

Fig. 5.20   Interatrial septum (IAS) is aneurysmal (*pink arrow*), and there is a small fenestration (*green arrow*) in it by TEE short-axis view **a**, small flow through that fenestration (*green arrow*) is evident by color Doppler study in this view **b**

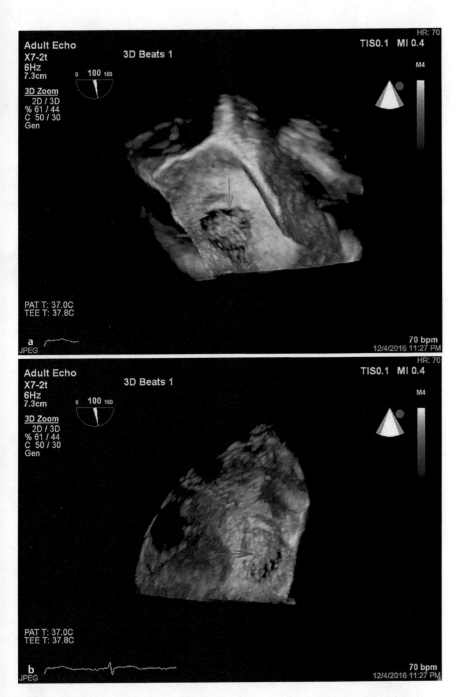

Fig. 5.21 IAS in the site of foramen ovale is visualized in this TEE 100° from left atrial side (*pink arrow*) **a** by 3D zoom and from right atrial side (*pink arrow*) **b**, small fenestrations are evident by this view (*green arrows*) **a**

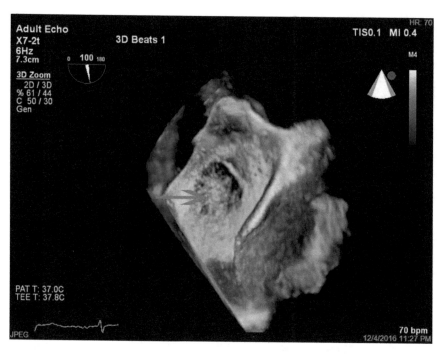

◻ Fig. 5.22 IAS is prominent toward left atrium (*arrow*) by TEE 100° view 3D zoom from left atrial side

Diagnosis   Moderate valvular pulmonary stenosis (PG = 57 mmHg), annulus of pulmonary valve = 21–22 mm, small fenestration in IAS, aneurysmal IAS, and RV systolic dysfunction.

Comment   The patient was referred for valvuloplasty of pulmonary valve.

Lesson   Global longitudinal right ventricular strain is −25.8 ± 3% in normal population [3]. In this patient, global longitudinal right ventricular strain measures −13.5% and is reduced.

Global right ventricular ejection fraction in normal population is 59 ± 6% by 4D echocardiography [3]. In this patient, global right ventricular ejection fraction measures 33% and so is reduced.

Right ventricular end-diastolic volume (RVEDV) in normal population is 95 cm^3, and end-systolic volume (RVESV) is 39 cm^3 [3]. In this patient, these figures are 89 cm^3 and 57 cm^3, respectively, due to pulmonary stenosis; RVEDV is not increased, but RVESV is increased because of right ventricular failure.

5.5   Case 4: Severe PI Due to Infective Endocarditis

A 55-year-old man presented with ascites. He was a known case of severe pulmonary stenosis who underwent cardiac surgery and valvotomy of the pulmonary valve some years ago.

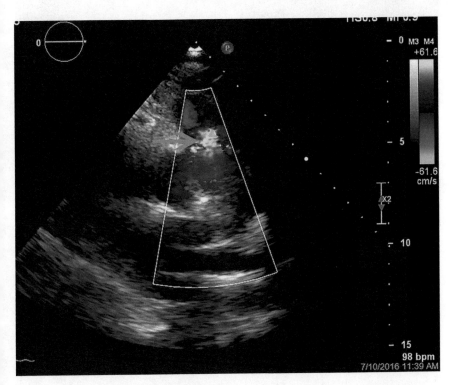

◻ Fig. 5.23   Severe pulmonary insufficiency is visualized in parasternal short-axis view (*arrow*)

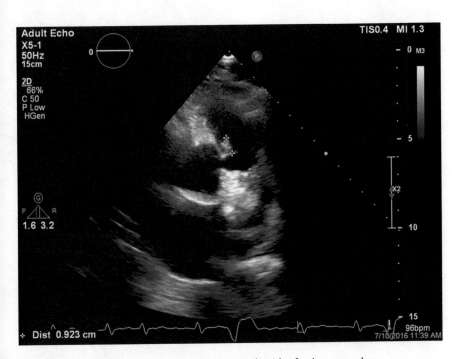

◻ Fig. 5.24   There is a mass 9 mm in size on ventricular side of pulmonary valve

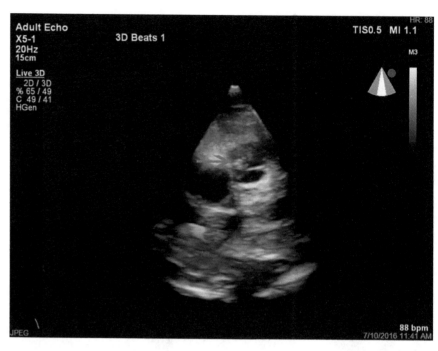

■ **Fig. 5.25**   This mass is fully visualized by live 3D (*arrow*) of pulmonary valve

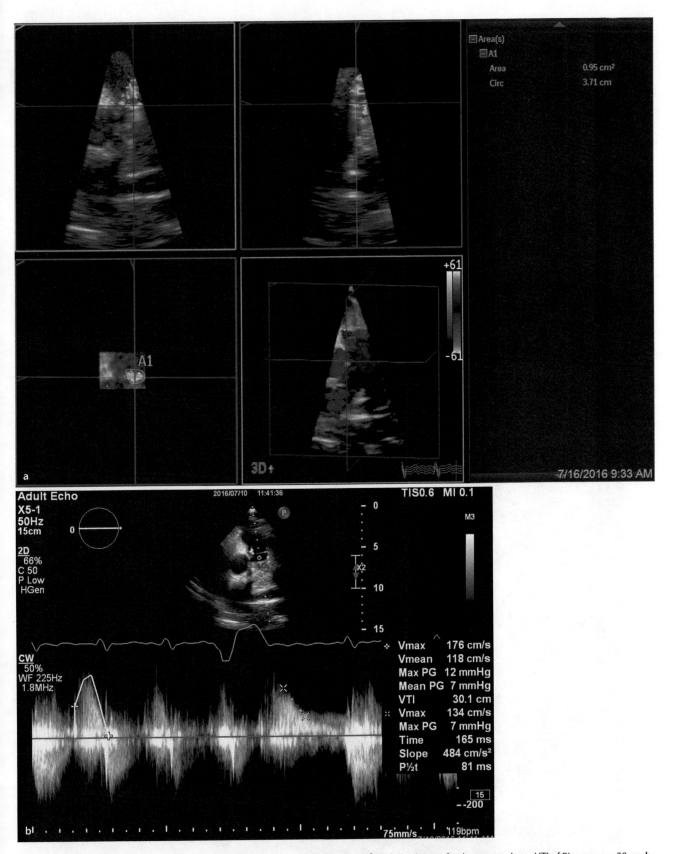

Fig. 5.26 Vena contracta area of pulmonary regurgitation measures 0.95 cm² by full volume of pulmonary valve **a**, VTI of PI measures 30 cm **b**, PI regurgitation volume measures as follows: 0.95*31 = 29.45 cm³

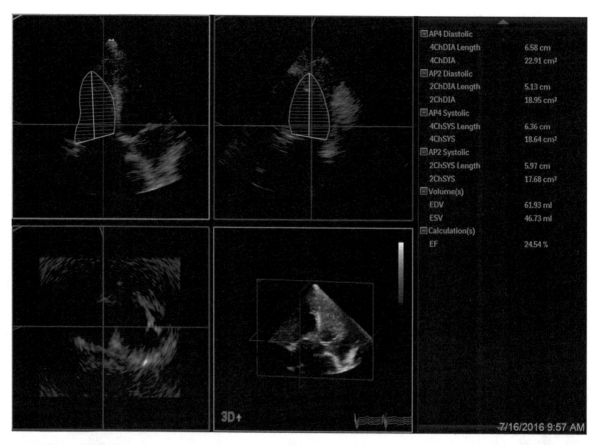

Fig. 5.27 RVEDV = 62 cm³, RVESV = 47 cm³, RVEF = 25% by 4D

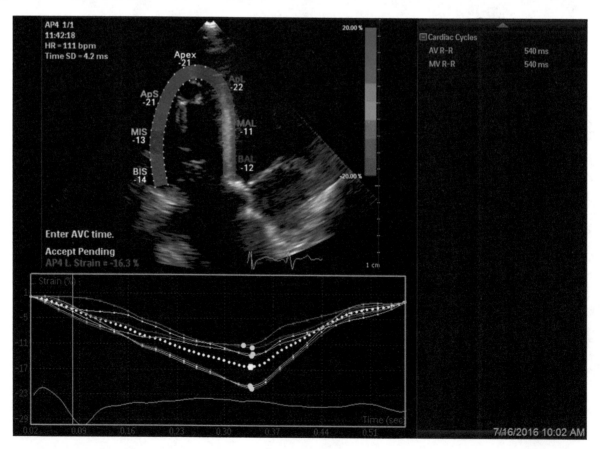

Fig. 5.28 RV longitudinal strain = −16%

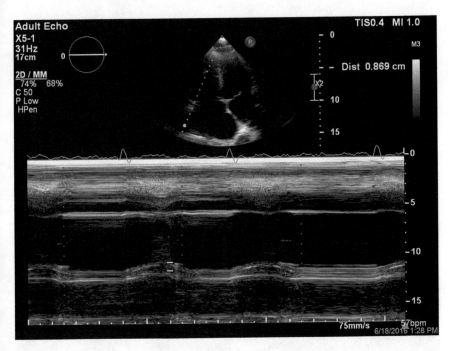

◘ **Fig. 5.29** TAPSE = 9 mm in favor of severe RV systolic dysfunction

Diagnosis   Infective endocarditis on pulmonary valve with severe PI.

Comment   PVR after medical treatment.

Lesson   Because of severe free PI, RVEDV did not increase, but RVESV increased.

5.6   Case 5: Bicuspid Pulmonic Valve with Mild PS

A 65-year-old man presented with a history of aortic valve replacement about 2 weeks previously. He was referred to the echocardiography laboratory for evaluation of aortic prosthetic valve; in physical examination he had a systolic murmur in pulmonic area.

Transthoracic echocardiography showed normal aortic prosthetic valve function and good left ventricular systolic function.

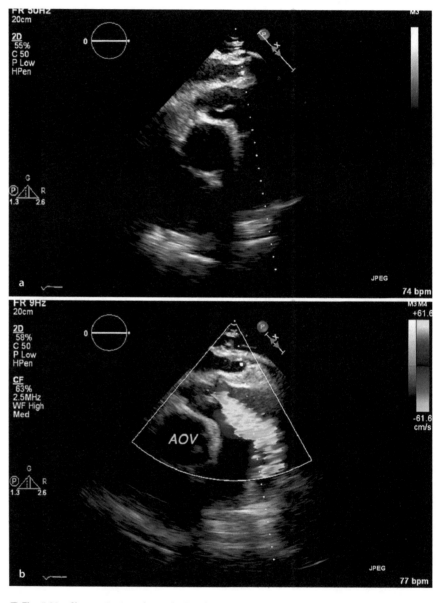

■ **Fig. 5.30**   Short-axis view shows thick pulmonary leaflets **a** and a systolic turbulency in pulmonary artery which originates from pulmonic valve **b**

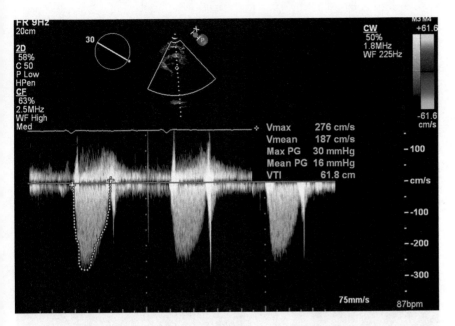

Fig. 5.31 Color Doppler flow study of pulmonic valve demonstrates peak gradient across pulmonic valve and is about 30 mmHg, and mean gradient is about 16 mmHg indicative for mild pulmonary stenosis

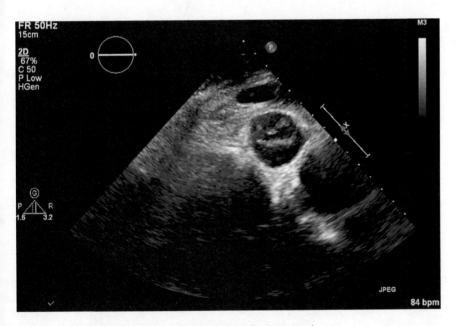

Fig. 5.32 Off-axis short-axis view depicts bicuspid pulmonic valve

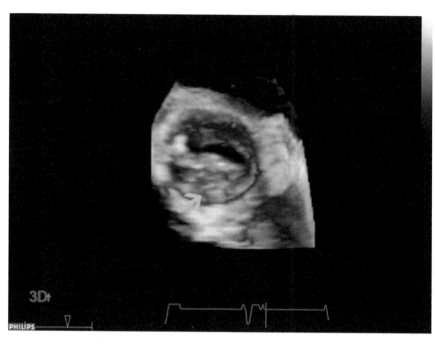

☐ **Fig. 5.33** 3D zoom view confirms bicuspid pulmonic valve and depicts raphe of bicuspid pulmonic valve

Diagnosis Bicuspid pulmonic valve with mild valvular PS.

Comment With respect to moderate PS only, follow-up is recommended. Bicuspid pulmonic valve is a rare congenital anomaly.

References

1. Baumgartner H, Bonhoeffer P, De Groot NM, de Haan F, Deanfield JE, Galie N, et al. ESC guidelines for the management of grown-up congenital heart disease (new version 2010). Eur Heart J. 2010;31(23):2915–57.
2. Nishimura RA, Otto CM, Bonow RO, Carabello BA, Erwin 3rd JP, Guyton RA, et al. 2014 AHA/ACC guideline for the Management of Patients with Valvular Heart Disease: executive summary: a report of the American College of Cardiology/American Heart Association task force on practice guidelines. Circulation. 2014;129(23):2440–92.
3. Muraru D, Onciul S, Peluso D, Soriani N, Cucchini U, Aruta P, et al. Sex- and method-specific reference values for right ventricular strain by 2-dimensional speckle-tracking echocardiography. Circ Cardiovasc Imaging. 2016;9(2):e003866.

Malfunction and Other Complications After Heart Valve Surgery

Videos can be found in the electronic supplementary material in the online version of the chapter.
On http://springerlink.com enter the DOI number given on the bottom of the chapter opening page.
Scroll down to the Supplementary material tab and click on the respective videos link.

© Springer International Publishing AG 2017
H. Sadeghian, Z. Savand-Roomi, *3D Echocardiography of Structural Heart Disease*,
DOI 10.1007/978-3-319-54039-9_6

6.1 Case 1: MVR with Bileaflet Prosthetic Mitral Valve and TVR with Bioprosthetic

A 55-year-old woman presented with fatigue of 1-month duration. She underwent MVR with bileaflet prosthetic valve and TVR with bioprosthetic valve 8 years ago and 3 months after her first operation; the second surgery was performed on her due to infective endocarditis and fistula between LA and LV.

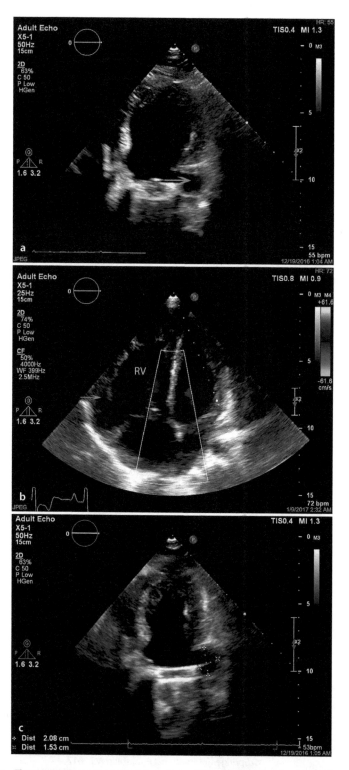

◻ **Fig. 6.1** There is an aneurysm in the base of lateral LV wall (*arrow*) **a**, there is no flow through this aneurysm toward LV (*arrow*) **b**, and this aneurysm measures 21*15 mm **c** in apical four-chamber view

6.1 · Case 1: MVR with Bileaflet Prosthetic Mitral Valve and TVR with Bioprosthetic

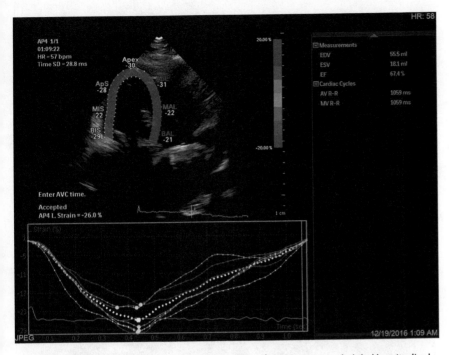

☐ **Fig. 6.2** RVEDV measures 55 cm^3 and RVESV = 18 cm^3; RVEF = 67% and global longitudinal RV strain in apical four-chamber view is -26%, all in normal limits

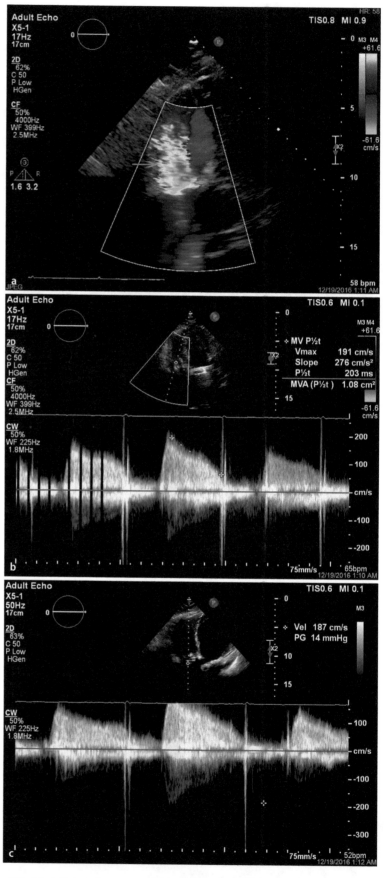

Fig. 6.3 Diastolic turbulency across bioprosthetic TV is visualized in this apical four-chamber view (*arrow*) **a** and TVA measures 1.08 cm² by PHT **b**. Peak and mean bioprosthetic tricuspid gradients are 10 and 5 mmHg, respectively, and TRG measures 14 mmHg **c**

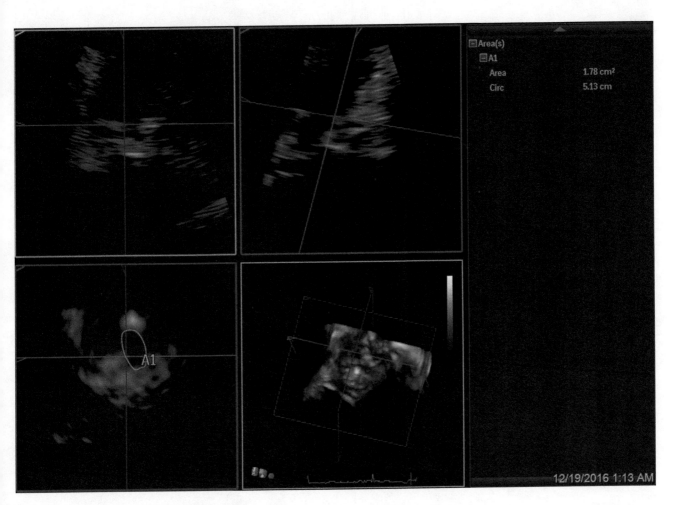

Fig. 6.4 TVA measures 1.78 cm² by 3DQ method

Diagnosis   Good function of prosthetic MV and moderate TS on bioprosthetic TV in addition to long pauses on Holter monitoring.

Comment   If symptomatic on medical treatment, valve-in-valve replacement [1] on TV and pacemaker epicardial lead implantation.

Lesson
(1) Due to bioprosthetic tricuspid valve, endocardial pace implantation is not recommended due to the danger of bioprosthetic valve dislodgment.
(2) For prosthetic tricuspid valves, mean gradient more than 6 mmHg and pressure half-time >230 ms are considered as significant obstruction [2].

6.2   Case 2: Valve in Ring for TV

A 46-year-old woman undergone valve-in-ring procedure on her tricuspid valve due to severe tricuspid regurgitation post-TV ring annuloplasty 4 years ago.

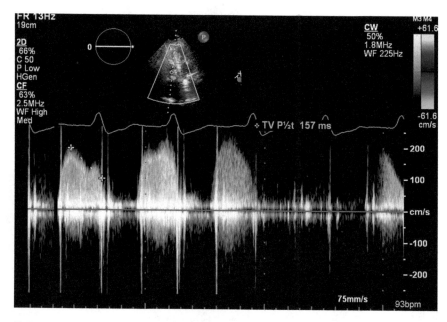

■ **Fig. 6.5**   TVA measures 157 ms by PHT; TVA will be calculated as follows: 190/157 = 1.2 cm². PG across tricuspid valve is 16 mmHg, and MG is 8 mmHg

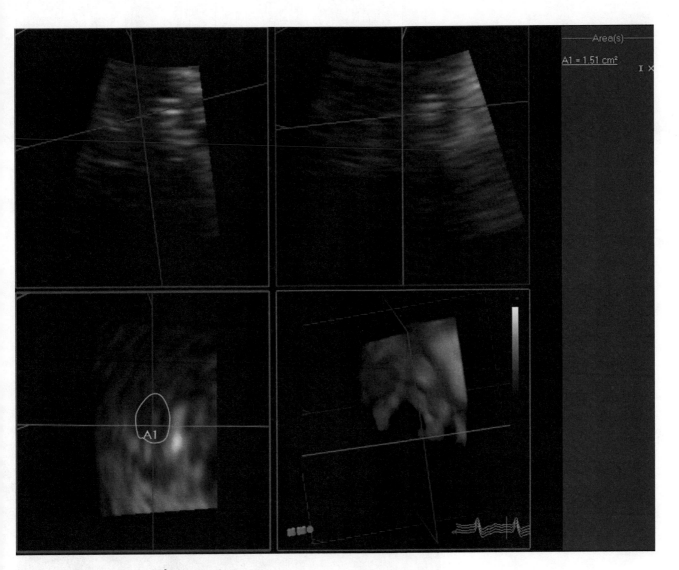

Area(s)

A1 = 1.51 cm²   I ×

A1

Fig. 6.6   TVA measures 1.5 cm² by 3DQ with 3D zoom

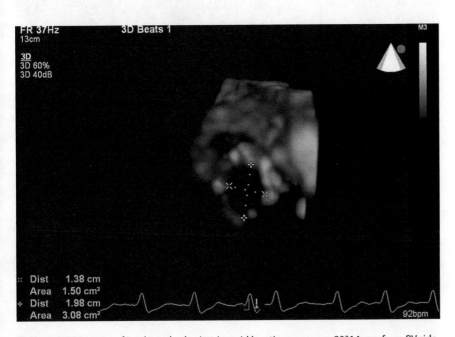

FR 37Hz   3D Beats 1   M3
13cm

3D
3D 60%
3D 40dB

Dist   1.38 cm
Area   1.50 cm²
Dist   1.98 cm
Area   3.08 cm²

92bpm

Fig. 6.7   Diameter of implanted valve in tricuspid location measures 20*14 mm from RV side by direct measurement

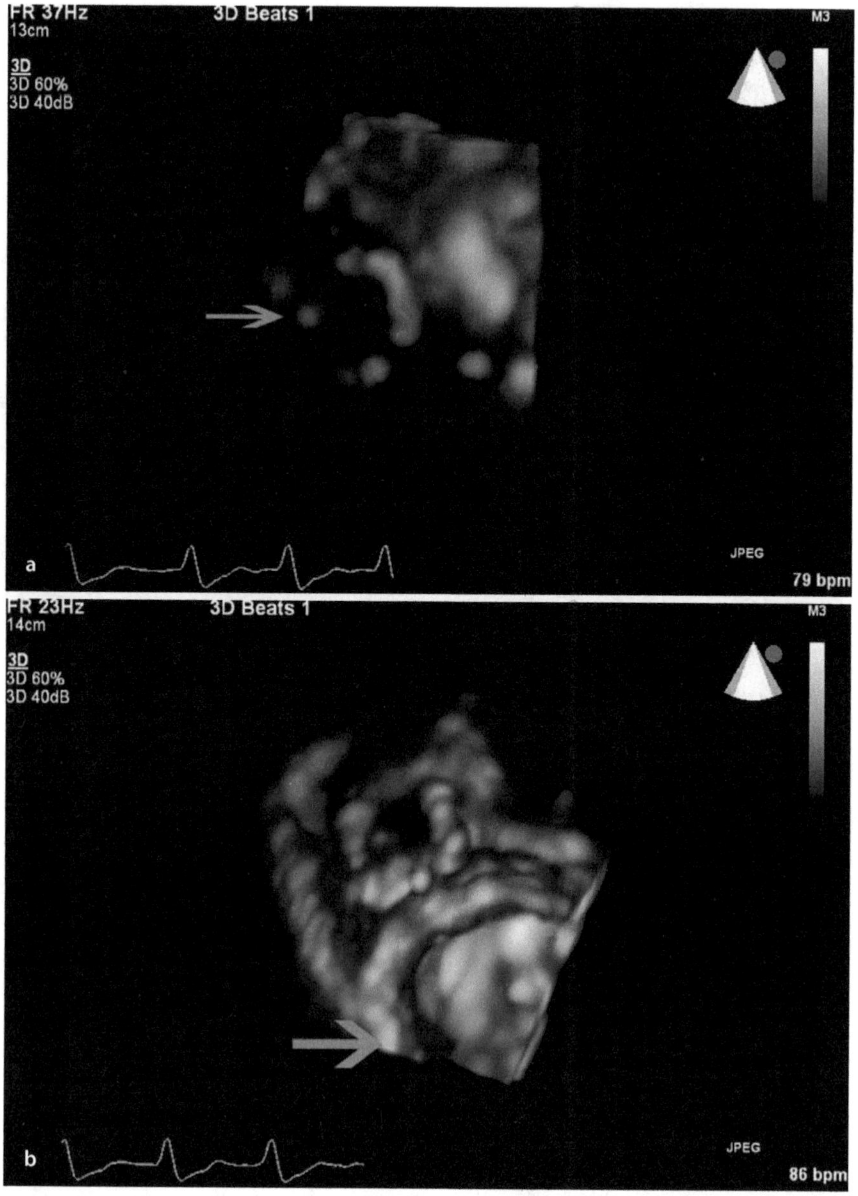

□ **Fig. 6.8** Valve in ring in tricuspid position from RV side **a** and RA side **b** with 3D zoom

Diagnosis Moderate stenosis of percutaneous implanted valve-in-ring tricuspid valve.

Comment Medical treatment and follow-up.

Lesson Valve-in-ring procedure is possible when there is a ring in tricuspid position. Indeed in this patient, TR is changed to TS.

6.3   Case 3: Severe TR on TV Ring Annuloplasty

A 67-year-old woman who had undergone MVR + AVR + TV repair with ring annuloplasty (size of ring = 28 mm) is referred to us because of dyspnea on exertion functional class III of 1-year duration. Transthoracic echocardiography showed normal left ventricular size and function; LVEF = 50–55%; peak and mean transmitral gradients were 8 and 4 mmHg, respectively; PHT was 72 ms; peak and mean transaortic gradients were 15 and 7 mmHg, respectively; activation time of aortic valve was 80 ms; there is good mobility of mitral and aortic prosthetic mitral leaflets; the right ventricle was mildly dilated with mild RV systolic dysfunction and severe TR; and TRG was equal to 30 mmHg.

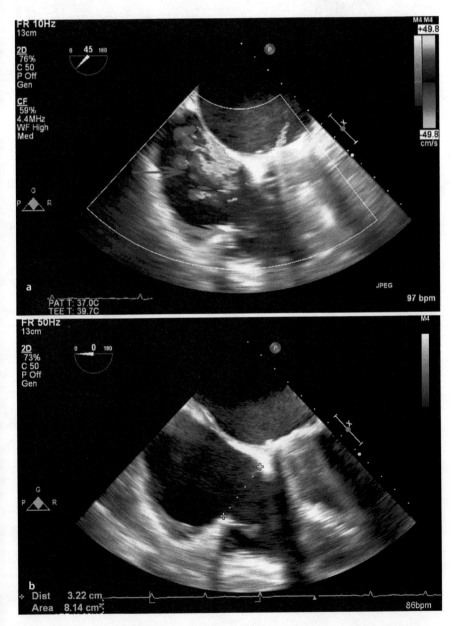

◻ **Fig. 6.9** Severe TR is evident in TEE short-axis views (*pink arrow*) **a**, the shadow of TV ring annuloplasty is evident in this view (*green arrow*) **a**, and annulus measures 32 mm in TEE 0° view **b**

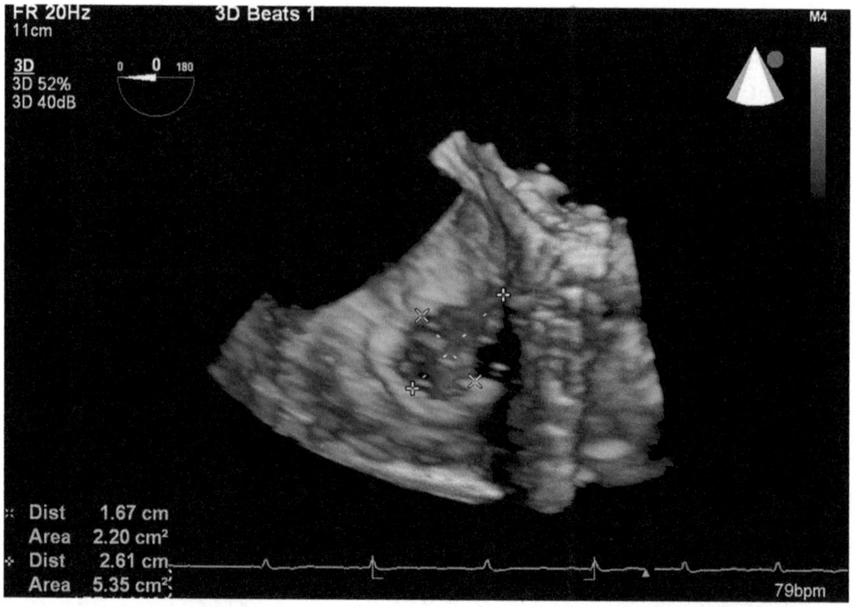

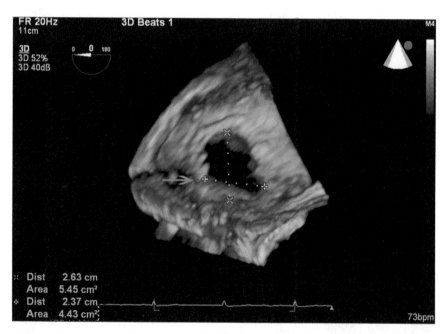

■ **Fig. 6.10**   TV ring measures 26*17 mm by TEE 4D reconstruction with 3D zoom from RA side

■ **Fig. 6.11**   TEE from RA side with Z rotation (rotation on the plane for positioning the septum in the lower part of the surface or 6 o'clock) shows clearly two ends of TV ring (*arrows*); TV ring measures 26*24 mm in this view

Diagnosis   Severe TR after TV ring annuloplasty.

Comment   Valve in ring for tricuspid valve is recommended.

6.4   Case 4: MVR and AVR and TV Ring Annuloplasty with Moderate TR

A 55-year-old woman presented with dyspnea on exertion functional class I of 6-month duration.

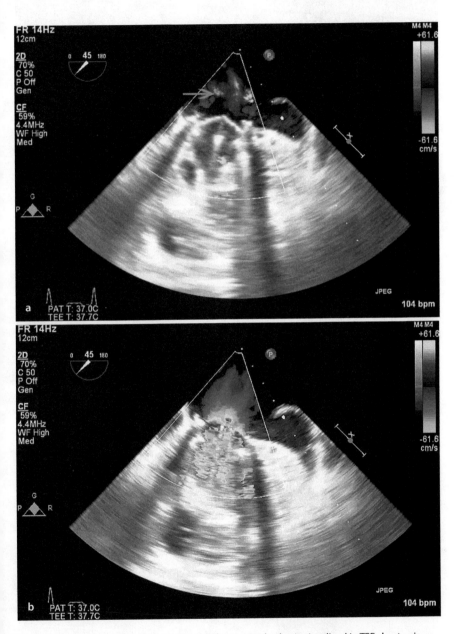

◻ **Fig. 6.12** Good mobility of bileaflet prosthetic mitral valve is visualized in TEE short-axis view with intravalvular MR (*arrow*) **a** and no paravalvular leak in systole **a** and diastole **b**

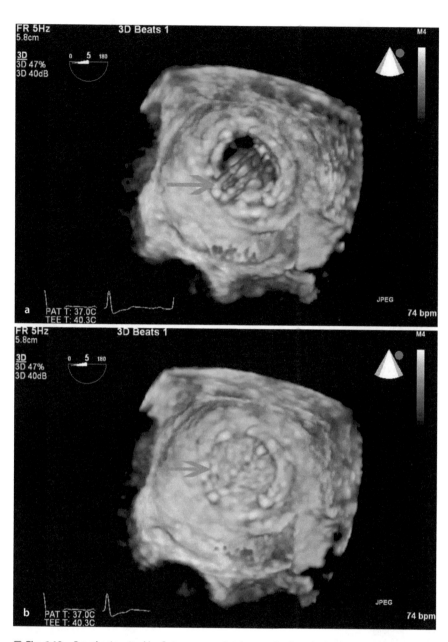

Fig. 6.13 Prosthetic mitral leaflets are completely open in diastole (*arrow*) **a** and completely closed in systole (*arrow*) **b**

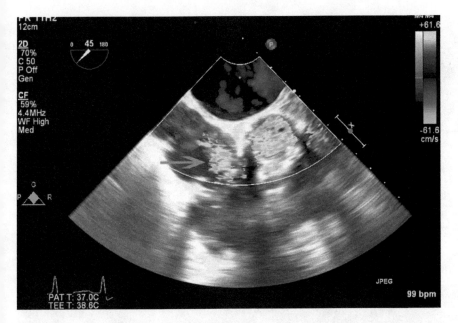

☐ **Fig. 6.14** Moderate TR is shown in TEE short-axis view in systole (*arrow*)

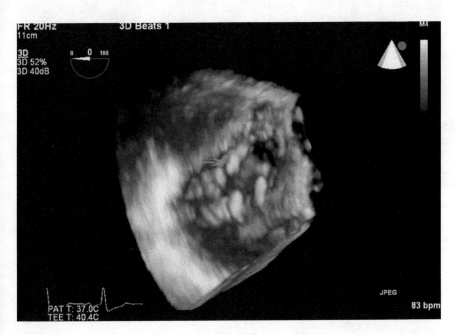

☐ **Fig. 6.15** Live 3D TEE 0° fully depicts TV ring annuloplasty from RA side (*arrow*)

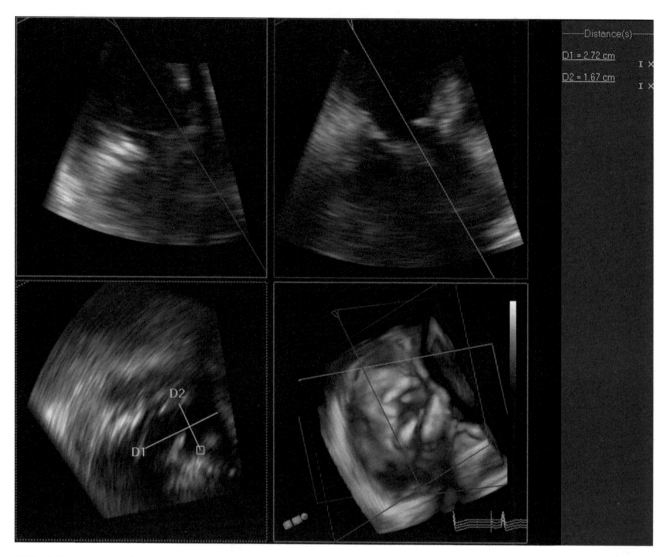

Fig. 6.16 TV ring annuloplasty measures 27*17 mm by 3DQ method

Diagnosis   Good function of bileaflet prosthetic mitral and aortic valves and moderate TR on TV ring annuloplasty.

Comment   Medical treatment and follow-up.

6.5   Case 5: Incomplete MV Ring Annuloplasty

A 69-year-old man presented with dyspnea on exertion functional class IV of recent exacerbation. He underwent mitral valve ring annuloplasty 1 year ago.

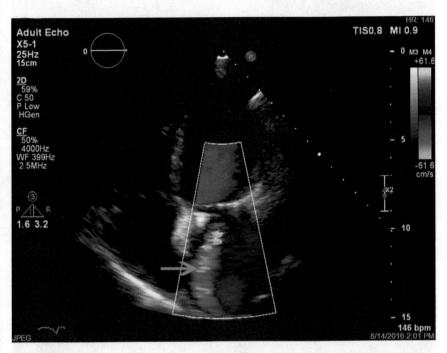

☐ **Fig. 6.17**   Severe eccentric mitral regurgitation is relevant in apical four-chamber view (*arrow*)

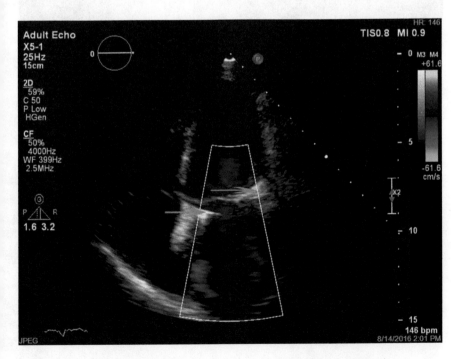

☐ **Fig. 6.18**   MV ring annuloplasty is seen in this apical four-chamber view (*arrows*)

☐ **Fig. 6.19** Mitral valve reconstruction by 3D zoom of mitral valve from left ventricular **a** and left atrial **b** sides shows incomplete ring annuloplasty (*arrows*)

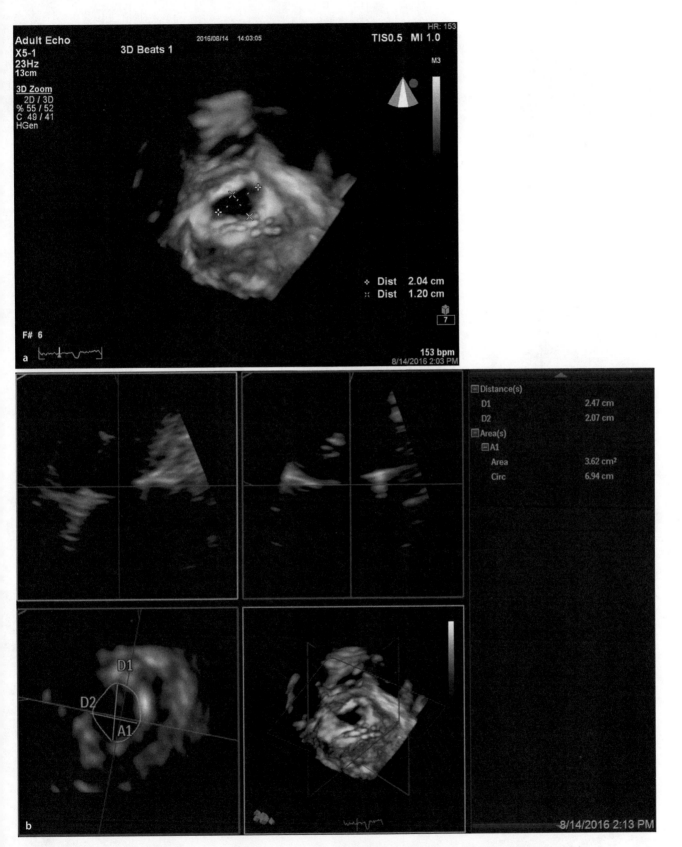

Fig. 6.20 Mitral ring measures 20*12 mm by direct measurement on 3D zoom from left ventricular side **a** and 25*21 by 3DQ **b**

Diagnosis   Severe MR after mitral ring annuloplasty, LVEF = 50%, PAPs = 55 mmHg.

Comment   The patient is referred for valve-in-ring procedure.

6.6   Case 6: Severe MS on MV Ring Annuloplasty

A 35-year-old woman presented with dyspnea on exertion functional class III of 6 months of exacerbation. She underwent mitral valve ring annuloplasty 6 years ago.

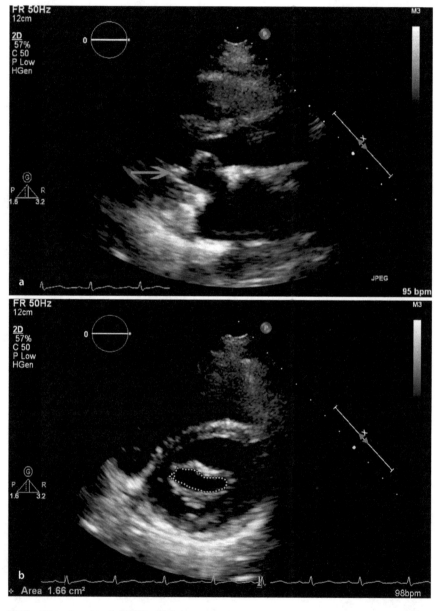

☐ **Fig. 6.21**   Restricted mitral leaflets opening and doming of leaflets are shown in parasternal long-axis view **a**; mitral valve area measures 1.66 cm² by planimetry in parasternal short-axis view **b**

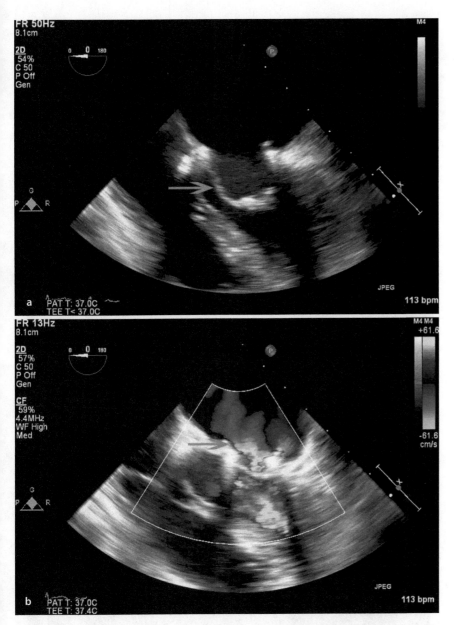

Fig. 6.22 TEE 0° view shows doming of anterior mitral leaflet (*arrow*) **a** in favor of mitral stenosis and diastolic turbulency across the mitral valve with color Doppler study (*arrow*) **b**

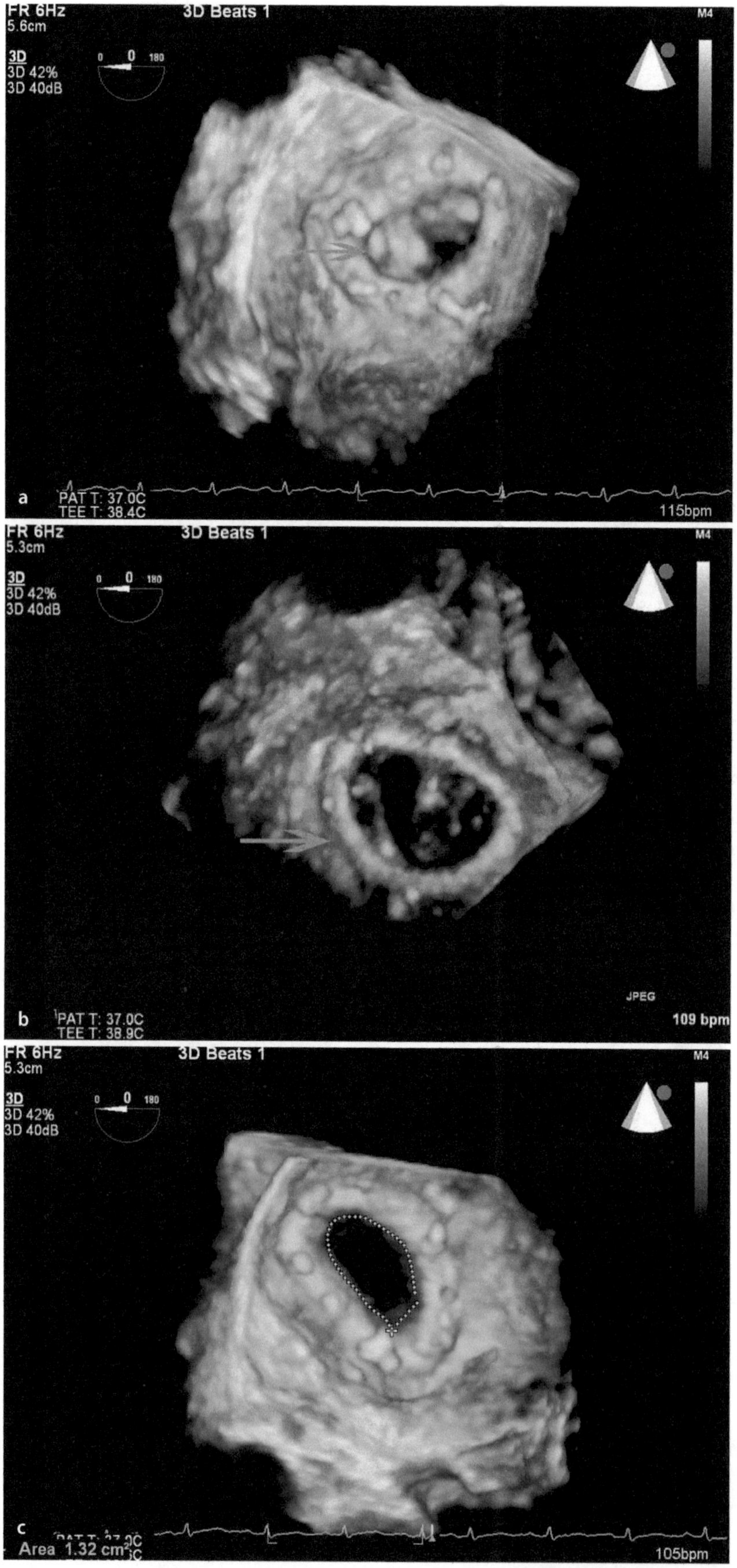

Fig. 6.23 Complete ring of mitral valve from atrial side (*arrow*) (**a**, before Z rotation; **b**, after Z rotation with placement of aortic valve in 12 o'clock), mitral valve area measures 1.3 cm² **c** by direct planimetry

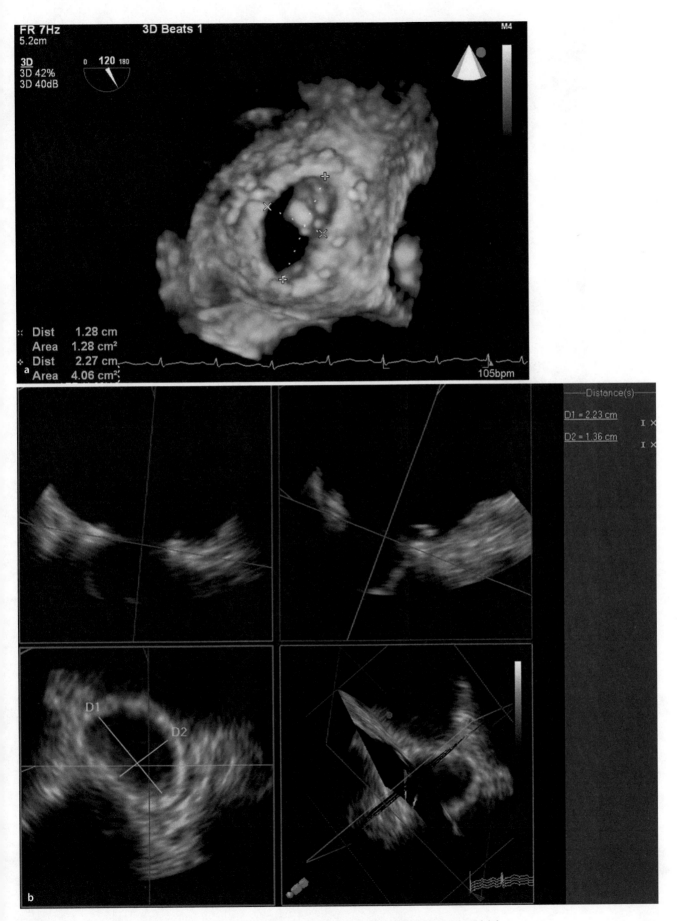

Fig. 6.24 Mitral ring measures 23*13 mm by direct measurement from LA side **a** and 22*14 mm by Q lab **b**

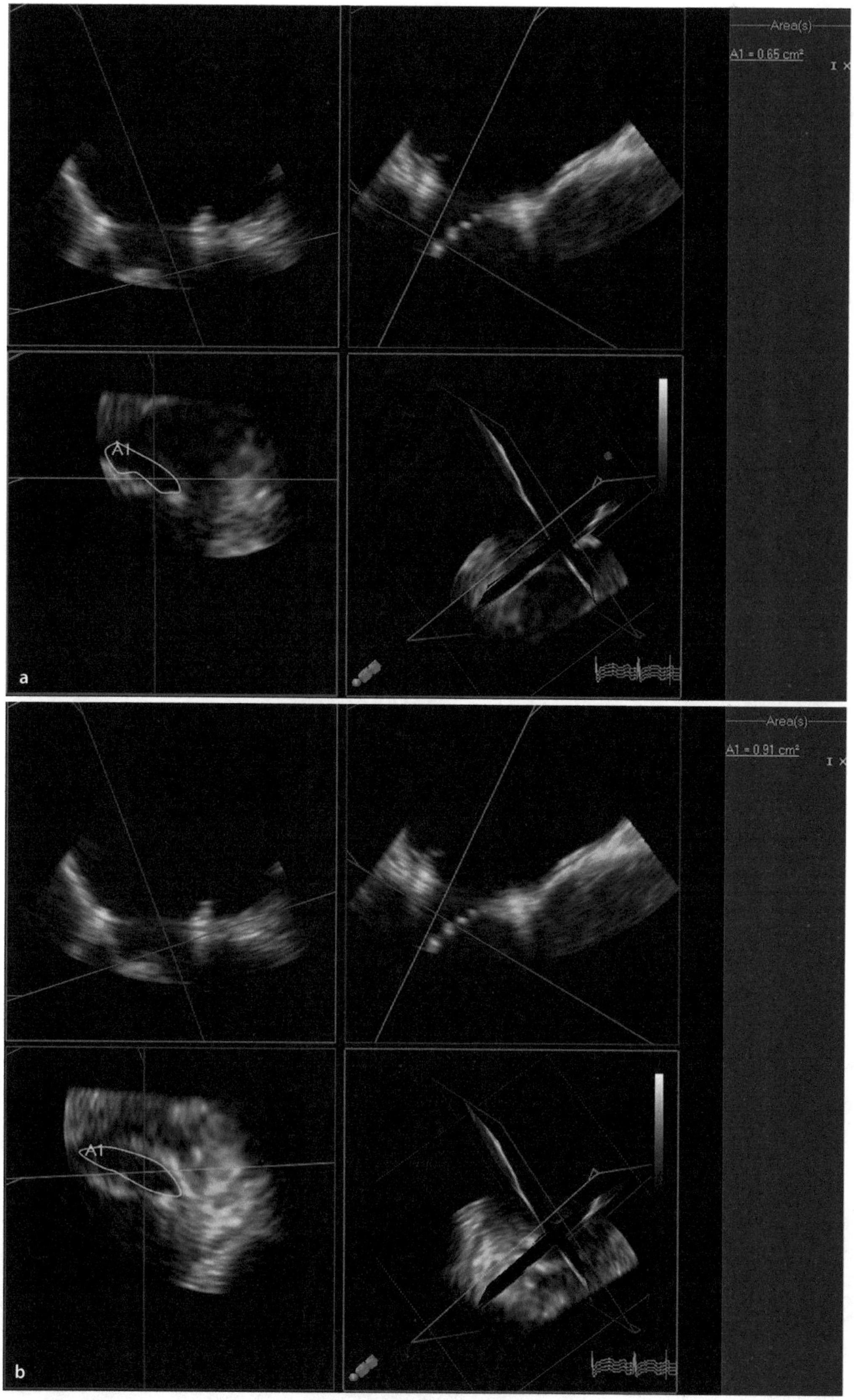

Fig. 6.25 Mitral valve area measures 0.66 cm² in tip of annulus **a** and 0.9 cm² in mid-leaflets **b**

Conclusion   Severe MS and trivial MR on MV ring annuloplasty, PAPs = 45 mmHg.

Comment   Valve in ring or MVR.

6.7   Case 7: MVR with Bioprosthetic MV with a Clot in LA

A 65-year-old man is referred for follow-up echocardiography after bioprosthetic MVR.

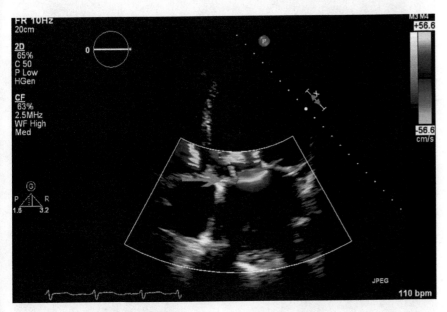

■ **Fig. 6.26**   Bioprosthetic MV is seen in apical four-chamber view (*arrow*)

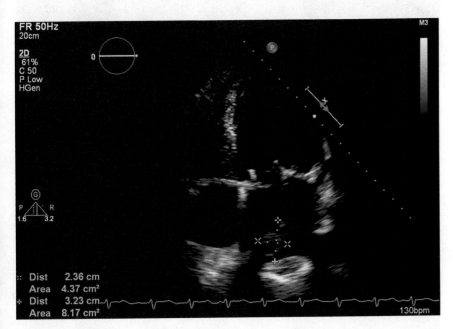

■ **Fig. 6.27**   There is a clot measuring 32*24 mm attached to atrial roof in apical four-chamber view

☐ **Fig. 6.28** Bioprosthetic MV is seen from LA side (*arrow*) **a** and LV side **b** with 3D zoom; three pedicles of bioprosthetic MV are seen from LV side (*arrows*) **b**

Diagnosis   Bioprosthetic MV with a clot in LA roof.

Comment   Full anticoagulation therapy and repeat echocardiography.

6.8   Case 8: Ross Operation

A 54-year-old woman presented with dyspnea on exertion functional class III of recent duration. She underwent Ross operation 20 years ago; coronary angiography revealed right coronary artery significant lesion in proximal part.

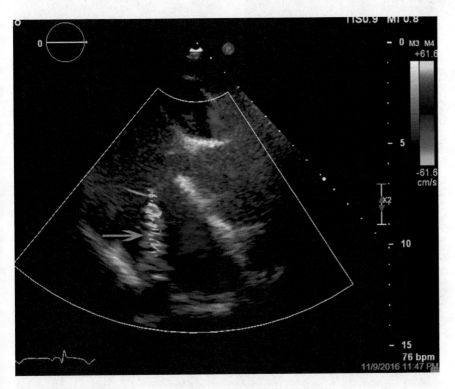

🔲 **Fig. 6.29**   Moderate MR is seen in parasternal long-axis view (*arrow*)

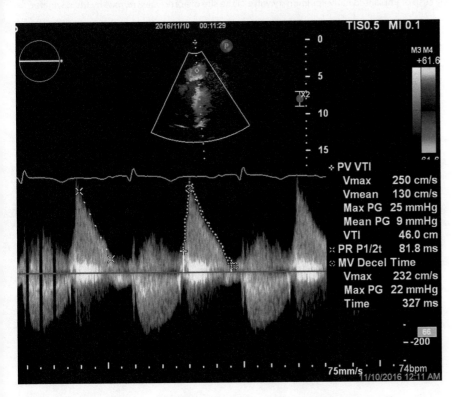

🔲 **Fig. 6.30**   Severe PI is shown on bioprosthetic PV in parasternal short-axis view, PI PHT = 81 ms

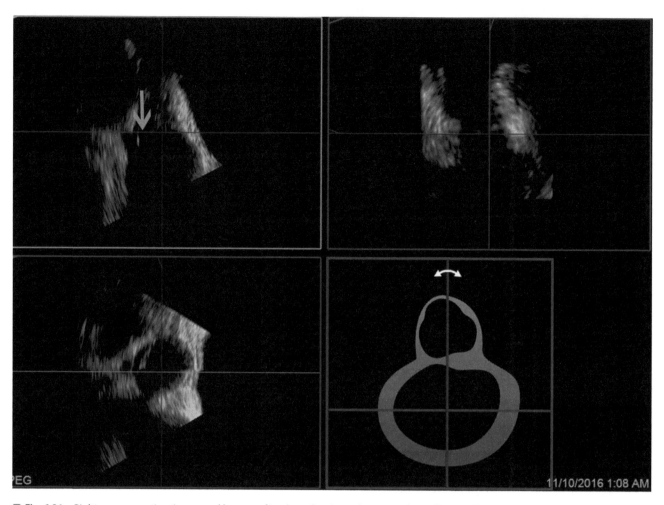

■ **Fig. 6.31** Right coronary ostium is engaged by cusp of implanted native pulmonary valve in the site of aortic valve (*arrow*) by MV navigator method full volume of aortic valve

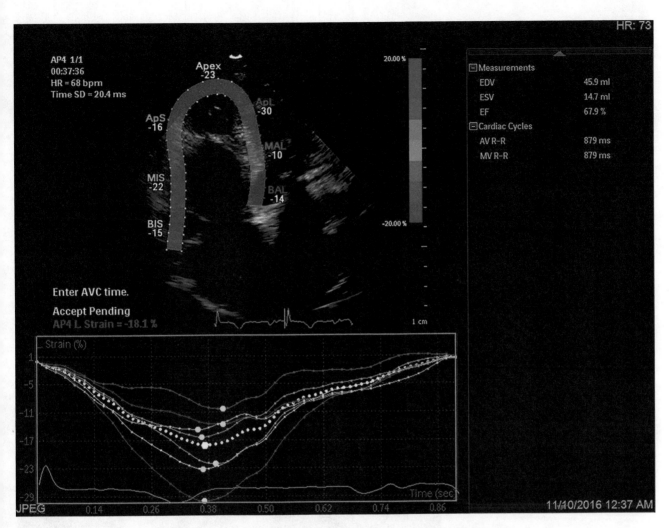

■ **Fig. 6.32** Right ventricular global longitudinal strain measures -18% in apical four-chamber view (mildly reduced)

Diagnosis   No AS and mild AI after Ross operation with severe PI and moderate MR.

Comment   Medical treatment and follow-up.

6.9 Case 9: Pannus Formation on Bileaflet Prosthetic Mitral and Aortic Valve

A 45-year-old woman presented with dyspnea on exertion functional class II of 1-year duration; she undergone MVR and AVR 7 years ago and was asymptomatic previously. Physical examination revealed normal prosthetic valve sounds and systolic murmur at aortic area. Transthoracic echocardiography showed normal left ventricular size and systolic function, LVEF = 50–55%, good mobility of prosthetic mitral valve with PG = 12 and MG = 5 mmHg but mildly increased PHT (112 ms), increased gradients across prosthetic aortic valve, annulus = 21, PG = 60, and MG = 35 mmHg but acceptable activation time (89 ms).

Transthoracic echocardiography from 1 year ago revealed increased gradients of prosthetic aortic valve, and mean gradient was 30 mmHg.

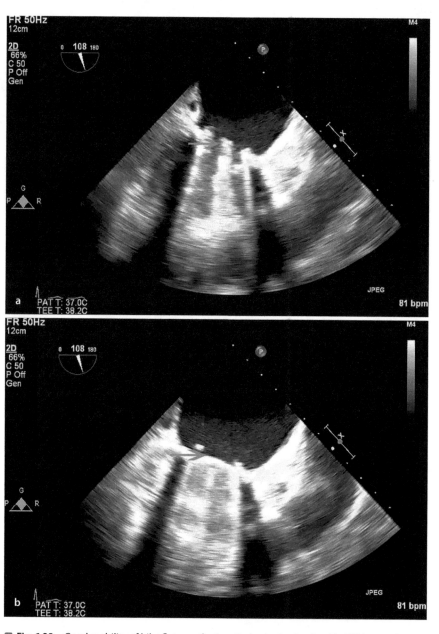

◘ Fig. 6.33 Good mobility of bileaflet prosthetic mitral valve is visualized in TEE long-axis view (**a**, diastole; **b**, systole)

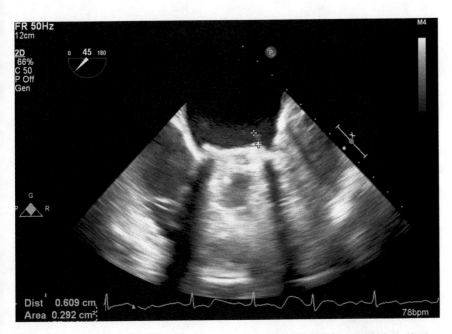

Fig. 6.34 TEE short-axis view shows that there is a mobile mass on lateral side of prosthetic mitral valve about 6 mm

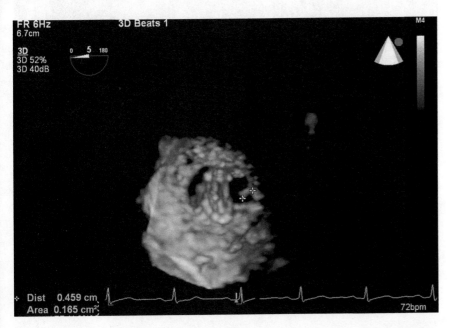

Fig. 6.35 TEE reconstruction of bileaflet prosthetic mitral valve with 3D zoom from LA side shows that mass on the lateral side of swing ring is about 5 mm

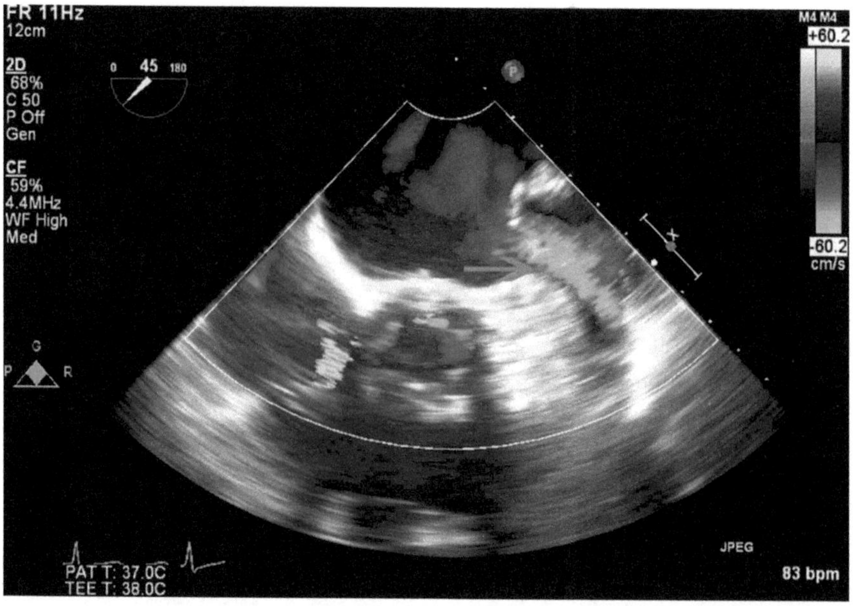

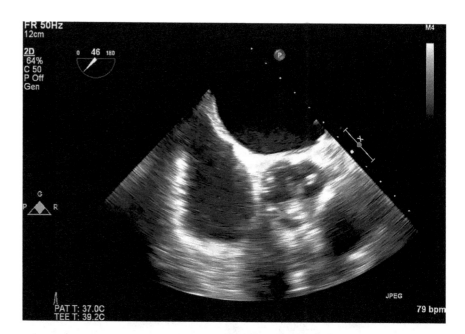

Fig. 6.36   LAA has partially closed in the previous surgery in TEE short-axis view (*arrow*)

Fig. 6.37   Pannus formation on bileaflet prosthetic aortic valve (*arrow*) by TEE short-axis view

Diagnosis   There is pannus formation about 5–6 mm on swing ring of prosthetic aortic valve, and peak and mean aortic gradients gradually increase most probably due to pannus formation.

Comment   Intensive anticoagulant therapy and follow-up echocardiography were recommended.

Lesson   How to differentiate thrombosis from pannus formation:
(1) Thrombosis is often larger and produces short duration of symptoms and interferes with valve function and is associated with lower INR and recent symptoms.
(2) About 30% of pannus formation may not be visualized; pannus formation is more common on prosthetic aortic position [2].

6.10   Case 10: Malfunction of Prosthetic Tricuspid Valve— Thrombosis

A 35-year-old man presented with a history of dyspnea on exertion from 2 weeks ago, and he had history of TVR 2 years ago. In physical examination, a muffle metallic sound and a systolic murmur in left sternal border were heard and INR was 2.8.

Transthoracic echo shows normal left systolic function and dilated right ventricle with normal systolic function; a metallic tricuspid valve is visible in tricuspid area, and gradients across tricuspid valve were too high, so transesophageal echocardiography was performed for more evaluation of tricuspid valve.

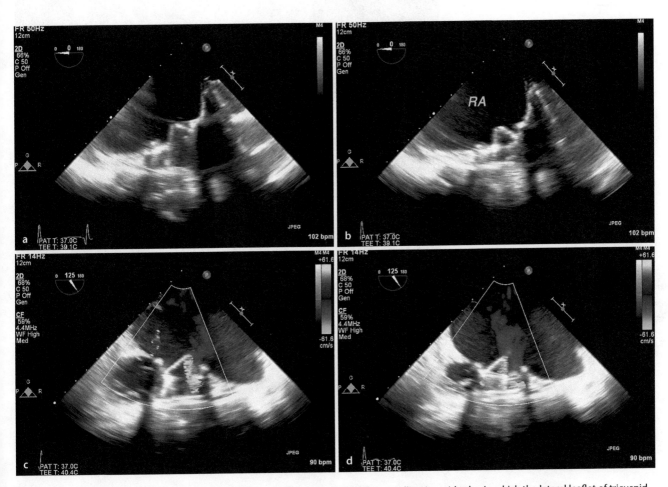

◻ **Fig. 6.38**   Transesophageal 0° view 2D and color Doppler views depict bileaflet metallic tricuspid valve in which the lateral leaflet of tricuspid valve has severely restricted range of motion and it seems closed during diastolic time (**a**, **c** during systole; **b**, **d** during diastole)

◻ **Fig. 6.39**   3D zoom view from right atrial side of tricuspid valve shows bileaflet metallic valve (*arrow*) **a**, and there is a thrombus on it (*arrow*) **b**

Diagnosis   TV prosthetic valve thrombosis.

Treatment   Fibrinolytic therapy was started and the patient was reevaluated after that. Transthoracic echocardiography depicts good mobility of restricted TV leaflet, and tricuspid valve gradients decreased significantly in favor of good response to fibrinolytic therapy.

What is the first-step treatment for prosthetic tricuspid valve dysfunction?

Fibrinolytic therapy is class IIa for thrombosed right-sided prosthetic heart valve.

6.11   Case 11: Unsuccessful MV Repair

A 60-year-old woman presented with a history of dyspnea on exertion for 2 months; she undergone mitral valve repair 2 years ago. Physical examination showed systolic murmur grade IV/VI in mitral area.

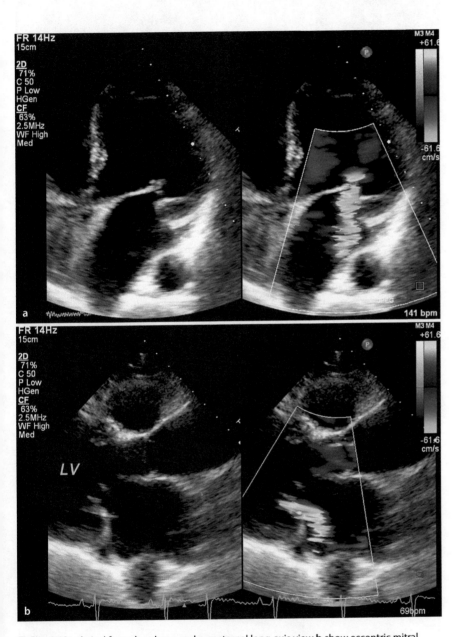

☐ **Fig. 6.40**   Apical four-chamber **a** and parasternal long-axis view **b** show eccentric mitral regurgitation to lateral wall of the left atrium

Transesophageal echocardiography was performed for evaluation of the cause and severity of MR.

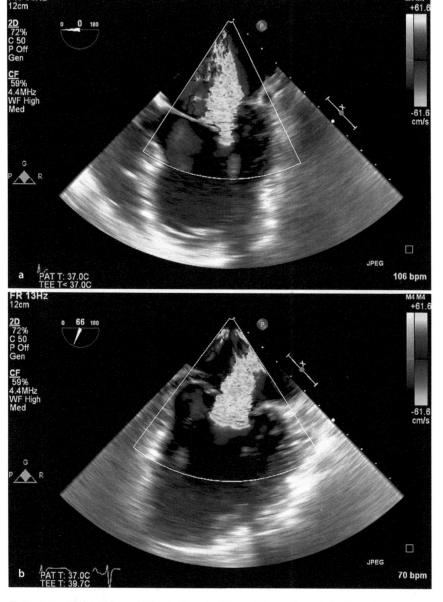

◘ **Fig. 6.41**   Mid-esophageal 2D color Doppler 0° **a** and bicommissural view **b** depict severe mitral regurgitation with wide vena contracta

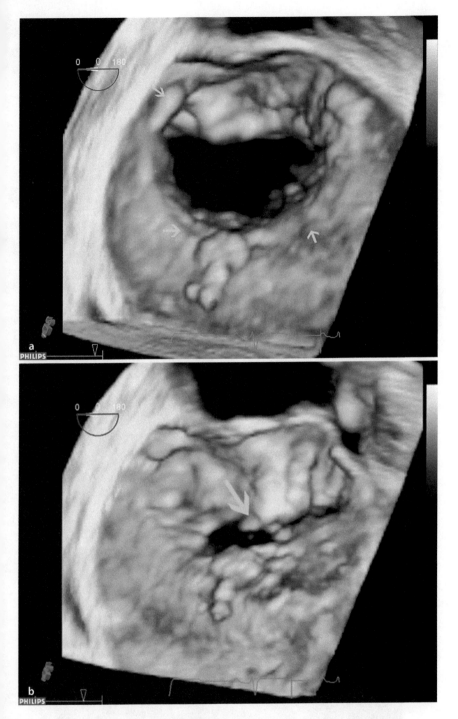

☐ **Fig. 6.42** 3D en face view of mitral valve from left atrial side during diastolic **a** shows incomplete ring of mitral repair (*arrow*) and during systolic time **b** demonstrates incomplete closure of leaflets and a wide non-coaptation area (**a**, *arrow*) in favor of failed mitral valve repair

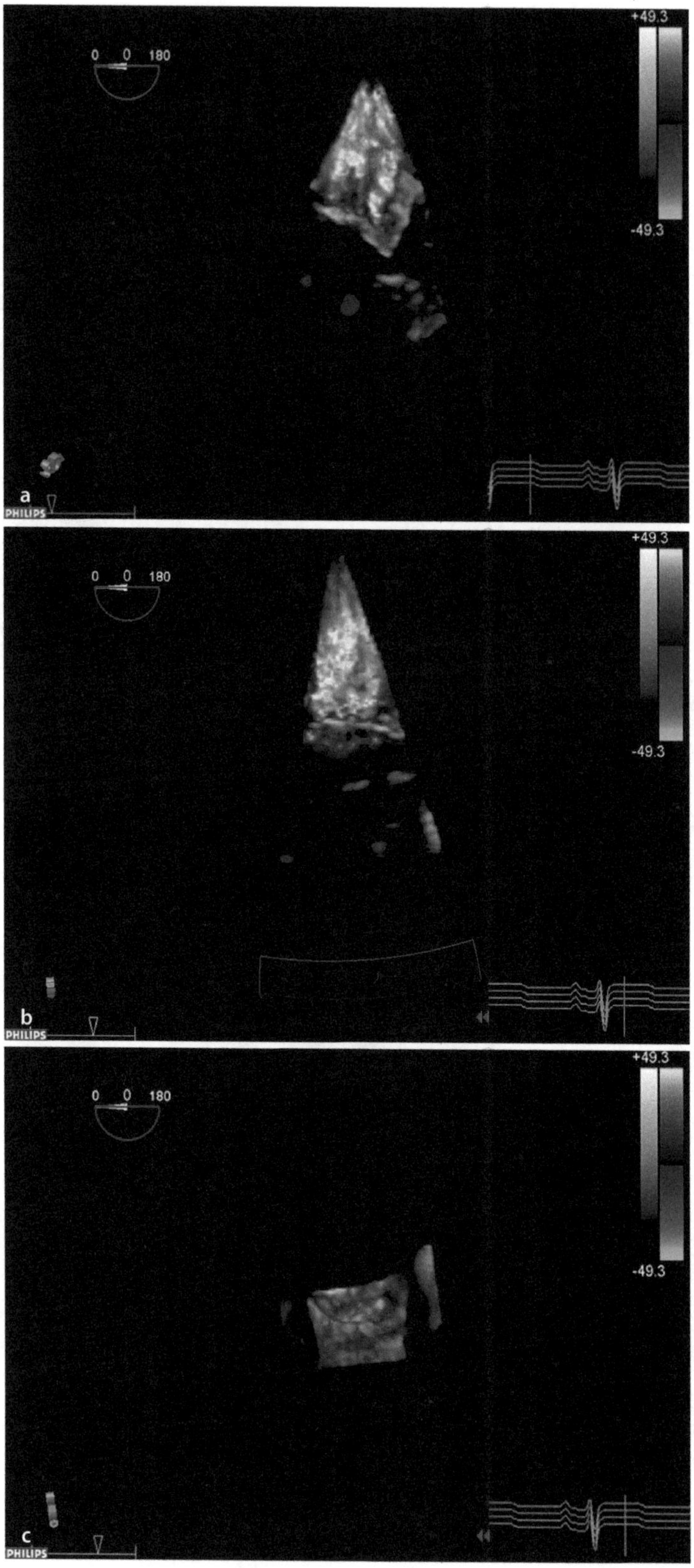

6

◘ Fig. 6.43   3D full-volume color study **a–c** demonstrates that mitral regurgitation is along the cooptation area and an asymmetric PISA zone along the commissure

Diagnosis   An unsuccessful mitral valve repair with severe mitral regurgitation.

Whit respect to severity of mitral valve regurgitation and symptoms of the patient, she was sent for MVR.

6.12   Case 12: Severe TR on Bioprosthetic TV

A 25-year-old woman presented with a history of lower extremity edema and easy fatigability for a 3-month duration. She had a history of infective endocarditis, and then she underwent tricuspid valve replacement. Physical examination revealed a systolic murmur in left sternal border.

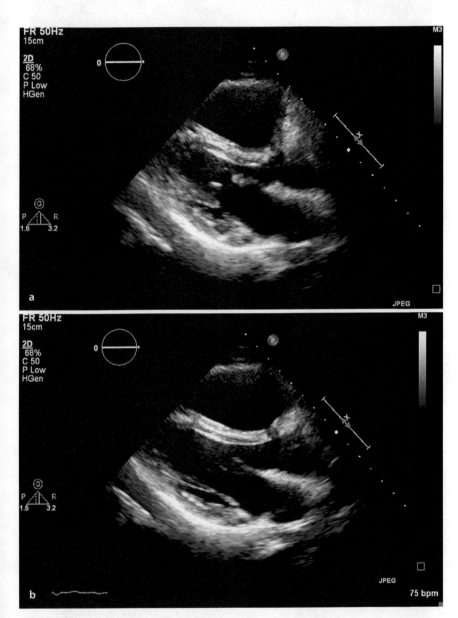

☐ **Fig. 6.44**   Parasternal long-axis view shows dilated right ventricular outflow tract (**a**, systole; **b**, diastole)

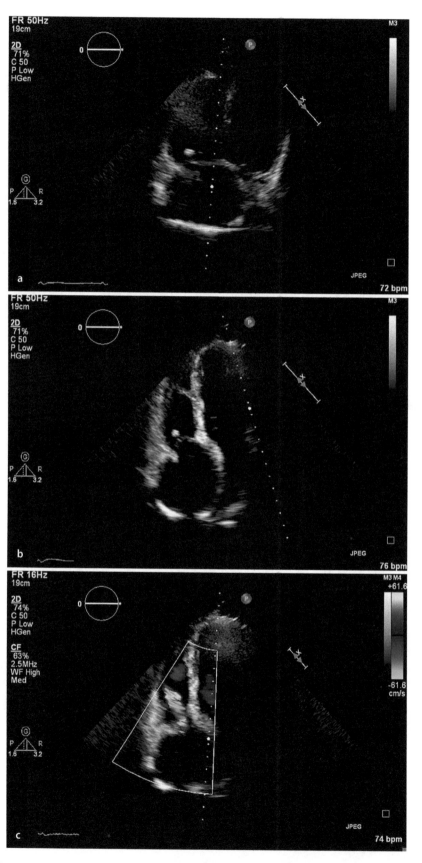

◻ Fig. 6.45   Apical four-chamber view depicts dilated right ventricle **a** and deviated interatrial septum toward left side **b** in favor of high right atrial pressure, and color study shows diastolic turbulency on tricuspid valve suggestive for severe tricuspid stenosis **c**

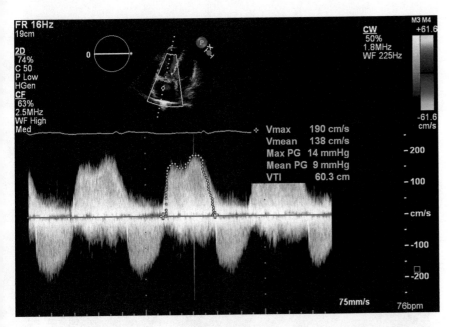

Fig. 6.46 Color Doppler flow study demonstrates high gradients across bioprosthetic tricuspid valve (peak and mean gradients are measured about 14 and 9 mmHg, respectively)

Transesophageal echocardiography was performed for evaluation of tricuspid valve.

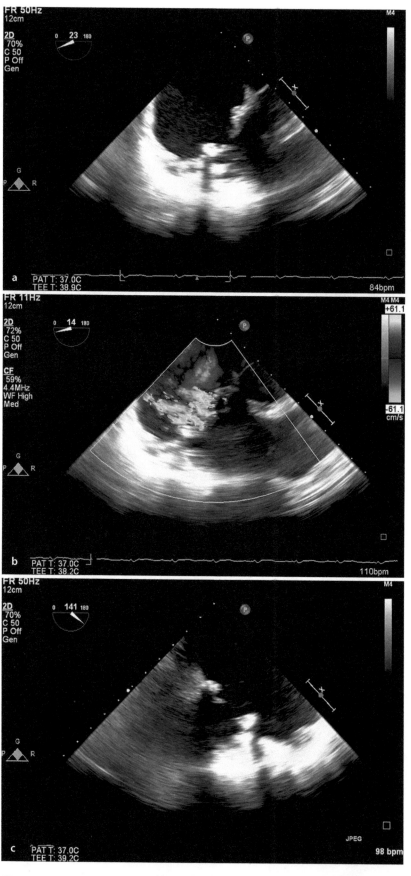

☐ **Fig. 6.47** Mid-esophageal 14° view depicts thick bioprosthetic leaflets **a** with severe tricuspid valve regurgitation **b** and mid-esophageal 114° view demonstrates malcoaptation of tricuspid valve leaflets **c**

6.12 · Case 12: Severe TR on Bioprosthetic TV

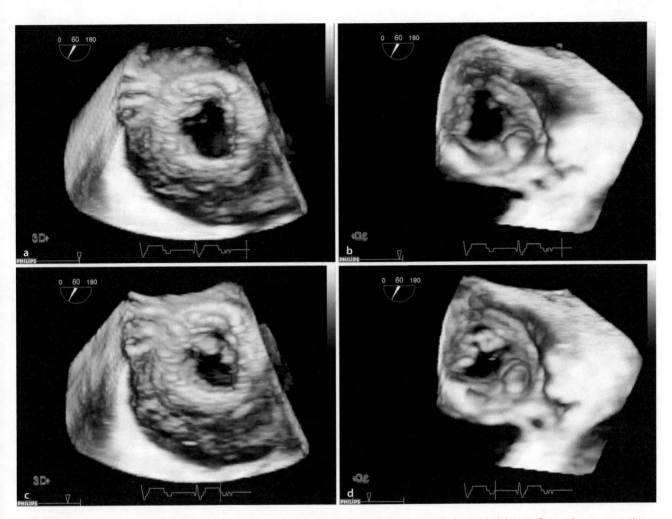

◼ **Fig. 6.48** 3D zoom en face view of tricuspid valve from right atrium **a** and right ventricular side **b** revealed thick leaflets and non-cooptation of leaflets during systolic time **c**, **d**, and one leaflet seems fixed

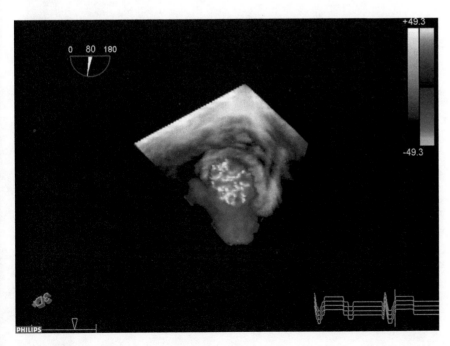

◼ **Fig. 6.49** Color full-volume en face view of tricuspid bioprosthetic shows severe tricuspid valve regurgitation (*arrow*)

Diagnosis   Malfunction of bioprosthetic valve only after a 2-year duration.

Recommendation   With respect to right ventricular dilation and severe tricuspid valve dysfunction, redo TVR or valve in valve is recommended.

References

1. Webb JG, Wood DA, Ye J, Gurvitch R, Masson JB, Rodes-Cabau J, et al. Transcatheter valve-in-valve implantation for failed bioprosthetic heart valves. Circulation. 2010;121(16):1848–57.
2. Zoghbi WA, Chambers JB, Dumesnil JG, Foster E, Gottdiener JS, Grayburn PA, et al. Recommendations for evaluation of prosthetic valves with echocardiography and Doppler ultrasound: a report from the American Society of Echocardiography's Guidelines and Standards Committee and the Task Force on Prosthetic Valves, developed in conjunction with the American College of Cardiology Cardiovascular Imaging Committee, Cardiac Imaging Committee of the American Heart Association, the European Association of Echocardiography, a registered branch of the European Society of Cardiology, the Japanese Society of Echocardiography and the Canadian Society of Echocardiography, endorsed by the American College of Cardiology Foundation, American Heart Association, European Association of Echocardiography, a registered branch of the European Society of Cardiology, the Japanese Society of Echocardiography, and Canadian Society of Echocardiography. J Amsoc Echocardiogr. 2009;22(9):975–1014. quiz 82-4

Paravalvular Leak of Prosthetic Valves

Videos can be found in the electronic supplementary material in the online version of the chapter.
On http://springerlink.com enter the DOI number given on the bottom of the chapter opening page.
Scroll down to the Supplementary material tab and click on the respective videos link.

© Springer International Publishing AG 2017
H. Sadeghian, Z. Savand-Roomi, *3D Echocardiography of Structural Heart Disease*,
DOI 10.1007/978-3-319-54039-9_7

Paravalvular leak of prosthetic valve occurs between 5–17% [1] in some studies and 3–6% in other reports [2]. Most of paravalvular leaks are mild and do not need interventions. If paravalvular leak produces symptoms of heart failure or hemolysis, it needs intervention.

Paravalvular leak in aortic position produces more hemolysis even in small sizes due to high jet velocity.

In cases of paravalvular leak with NYHA functional class III–IV or significant hemolysis anemia, moderately severe or severe paravalvular leak, and absence of infective endocarditis, percutaneous paravalvular leak closure can be considered, although surgery is a standard method of treatment [1, 2].

7.1   Case 1: Dehiscence of Prosthetic Aortic Valve

A 33-year-old man presented with dyspnea on exertion functional class II–III of recent exacerbation. He was a known case of AVR a few years ago. Physical examination revealed early diastolic murmur at aortic area.

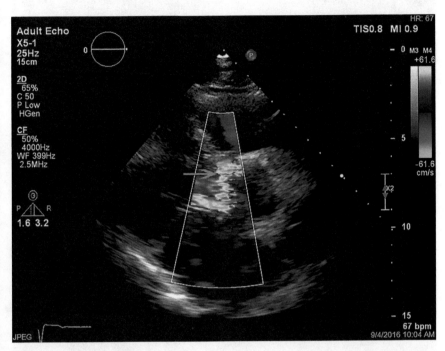

Fig. 7.1 Severe paravalvular leak is relevant in parasternal long-axis view (*arrow*) from right coronary cusp

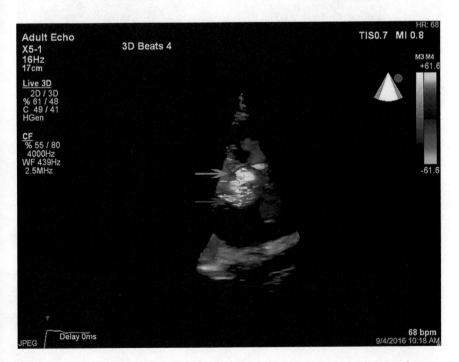

Fig. 7.2 Live 3D mode of aortic valve in parasternal short-axis view shows that site of paravalvular leak is from right (*green arrow*) and non-coronary (*pink arrow*) cusps

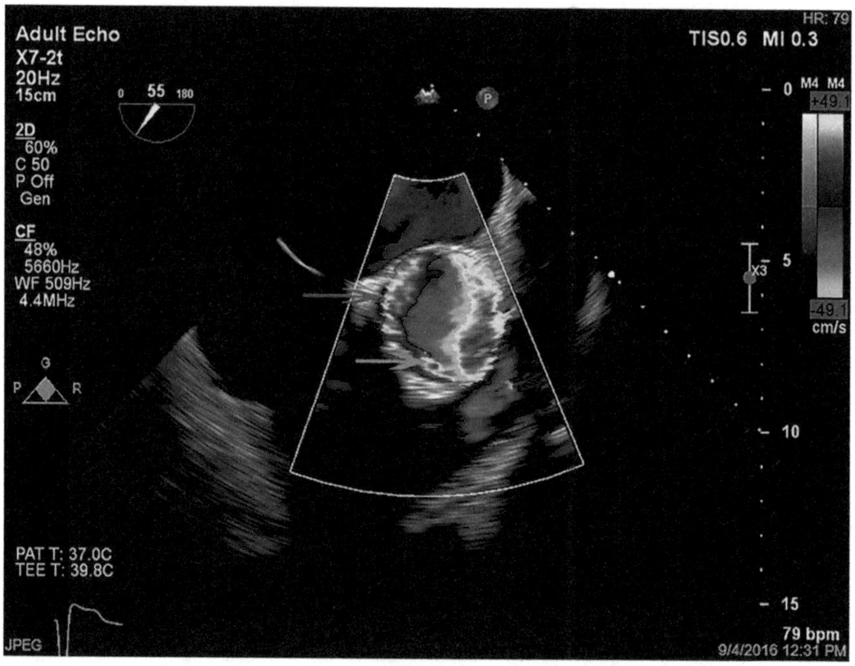

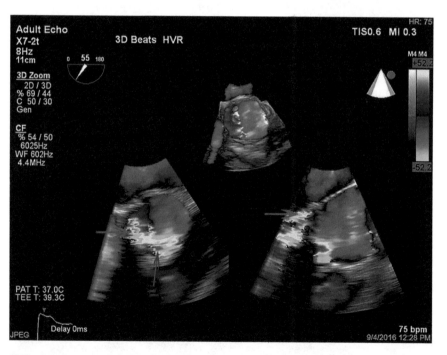

● **Fig. 7.3**   Transesophageal short-axis view reveals that paravalvular leak is from right (*green arrow*) and non-coronary (*pink arrow*) cusps; this leak contains about 50% of aortic circumference

● **Fig. 7.4**   Live 3D echocardiography by TEE short-axis view shows that paravalvular leak is from non-coronary cusp (*pink arrow*) and right coronary cusp (*green arrow*)

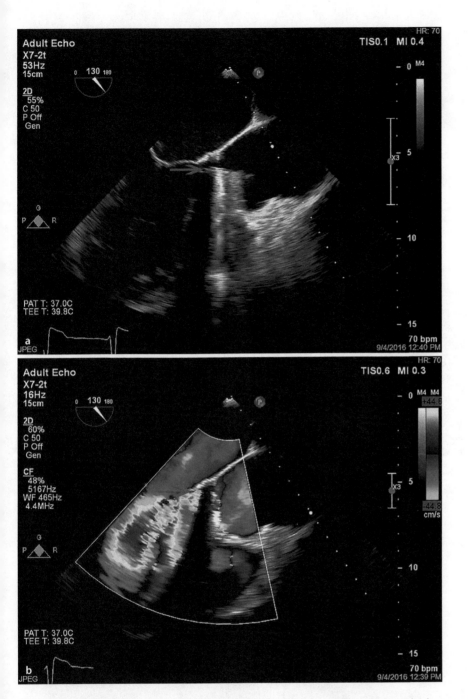

◨ **Fig. 7.5** TEETEE long-axis view shows site of paravalvular leak from non-coronary cusp (*pink arrows*) by 2D echocardiography **a** and color Doppler study **b**

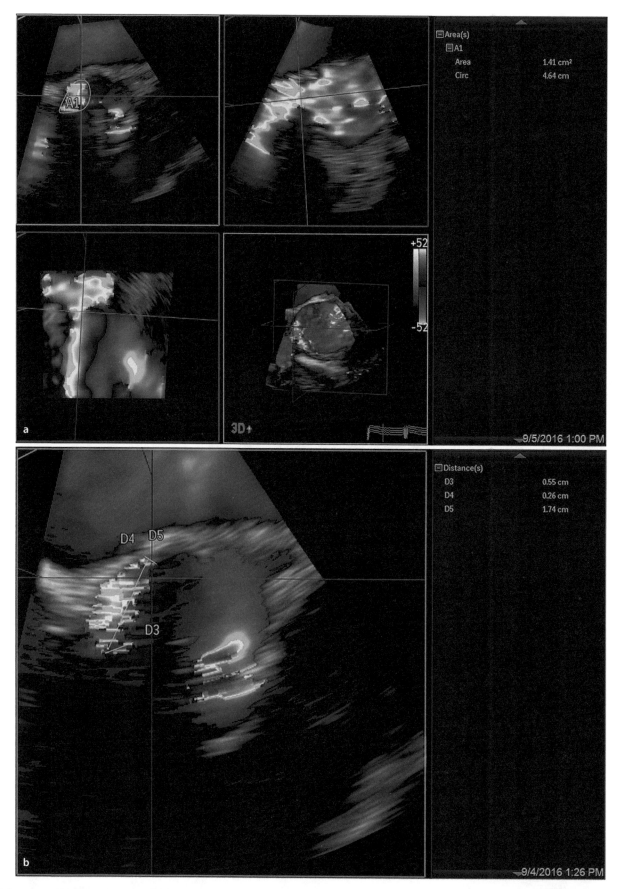

◘ Fig. 7.6   Full volume of aortic valve by color Doppler study shows that vena contracta area measures 1.4 cm² **a**, and length of tract of paravalvular leak is 17 mm, D1 is 5.5 mm, and D2 is 2.6 mm **b**

Diagnosis   Severe paravalvular leak from right and non-coronary cusps.

Comment   The patient is referred for surgery (Bentall operation) as aortic root measures 42 mm and ascending aorta measures 49 mm (dilated).

Lesson

1. Due to dehiscence of mechanical aortic valve, the patient is referred for surgery, and because of dilation of ascending aorta, Bentall was recommended. Significant dehiscence of prosthetic valve is defined as dehiscence involving more than one fourth of the valve ring [1]; significant dehiscence and endocarditis are contraindications for percutaneous paraprosthetic regurgitation [1].
2. Prosthetic aortic valve regurgitation is classified as mild (<10% of swing ring), moderate (between 10% and 20% of swing ring), and severe (>20% of swing ring). Rocking motion of prosthetic aortic valve is defined as dehiscence more than 40% of swing ring [3].

7.2 Case 2: Moderately Severe Paravalvular Leak on Prosthetic Mitral Valve

A 59-year-old woman presented with dyspnea on exertion functional class II and typical chest pain during the recent 3 months.

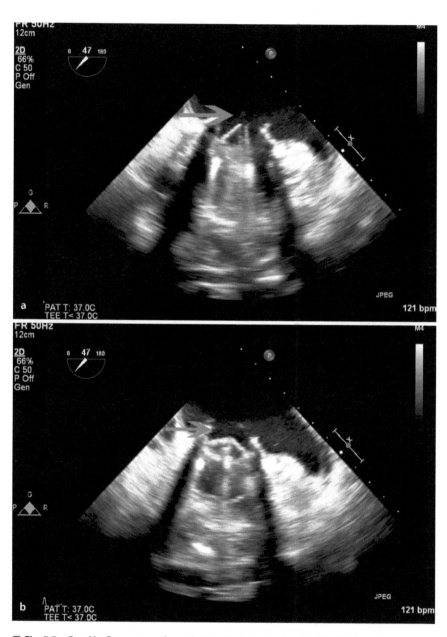

◘ **Fig. 7.7** Good leaflet motion of prosthetic mitral valve is visualized in TEE short-axis view (*arrows*) **a**, **b**

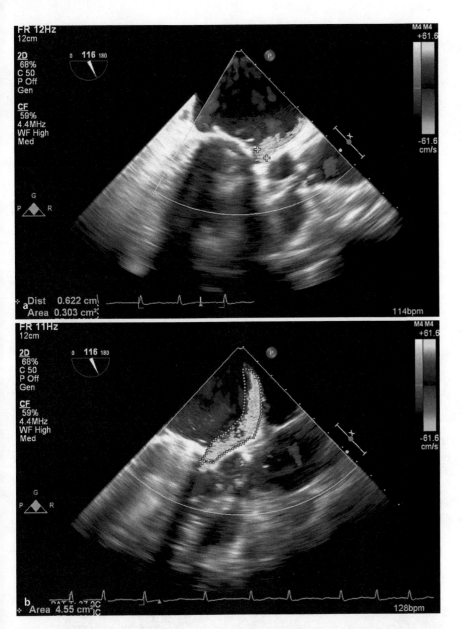

❑ **Fig. 7.8** Paravalvular leak of prosthetic mitral valve is shown in TEE long-axis view between prosthetic mitral valve and aortic valve; vena contracta measures 6.2 mm **a**; surface of MR para-valvular leak measures 4.5 cm² in this view **b**

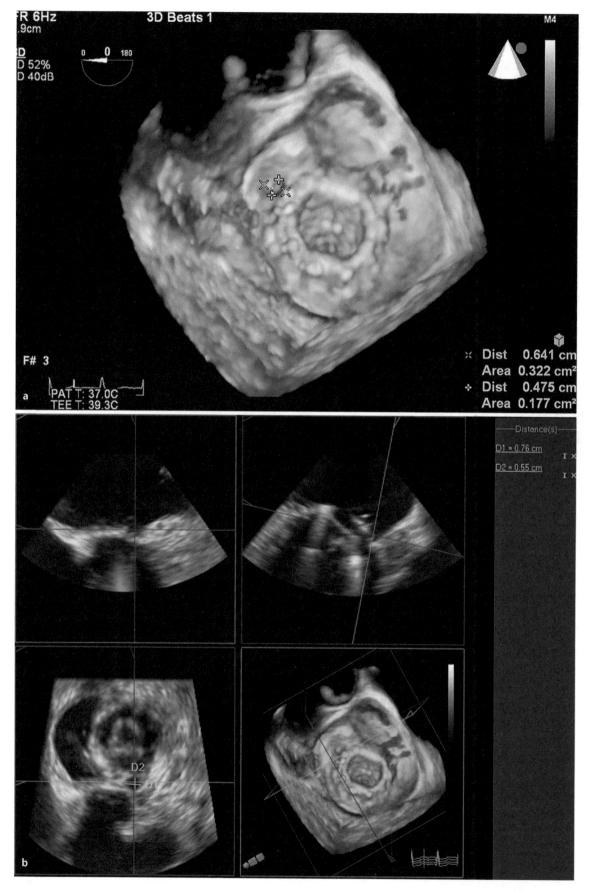

Fig. 7.9   3D zoom of prosthetic mitral valve shows site of paravalvular leak between mitral and aortic valve nearly at 10 o'clock, and its size measures 4.8*6.5 mm by direct measurement **a** and 7.5*5.5 mm by 3DQ method **b**

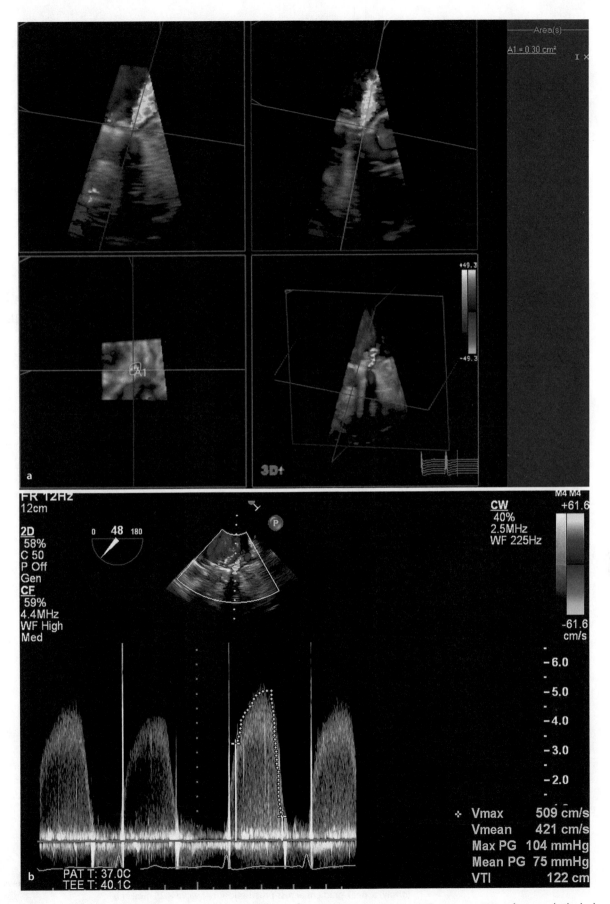

■ **Fig. 7.10** Vena contracta area of paravalvular leak measures 0.3 cm² **a**, and mitral regurgitation VTI measures 122 cm **b**; paravalvular leak volume measures as follows: Vena contracta area*VTI = 0.3*122 = 36.6 cm³

Diagnosis   Symptomatic patient with moderately severe paravalvular leak on prosthetic mitral valve, the paravalvular leak is oval shaped and its position is in 10 o'clock.

Comment   The patient is referred for paravalvular leak device closure.

Lesson

For prosthetic mitral valve paravalvular leak:

Vena contracta <2 mm: Mild

Vena contracta between 2 and 6: Moderate

Vena contracta ≥6 mm: Severe [3]

Amplatzer vascular plug I can be used for this lesion; this device is available in diameter 4–16 mm and length 7–8 mm.

7.3   Case 3: Moderate Paravalvular Leak of Prosthetic Aortic Valve and Moderate Paravalvular Leak of Prosthetic Mitral Valve

A 55-year-old woman presented with dyspnea on exertion functional class II. She underwent AVR and MVR 10 years ago.

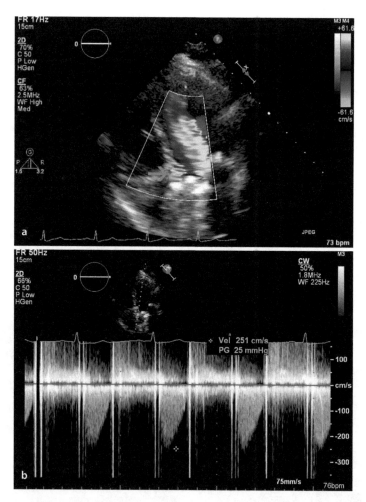

◼ **Fig. 7.11**   Moderate paravalvular aortic regurgitation is seen in apical five-chamber views (*arrow*) **a**; peak gradient across prosthetic aortic valve is 25 mmHg **b**

381 7

7.3 · Case 3: Moderate Paravalvular Leak of Prosthetic Aortic Valve and Moderate Paravalvular Leak of Prosthetic Mitral Valve

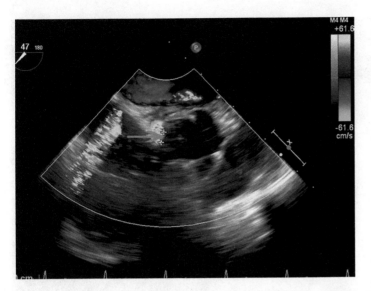

Fig. 7.12 TEE short-axis view shows that paravalvular leak is from non-coronary cusp (*arrow*)

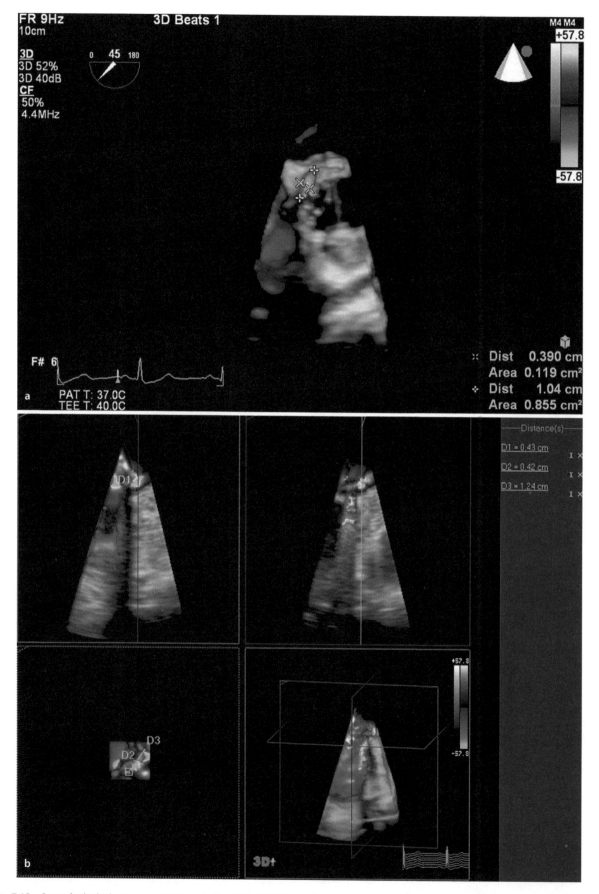

Fig. 7.13 Paravalvular leak measures 4*10 mm by live 3D by TEE short-axis of aortic valve **a**; 3DQ measurement of paravalvular leak shows that the diameter of paravalvular leak is 5 mm, and its length is 12 mm **b**

383   7

7.3 · Case 3: Moderate Paravalvular Leak of Prosthetic Aortic Valve and Moderate Paravalvular Leak of Prosthetic Mitral Valve

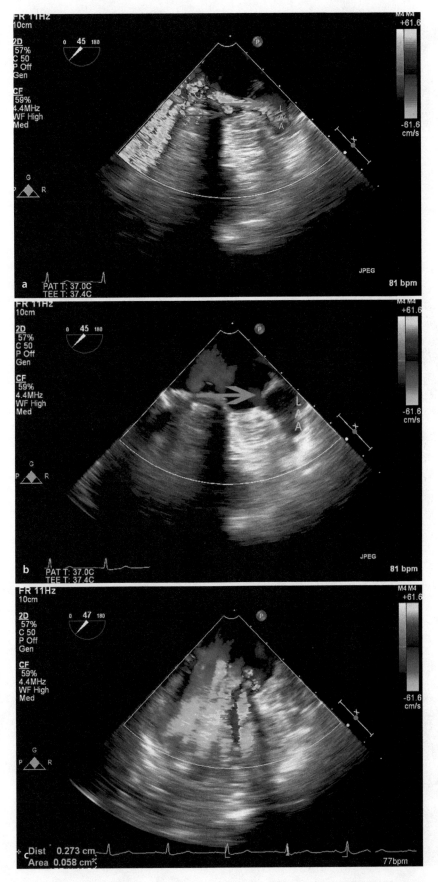

◨ **Fig. 7.14** TEE short-axis view also reveals that there is mild paravalvular leak between prosthetic MV and LAA (*pink arrow*); LAA is partially closed in previous surgery and flow across it is
visible (*green arrow*) **a**, **b**; this site of leak measures 2.7 mm in this view **c**

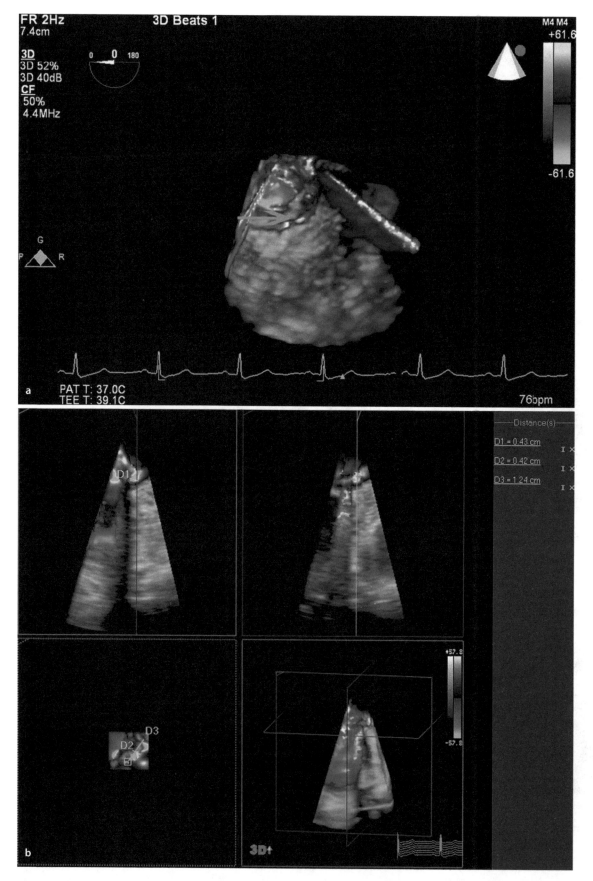

Fig. 7.15 Paravalvular leak of lateral side of prosthetic MV is crescent shaped by 3D zoom mode **a**, but it is of notice that with this modality (3D zoom color), frequency of image is 2 Hz and so very low. Diameter of paravalvular leak of mitral valve is 4.2 and 4.3 mm on its ends, and its length measures 12 mm by 3DQ full-volume color modality **b**

Diagnosis Moderate paravalvular leak of prosthetic aortic valve and moderate paravalvular leak of prosthetic mitral valve, the position of paramitral leak is between 9 and 10 o'clock.

Comment Medical treatment and follow-up.

Lesson
1. There were two jets of regurgitation for prosthetic aortic valve: One jet is paravalvular from NCC, and another jet is intravalvular.
2. 3D echo with color Doppler should be obtained by full-volume or live 3D; by 3D zoom due the problem of temporal resolution, the quality of image would not be acceptable.
3. Indication for intervention in paravalvular leak is more than moderate paravalvular leak which produces symptoms of heart failure FC III–IV or intractable hemolysis; surgery is of class I, and if the patient is high risk for surgery, paravalvular leak by device closure is of class IIa [4].
4. Lower size of available device is 3 mm.
5. Amplatzer vascular plug II is the more preferable device.

7.4 Case 4: Severe Paravalvular Leak of Prosthetic Mitral Valve

A 65-year-old woman presented with a history of dyspnea (functional class III) with 3-month duration. Physical examination shows metallic sound and systolic murmur grad III/VI in mitral area and left sternal border and a diastolic murmur grad II/VI in aortic area.

Transthoracic echocardiography showed good left ventricular size and function.

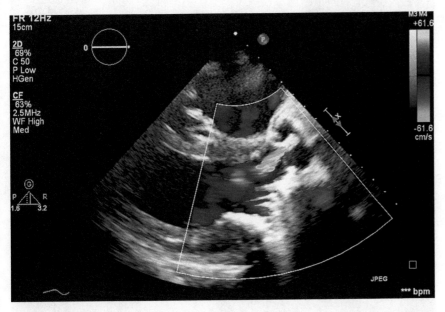

◻ **Fig. 7.16** Parasternal long-axis view shows metallic prosthetic valve in mitral area (*arrow*) and mild aortic regurgitation

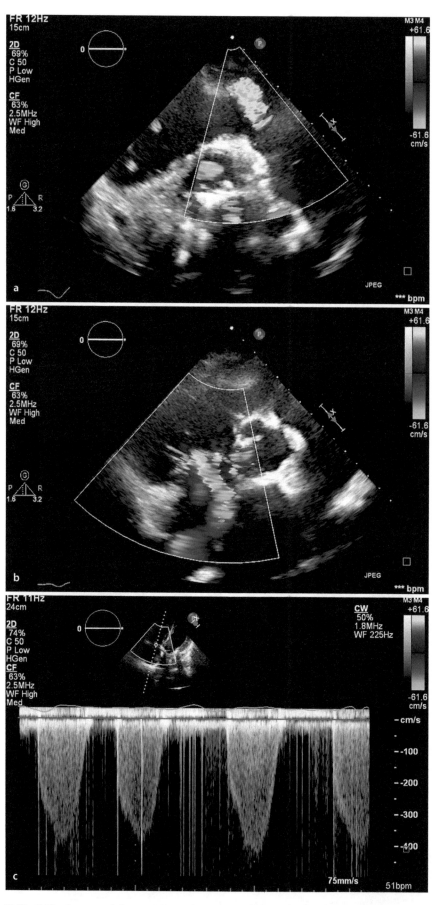

■ **Fig. 7.17** Parasternal short-axis view of great vessels reveals moderate pulmonic regurgitation **a** and moderate tricuspid regurgitation **b** with high systolic pulmonary pressure **c**

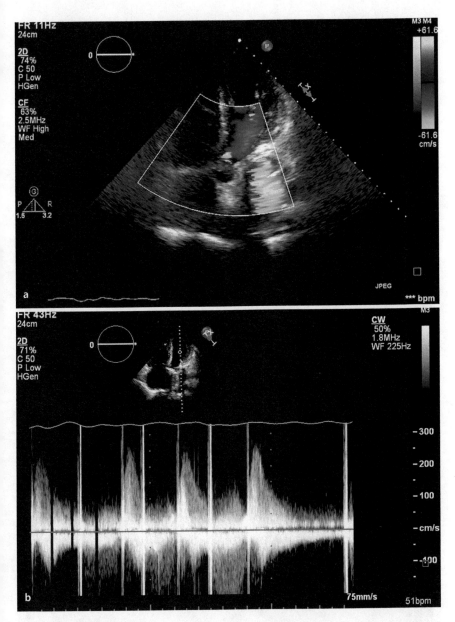

Fig. 7.18 Apical four-chamber view depicts systolic turbulent flow in left atrium **a**, and color Doppler flow study across mitral valve demonstrates high gradient **b** with very steep A wave, and MV VTI/LVOT VTI is measured more than 2.2 in favor of regurgitation (doesn't show in this view)

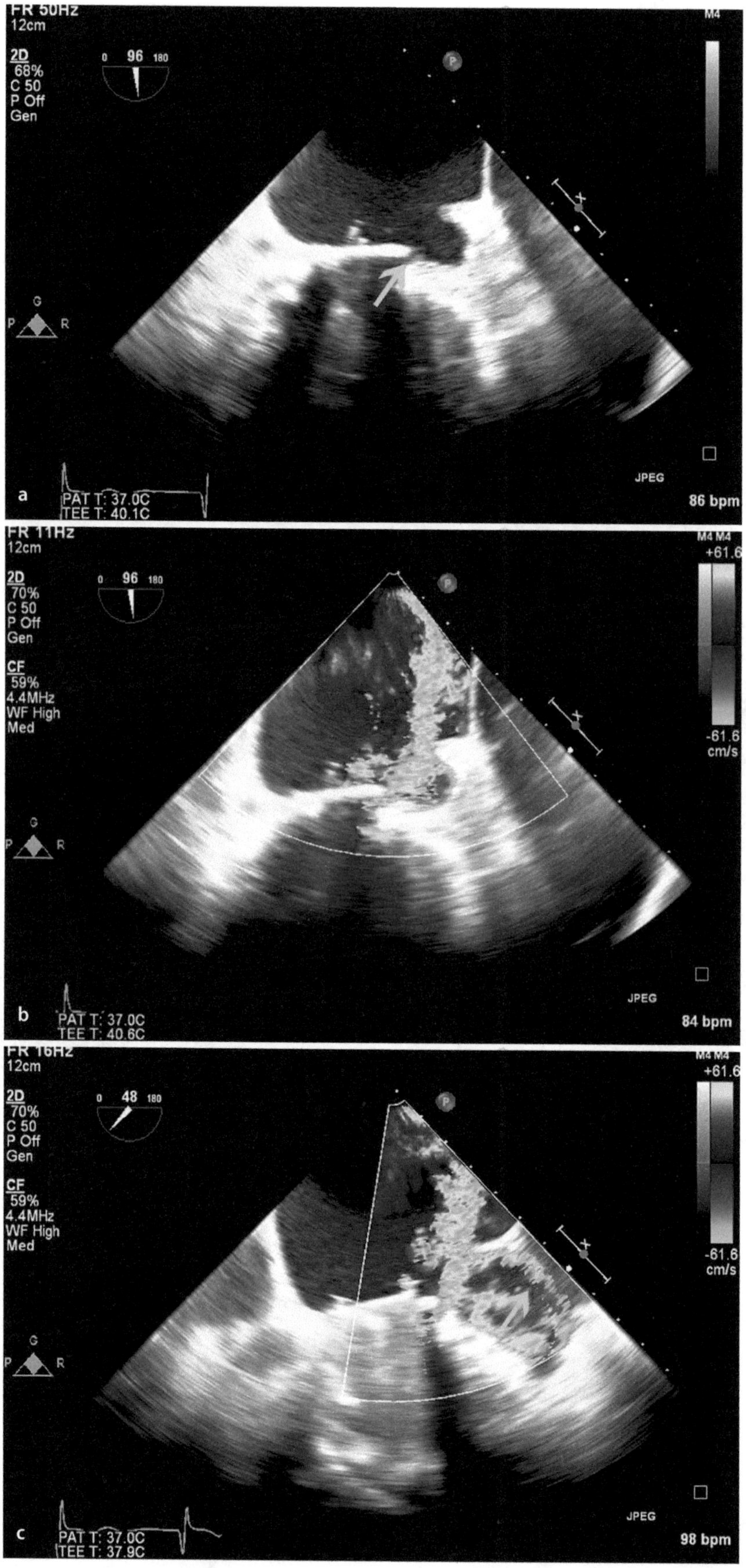

■ **Fig. 7.19**   Mid-esophageal 96° depicts a defect in lateral wall of swing ring near to left atrial appendage (*arrow*, **a**), and color Doppler study confirms paravalvular leakage **b**, and it shows swirling of paravalvular leakage to left atrial appendage (*arrow*, **c**)

Transesophageal echocardiography was performed for more evaluation of mitral prosthetic valve.

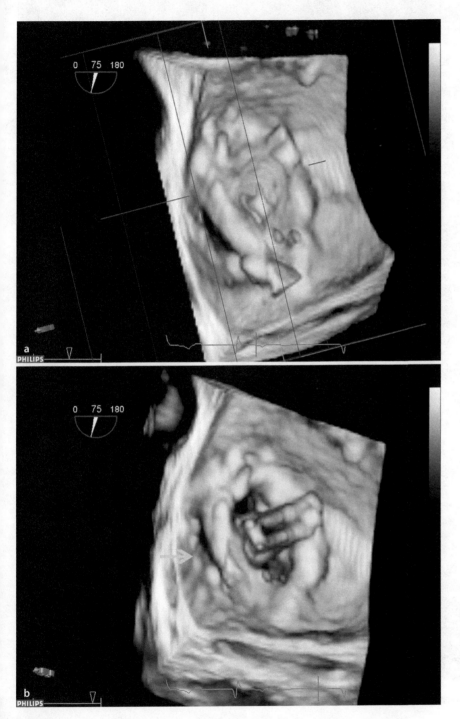

☐ **Fig. 7.20**   3D zoom view from left atrial side shows good leaflet mobility in systolic **a** and diastolic **b** time and a crescent-shaped defect in 9 o'clock (near to left atrial appendage site)

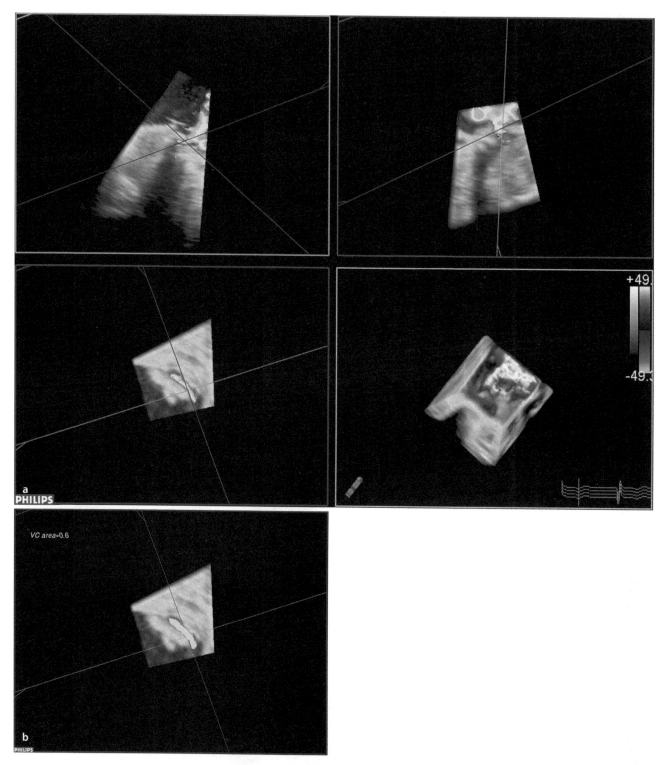

Fig. 7.21 3D full-volume color study demonstrates a crescent-shaped vena contracta with area about 0.6 cm^2 in favor of severe mitral regurgitation **a, b**

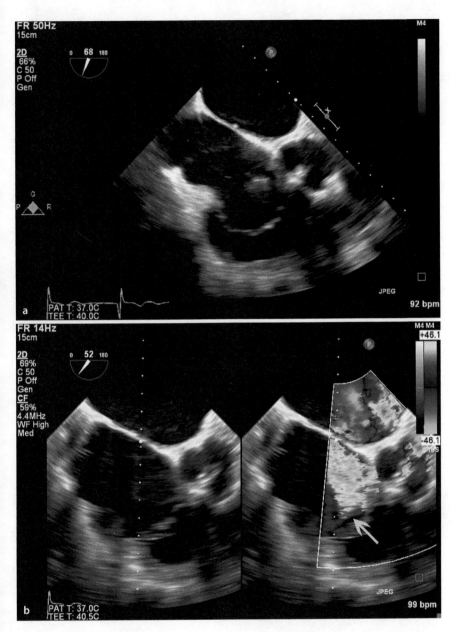

□ **Fig. 7.22** Mid-esophageal short-axis view of tricuspid valve shows thick tricuspid valve **a** with moderate tricuspid regurgitation (**b**, *arrow*), without tricuspid stenosis, and with tricuspid annulus diameter about 33 mm (17 mm/m²) (doesn't show in this view)

Diagnosis   Severe mitral paravalvular leakage and moderate tricuspid regurgitation without annular dilation and tricuspid stenosis.

Recommendation   The patient was sent for paravalvular device closure.

References

1. Rihal CS, Sorajja P, Booker JD, Hagler DJ, Cabalka AK. Principles of percutaneous paravalvular leak closure. JACC Cardiovasc Interv. 2012;5(2):121–30.

2. Sorajja P, Cabalka AK, Hagler DJ, Rihal CS. Percutaneous repair of paravalvular prosthetic regurgitation: acute and 30-day outcomes in 115 patients. Circ Cardiovasc Interv. 2011;4(4):314–21.

3. Zoghbi WA, Chambers JB, Dumesnil JG, Foster E, Gottdiener JS, Grayburn PA, et al. Recommendations for evaluation of prosthetic valves with echocardiography and Doppler ultrasound: a report from the American Society of Echocardiography's guidelines and standards committee and the task force on prosthetic valves, developed in conjunction with the American College of Cardiology Cardiovascular Imaging Committee, cardiac imaging Committee of the American Heart Association, the European Association of Echocardiography, a registered branch of the European Society of Cardiology, the Japanese Society of Echocardiography and the Canadian Society of Echocardiography, endorsed by the American College of Cardiology Foundation, American Heart Association, European Association of Echocardiography, a registered branch of the European Society of Cardiology, the Japanese Society of Echocardiography, and Canadian Society of Echocardiography. J Am Soc Echocardiogr. 2009;22(9):975–1014. quiz 82-4

4. Nishimura RA, Otto CM, Bonow RO, Carabello BA, Erwin 3rd JP, Guyton RA, et al. 2014 AHA/ACC guideline for the Management of Patients with Valvular Heart Disease: executive summary: a report of the American College of Cardiology/American Heart Association Task Force on Practice Guidelines. Circulation. 2014;129(23):2440–92.

Infective Endocarditis (IE)

Videos can be found in the electronic supplementary material in the online version of the chapter.
On http://springerlink.com enter the DOI number given on the bottom of the chapter opening page.
Scroll down to the Supplementary material tab and click on the respective videos link.

© Springer International Publishing AG 2017
H. Sadeghian, Z. Savand-Roomi, *3D Echocardiography of Structural Heart Disease*,
DOI 10.1007/978-3-319-54039-9_8

Infective endocarditis may involve native cardiac valves or prosthetic valves and devices.

Native valve with an underlying disease like bicuspid aortic valve, degenerative changes of mitral valve, or rheumatismal involvement of valves especially valvular regurgitations or congenital heart disease is predisposing cardiac lesions for IE.

Indications for surgery of IE include:

1. Heart failure due to valvular lesions
2. Abscess formation
3. Recurrent emboli despite antibiotic therapy
4. Severe valvular regurgitation and vegetation >10 mm (IIa) [1]

Complete removal of pacemaker lead is recommended if there is documented infection of leads [2].

8.1   Case 1: Infective Endocarditis on Pacemaker Lead

A 45-year-old woman presented with a history of diabetes mellitus and chronic renal failure on routine dialysis and new-onset chest pain who was admitted in CCU, and after coronary angiography, she was candidate for CABG and was sent to echo-lab for echocardiography before surgery. In physical examination, a faint systolic murmur was heard in the mitral area.

Transthoracic echocardiography showed mild systolic dysfunction and left ventricular hypertrophy and mild mitral regurgitation.

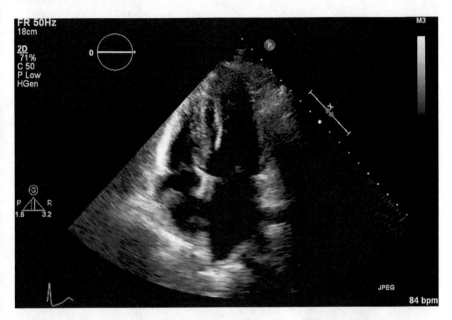

◻ **Fig. 8.1**   Apical four-chamber view shows a broad base and non-oscillating hyperecho density mass in the right atrium (*arrow*)

Transesophageal echocardiography was performed for further evaluation of right atrial mass.

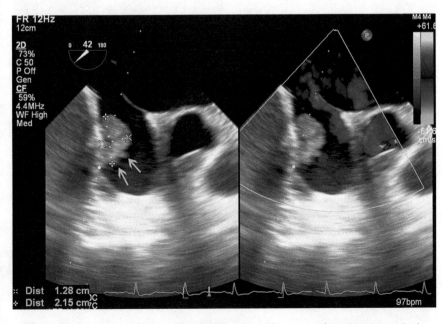

◻ **Fig. 8.2**   Mid-esophageal shot axis view shows a broad base mass about 21 × 14 mm in size, immobile (*arrow*) and with some small oscillating mass on it (*arrow heads*) indicative for a large vegetation versus mass

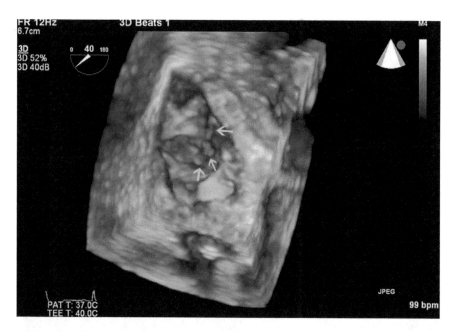

Fig. 8.3 3D zoom view confirms small mobile particle on mass (*arrow heads*)

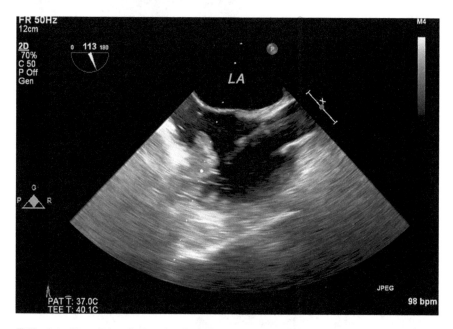

Fig. 8.4 Bicaval view depicts that the right atrial mass is near to a catheter which passes from the superior vena cava and tip of catheter is attached to the mass (*arrow*)

With respect to patient that was immune deficient due to chronic renal failure and diabetes mellitus, the possibility of vegetation was high; blood culture was sent, and catheter was removed, and *Staphylococcus aureus* was depicted, so treatment with antibiotic was started, and after 4 weeks, transesophageal echocardiography showed that the size of the vegetation decreased significantly, and then patient was referred for CABG and vegetation remnant resection.

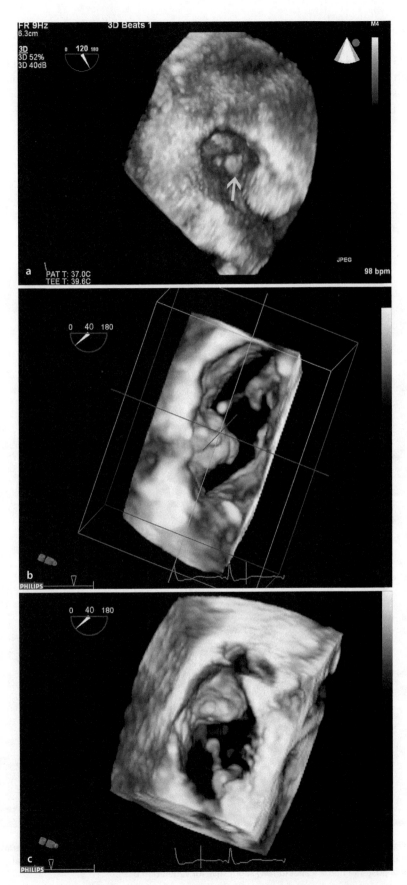

◘ **Fig. 8.5** 3D zoom view in 120° (*en face view*) shows the superior vena cava and a catheter in it **a**; cropping along *blue* axis **b** depicts the mass and catheter together in one view and demonstrates that mass and catheter are separated from each other completely **c**

8.2   Case 2: Infective Endocarditis on Mitral Valve

A 23-year-old man with a history of idiopathic thrombocytopenia (ITP) presented with fever, malaise, and weight loss from 2 weeks ago. In physical examination, a pansystolic murmur IV/VI in the mitral area was heard.

TTE showed normal LV size and systolic function.

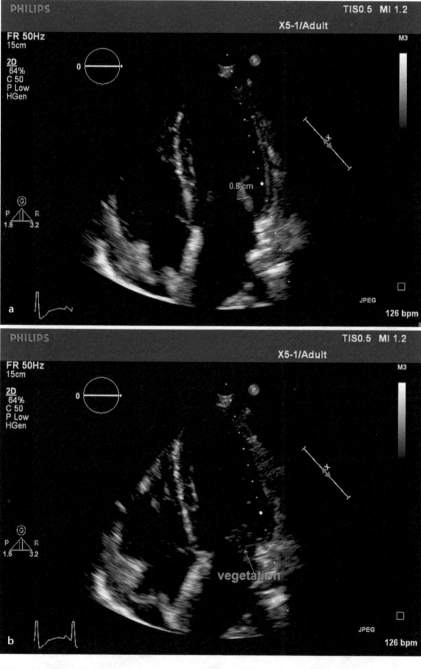

◘ **Fig. 8.6** Apical four-chamber view shows that the mitral valve is structurally thick, posterior mitral leaflet thickness is about 8 mm **a**, and there is an oscillating mass attached to the atrial side of posterior mitral leaflet (*arrow*) suggestive for vegetation **b**

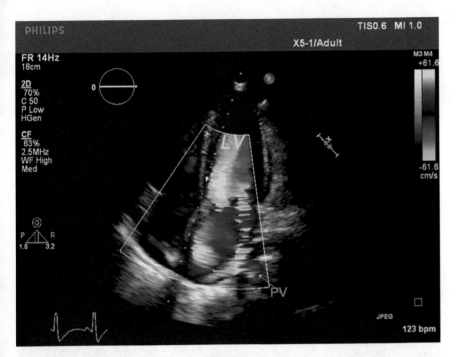

□ **Fig. 8.7** Apical four-chamber view shows an eccentric mitral regurgitation which is swirling toward the lateral wall of the left atrium and flow reversal in the pulmonary vein indicative for severe mitral regurgitation. *PV* pulmonary vein

TEE was performed for more evaluation of mitral valve and for rule-out of infective endocarditis and its complications such as abscess formation or leaflet perforation.

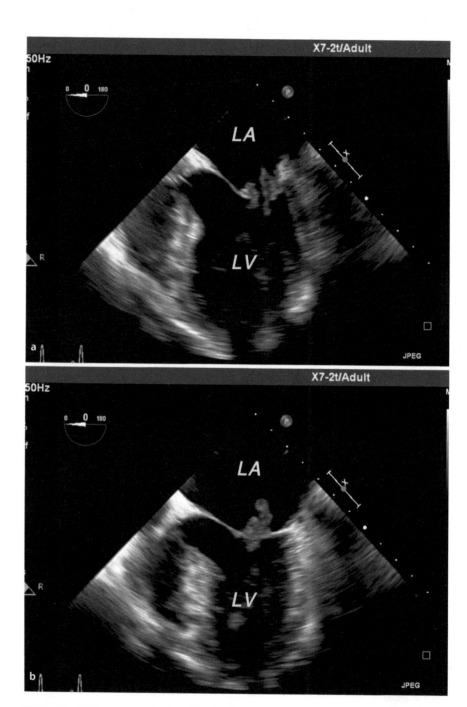

■ **Fig. 8.8** Mid-esophageal 0° **a**, **b** and X-plane long-axis views **c** and commissural view **d** depict a large vegetation attached to the atrial side of each leaflet; posterior mitral leaflet vegetation (*arrow*) is larger than anterior mitral leaflet vegetation **a**, **c**. *LA* left atrium, *LV* left ventricle

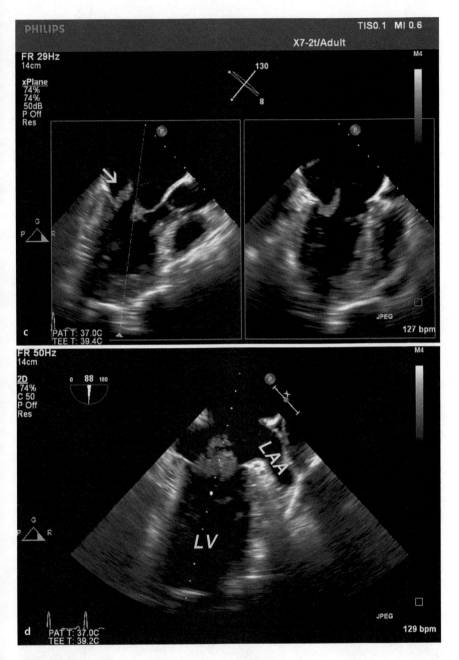

■ **Fig. 8.8** (continued)

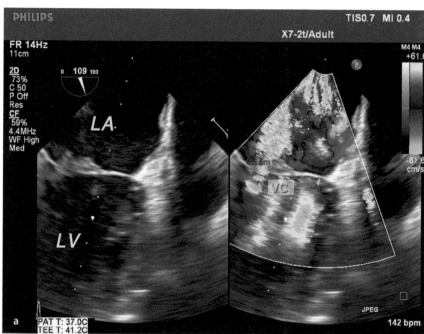

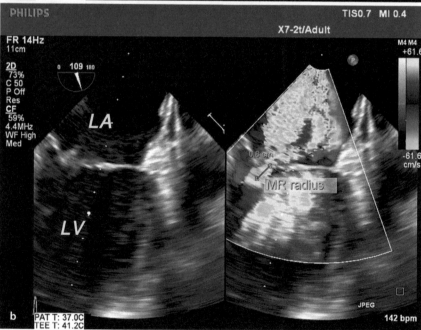

◨ **Fig. 8.9** Color Doppler flow study reveals severe mitral regurgitation; MRVC is about 6 mm **a** and MR radius is 8 mm **b** and MR volume by PISA method is measured more than 80 mL in which it is in favor of severe MR. *PISA* proximal isovelocity surface area, *MRVC* mitral regurgitation vena contracta

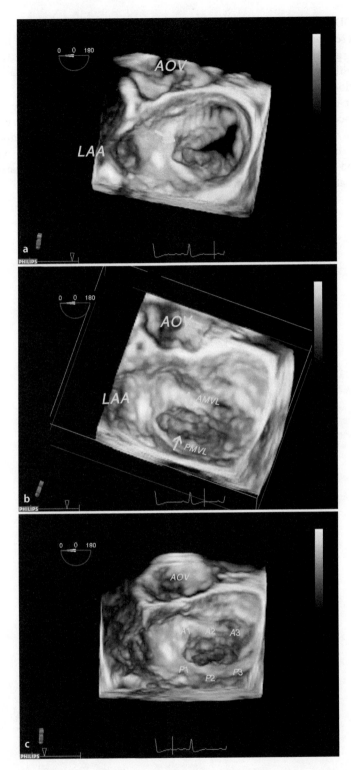

□ **Fig. 8.10** 3D zoom surgical view of MV shows involvement of anterolateral commissure and flail of MV in this area (*arrow*) **a** two purple masses (*arrows*) on all scallops of posterior and anterior mitral leaflet **b, c** indicative for large vegetation. *LAA* left atrial appendage, *AMVL* anterior mitral valve leaflet, *PMVL* posterior mitral valve leaflet, *AOV* aortic valve

For 3D zoom surgical view acquisition, select 3D zoom option. After selecting, you can see two 2D orthogonal views and a selecting green pan, put the least size selecting green pan on the mitral valve including annulus, and then select 3D zoom again; with z rotate option, you can put AOV to the top (in surgical view, AOV is in 12 o'clock and LAA is in 9 o'clock).

The patient was sent for infective endocarditis work-up; blood culture revealed enterococci microorganism; antibiotic therapy was started; after 2 weeks, echocardiography was performed again; there were no changes in second echocardiographic data compared to first study except for size of vegetation in which it increased up to 25 mm, and blood culture was persistently positive regardless of appropriate antibiotic therapy, so the patient was referred for surgery.

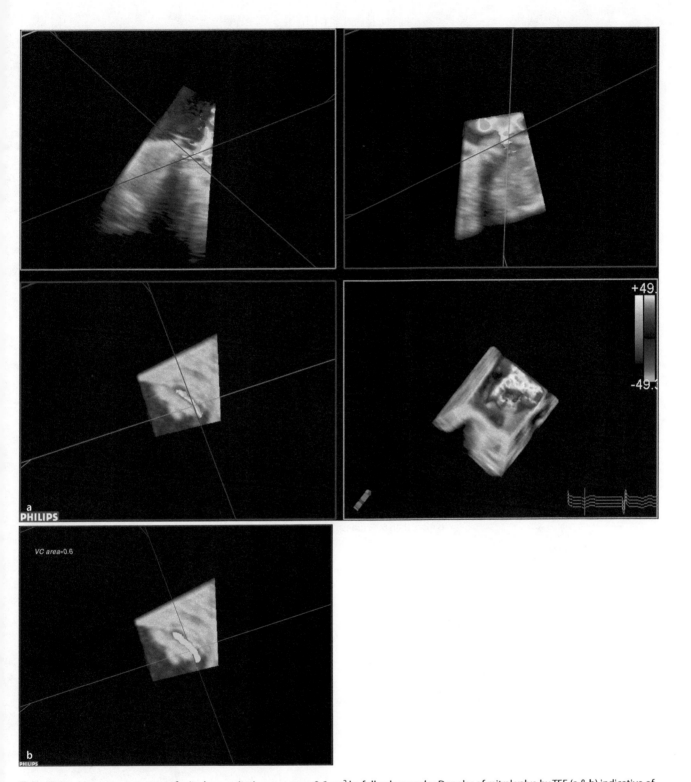

◪ **Fig. 8.11** Vena contracta area of mitral regurgitation measures 0.6 cm² by full volume color Doppler of mitral valve by TEE (**a** & **b**) indicative of severe mitral regurgitation

8.3   Case 3: Infective Endocarditis on the Aortic Valve

Patient is a 60-year-old man with history of fever and weight loss from 2 weeks ago who presented with dyspnea on excretion. In physical examination, a diastolic murmur grade III/VI was heard in aortic area.

Transthoracic echocardiography showed severe aortic regurgitation; transesophageal echocardiography was performed for evaluating the cause of aortic regurgitation.

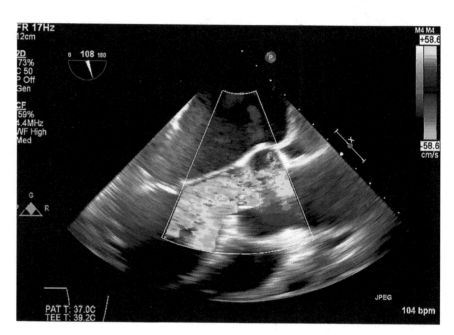

☐ **Fig. 8.12** Long-axis view shows severe aortic regurgitation, AIVC = 8 mm, and width AI/LVOT is more than 60% (doesn't show in this view)

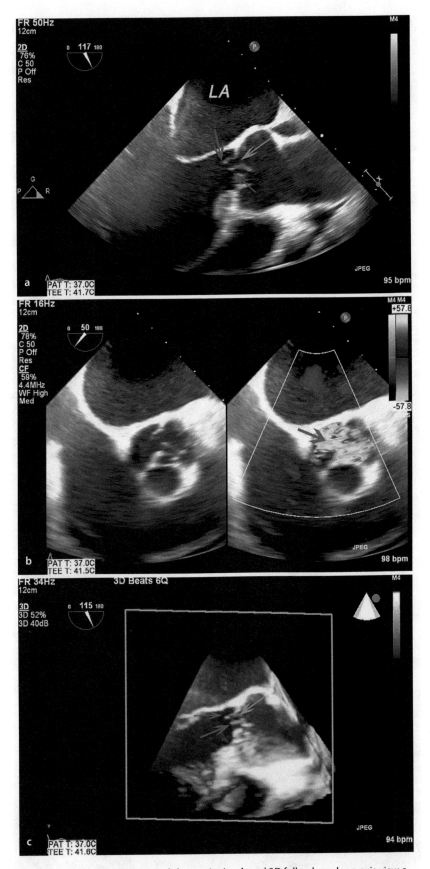

■ **Fig. 8.13** 2D long-axis view **a** and short-axis view **b** and 3D full-volume long-axis view **c** depict a defect of left coronary cusp (*green arrow*) **a, c** with some hypermobile oscillating mass (*pink arrows*) **a, c** on it suggestive for perforation of the left coronary cusp and vegetation on it; it is of notice that aortic regurgitation jet originates exactly from the site of perforation (*arrow*, **b**)

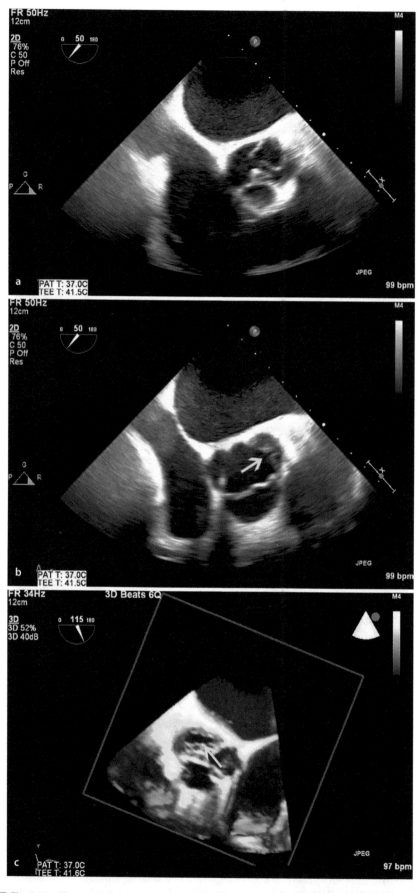

■ **Fig. 8.14** Short-axis view in systole **a** and diastole **b**, *arrow* and 3D zoom with cropping along red axis **c**, *arrow* show that site of perforation is on the left coronary cusp

The patient was admitted and evaluated for infective endocarditis and after 4-week antibiotic therapy was sent for aortic valve replacement.

References

1. Baddour LM, Wilson WR, Bayer AS, Fowler Jr VG, Tleyjeh IM, Rybak MJ, et al. Infective endocarditis in adults: diagnosis, antimicrobial therapy, and management of complications: a scientific statement for healthcare professionals from the American Heart Association. Circulation. 2015;132(15):1435–86.
2. Badour LM, Schildberg FW, Suri RM, Wilson WR. Cardiovascular infection. In: Mann DL, Zipes DP, Libby PP, Bonow RO, Braunwald E, editors. Braunwald's heart disease, vol. 2. 10th ed. Philadelphia, PA: Elsevier Saunders; 2015. p. 1524–50.

ASDs and PFO

Videos can be found in the electronic supplementary material in the online version of the chapter.
On http://springerlink.com enter the DOI number given on the bottom of the chapter opening page.
Scroll down to the Supplementary material tab and click on the respective videos link.

© Springer International Publishing AG 2017
H. Sadeghian, Z. Savand-Roomi, *3D Echocardiography of Structural Heart Disease*,
DOI 10.1007/978-3-319-54039-9_9

9.1   Atrial Septal Defects and PFO

Atrial septal defect (ASD) is the defect of interatrial septum, there are four types of ASD:

1. ASD ostium secundum type,
2. ASD ostium primum type,
3. ASD sinus venosus,
4. Unroofing coronary sinus.

9.1.1   ASD Ostium Secundum TYPE

ASD ostium secundum is the most common form of ASD (80%) [1], it is a defect in midportion of the interatrial septum, interatrial septum consists of two septums, septum primum and septum secundum, septum primum is the first interatrial septum that separates the common atria from each other, septum secundum originates from the roof and right side of the septum primum [2].

In fetal life, midportion of interatrial septum has a defect which consists of third of interatrial septum and there is a membrane named «membrane of vieuscence» or flap valve [2] from proximal part of this defect into left atrium, in fetal heart, the membrane of vieuscence is pathognomonic of diagnosis of left atrium. The direction of flow in fetal heart is from right atrium toward left atrium due to the fact that the lungs are not active in fetal life and pulmonary veins only export about 5–10% of blood flow of fetal circulation. The systemic venous flow which contains about 90% of flow of total circulation enters in the right atrium and then about 40% of this flow across through the defect of interatrial septum into the left atrium. After birth, with the first inspiration, the lungs and pulmonary circulation will be activated and the pulmonary veins export about 50% of flow and left atrial pressure will be 2–3 mmHg greater than right atrial pressure [3]. And normally, no flow will pass via interatrial septum [2]. The foramen ovalis which is just in the site of the first defect in interatrial septum is patent in up to 25% of normal population until adulthood but no flow passes via it except in the circumstances which right atrial pressure rise (like crying in neonates and infants or during valsalva maneuver in adult) and cause the blood passes via patent foramen ovalis from right atrium toward left atrium.

The ASD ostium secundum is a defect just in the site of fetal defect in interatrial septum and is due to excessive resorption of the septum primum or failure of adequate formation of septum secundum [2].

The patient may be completely asymptomatic until adulthood. In physical examination, fixed S2 splitting may be heard.

ECG is normal or shows right axis deviation and incomplete right bundle branch block [1].

The echocardiographic hallmark of diagnosis of ASD is right atrial and ventricular dilation. When ASD is large enough to produce a significant left to right shunt, it causes right atrial and ventricular dilation [3].

The ASD ostium secundum needs intervention when shunt is more than 1.5/1 or produces symptoms.

Only ASD ostium secundum type can be referred for ASD device closure in the presence of good rims of ASD to neighboring structures and not too large ASD.

The rims of ASD is the distance of ASD to neighboring valves or veins.

Anterior rims of ASD consist of two major valves:

1. Anterosuperior rim: Rim to aortic valve,
2. Anteroinferior rim: Rim to tricuspid valve.

Posterior rims of ASD consist of two major veins:

1. Posterosuperior rim: Rim to superior vena cava,
2. Posteroinferior rim: Rim to inferior vena cava [3].

Besides, rim to coronary sinus and rim to right pulmonary veins are important. The rim to coronary sinus is not always possible to measure due to the fact that the coronary sinus can be visualized in deep TEE 0° view and sometimes in this view, the ASD could not be visualized.

There are many published articles emphasize on the fact that rim to aortic valve is not important.

For other rims, it should be more than 5 or 7 mm in different studies and with different devices depending on the amount of opening of borders of device.

And about the size of ASD, the question is when ASD is too large?

The maximum size of ASD which can be closed is 36 mm on two-dimensional echocardiography or 41 mm with balloon sizing.

Balloon sizing diameter of ASD usually is greater than ASD size by two-dimensional echocardiography. Mean balloon diameter is 5 mm greater than ASD by two-dimensional echocardiography but it is of notice that for larger ASDs this difference is less. The final device size is 1–2 mm greater than ASD balloon sizing [4]. The exact device size can be calculated with this formula considering that final device size is 1–2 mm greater than balloon occlusive diameter (BOD):

BOD = 0.773 × ASD size by TEE + 8.562 [5].

About 3D echocardiography, Abdel-Massih ET colleagues found that mean ASD diameter by 3D echocardiography is 2 mm less than the size by balloon sizing. They reported that the mean maximal diameter measured by 3D–TEE was 20 ± 15 mm (range 10–28) while the mean BSD was 22 ± 4.8 mm (range 9–31) [6].

ASD ostium secundum is considered large when the diameter is more than 20 mm, ASD ostium secundum greater than 5 mm is an ASD in which intervention may be needed.

ASD ostium secundum referred for intervention with the following criteria:

1. Qp/Qs ≥ 1.5/1,
2. Significant RV dilation,
3. Elevated PAPs,
4. Paradoxical emboli,
5. The presence of symptoms.

9.2 ASD Pulmonary Hypertension

ASD rarely produces pulmonary hypertension. But if pulmonary hypertension occurs in ASD, it will go toward Isenmenger syndrome with lower PAP compared to other left to right shunts.

Why in ASD patients pulmonary hypertension occurs less than other left to right shunts?

1. In VSD, left to right shunt is a systemic phenomena, so blood enters from LV into RV in systole and directly to pulmonary artery, in consequence, the systemic pressure transfers to pulmonary artery.

2. In PDA patients, blood goes from aorta to pulmonary artery both in systole and in diastole, so pulmonary artery is in front of systemic pressure.

3. In ASD patients, left atrial pressure is 2–3 mmHg greater than right atrial pressure, so blood goes from LA to RA and RV which are the cavities that can accept volume overload. In consequence, RA and RV will be dilated with mildly elevated pulmonary artery pressure [3].

9.2.1 What is the Definition of Pulmonary Hypertension?

Pulmonary hypertension is defined as mean pulmonary artery pressure more than 25 mmHg [7]. It should be defined by cardiac catheterism. PAPs more than 36 mmHg is considered as mildly elevated and PAPs more than 50 mmHg is considered as significantly elevated.

In many references, pulmonary hypertension exists if pulmonary arterial pressure is more than 2/3 systemic arterial pressure and pulmonary vascular resistance is more than 2/3 of systemic vascular resistance.

9.2.2 How We Can Calculate Pulmonary and Systemic Vascular Resistance by Echocardiography?

Pulmonary vascular resistance is calculated as follows:

Mean pulmonary arterial pressure/pulmonary cardiac output.

Systemic vascular resistance is calculated as follows:

Mean systemic arterial pressure/systemic cardiac output.

In normal condition, mean pulmonary arterial pressure is about 10 mmHg and pulmonary cardiac output is about 5 L/min, so pulmonary vascular resistance would be 10/5 = 2 unit.

In addition, mean systemic arterial pressure is about 100 mmHg and systemic cardiac output is about 5 L/min, so systemic vascular resistance would be 100/5 = 20 unit.

It is obvious that systemic vascular resistance is tenfold more than pulmonary vascular resistance.

In most right to left shunts like VSD and PDA, pulmonary hypertension exits when pulmonary vascular resistance is more than 2/3 systemic vascular resistance, or the figure of pulmonary vascular resistance is more than 8 unit.

If pulmonary vascular resistance is more than 12 unit, it will be considered as Isenmenger syndrome.

Pulmonary vascular resistance between 8 and 12 unit needs more evaluation, if pulmonary vascular bed is reactive to oxygen or nitrite oxide, the patient can be referred for intervention in the presence of VSD and PDA.

Reactive pulmonary vascular bed is defined as: more than 10% decrease in pulmonary vascular resistance with 10 min oxygen or nitrite oxide or more than 40% decrease in mean pulmonary arterial pressure.

For ASD, the figure of pulmonary vascular resistance is 5 unit for considering elevated pulmonary vascular resistance [1].

One of the good markers of elevated pulmonary vascular resistance in ASD is the amount of shunt, if Qp/Qs is less than 1.5, it will be considered as high risk and needs more evaluation [1]. One of the possible considerations in such circumstances is use of fenestrated devices for ASD closure or surgery of ASD patch with a valve which permits of some passage of flow through it.

9.3 ASD Sinus Venosus

ASD sinus venosus lies below SVC in most cases, but there are some reports about ASD sinus venosus below IVC. Abnormal right pulmonary venous return almost always accompanies ASD sinus venosus [1]. Right pulmonary veins consist of three veins (upper, middle, and lower) in most patients. ASD sinus venosus should be operated at the time of diagnosis. Because of abnormal pulmonary venous return, shunt is almost always significant irrespective of size of ASD.

9.4 ASD Ostium Primum

ASD ostium primum is a defect in septum primum and indeed endocardial cushion defect, it may be associated by an inlet VSD, anterior mitral leaflet cleft is almost always accompanies this type of ASD. ASD ostium primum should be referred for surgery in case of significant left to right shunt or significant mitral regurgitation. MR of these patients may progress in future years despite repair of mitral valve cleft.

9.5   Unroofing Coronary Sinus

Unroofing coronary sinus is a rare anomaly which is associated with left persistent SVC.

Left persistent SVC is a rare anomaly in which left SVC is not absorbed.left SVC exists in fetal circulation and carries blood to coronary sinus. It causes that coronary sinus be dilated. If there is only left persistent SVC without associated anomalies, it produces no symptoms [3].

By transthoracic echocardiography, in the parasternal long-axis view, coronary sinus is dilated, with agitated saline injection in left arm, the bubbles first appears in coronary sinus and then in right atrium and right ventricle.

Dilated coronary sinus has three differential diagnoses:

1. Left persistent SVC,
2. Abnormal pulmonary venous return to coronary sinus (usually right pulmonary veins),
3. In association with unroofing coronary sinus [3].

In unroofing coronary sinus, there is defect in wall of coronary sinus and blood passes through the coronary sinus to the left atrium causing desaturation of blood in left atrium and right to left shunt, this defect may be at origin of the coronary sinus, at its end near right atrium or on its length or a combination form. Unroofing coronary sinus should be operated at the time of diagnosis.

9.6   Case 1: Two ASDs Ostium Secundum with PFO and Flap

A 38-year-old man presented with dyspnea on exertion functional class II. Right atrium and ventricle were moderately dilated by transthoracic echocardiography.

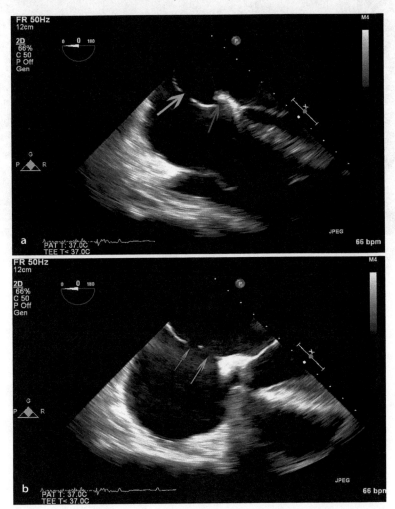

☐ **Fig. 9.1**   ASDs ostium secundum (*green arrows*) and PFO (*pink arrow*) are evident by TEE 0° view **a, b**

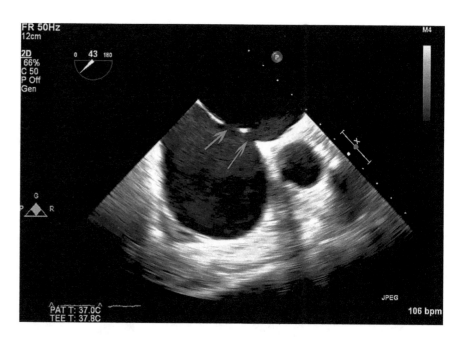

■ **Fig. 9.2**   ASDs are also evident by TEE short-axis view

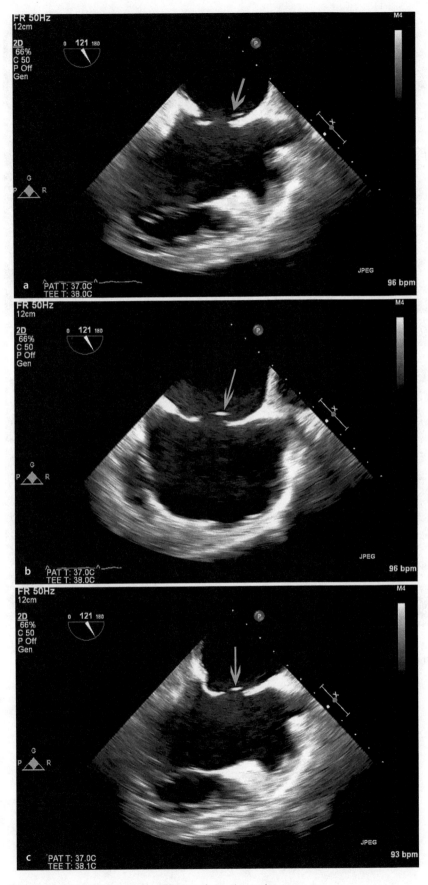

◘ Fig. 9.3 ASD flap is evident by TEE bicaval view (*arrows*) **a–c**

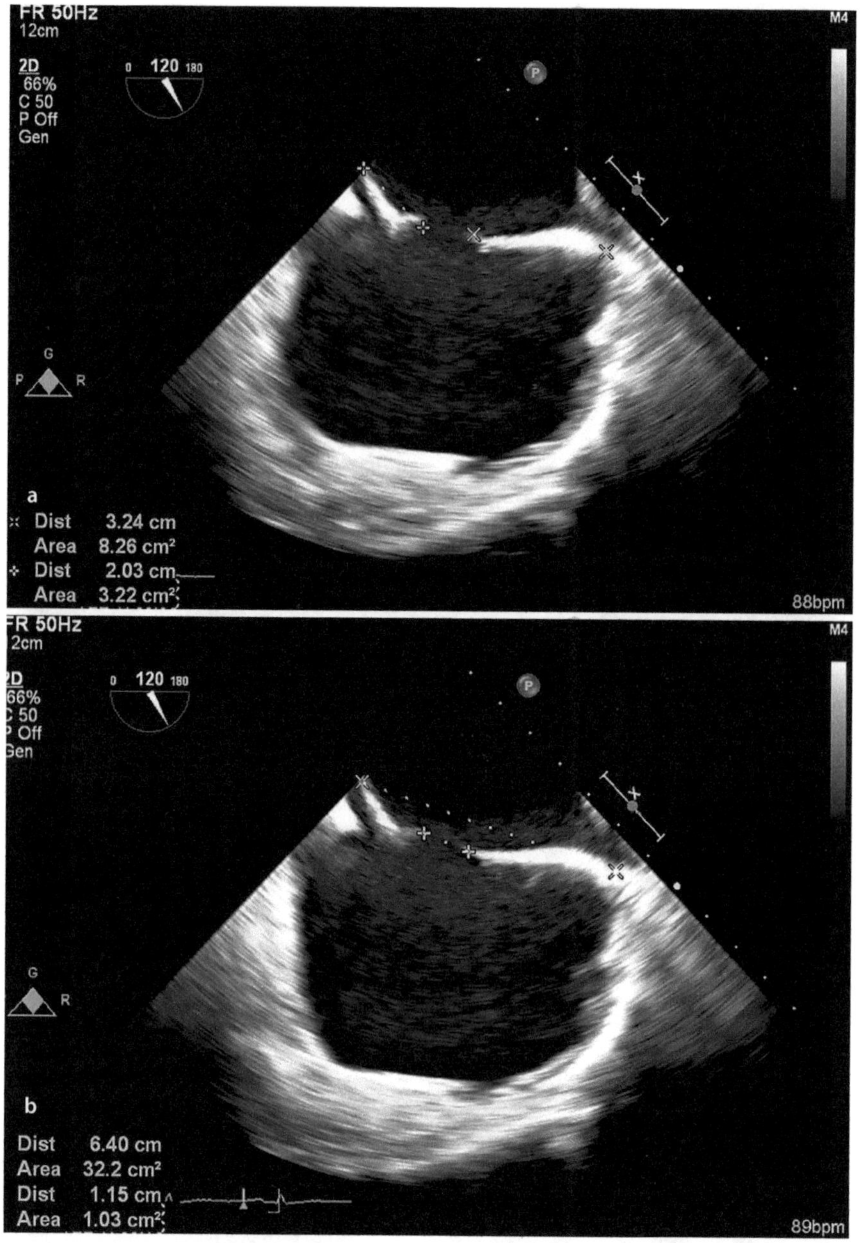

Fig. 9.4 ASD rim to SVC and IVC measure 32 and 20 mm, respectively, by TEE bicaval view **a**, the ratio of ASD/IAS measures 12/64 mm in this view **b**

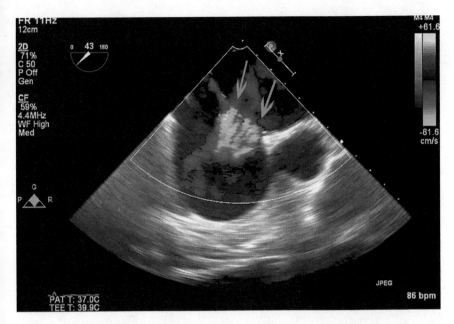

◼ **Fig. 9.5**   Left to right shunt of two ASDs is evident by TEE short-axis view (*arrows*)

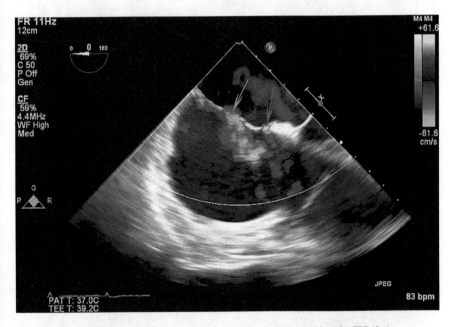

◼ **Fig. 9.6**   ASD flow (*green arrow*) and PFO flow (*pink arrow*) are evident by TEE 0° view

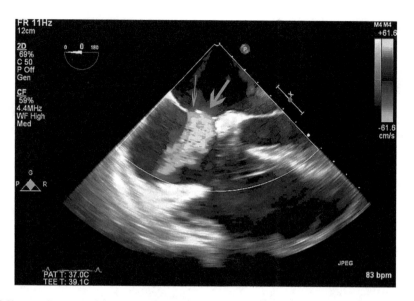

Fig. 9.7 Two ASDs flow are evident by TEE 0° view (*arrows*)

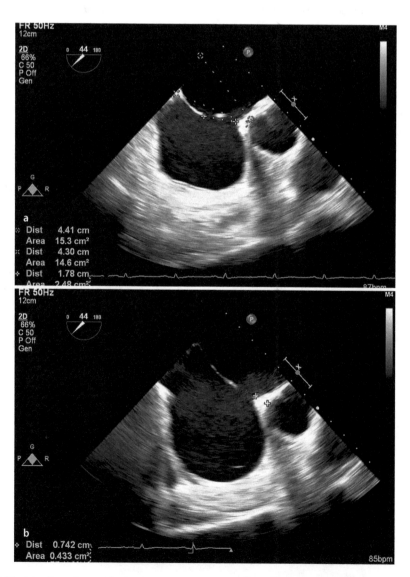

Fig. 9.8 Considering two ASDs together, the ratio of ASD/IAS measures 18/43 by TEE short-axis view, atrial depth measures 44 mm **a** and rim to aorta measures 7.4 mm in this view **b**

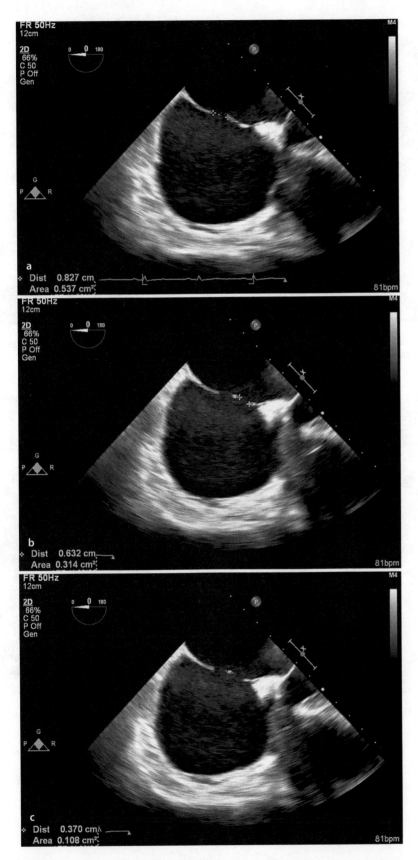

■ **Fig. 9.9** One ASD measures 8.3 mm **a** and another one measures 6.3 mm **b** in TEE 0° view, the flap between ASDs measures 3.7 mm **c**

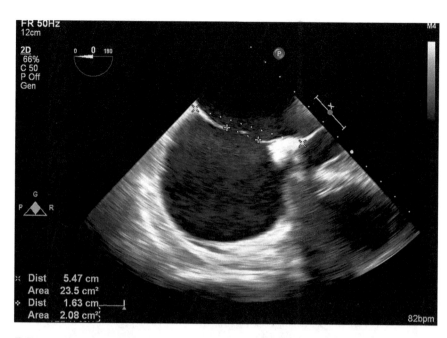

Fig. 9.10   Considering two ASDs together, the ratio of ASDs/IAS measures 16/55 mm in TEE 0° view

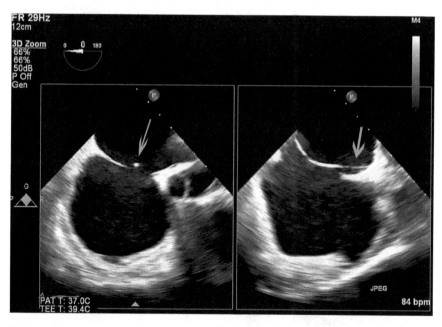

Fig. 9.11   Two orthogonal plane of ASD shows two ASDs and the flap (*arrows*) by 3D modality

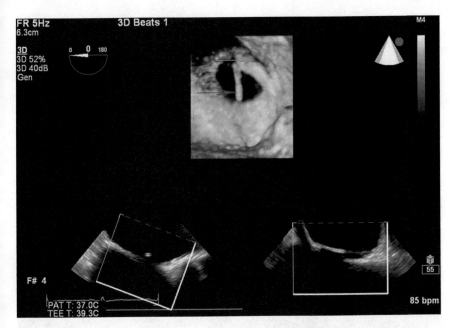

☐ **Fig. 9.12** There are two ASDs ostium secundum, which are separated by a flap (*pink arrow*), one is larger which is seen in the left side and another is smaller which is located in the right side with I crop from LA side, the PFO is marked by *green arrow*

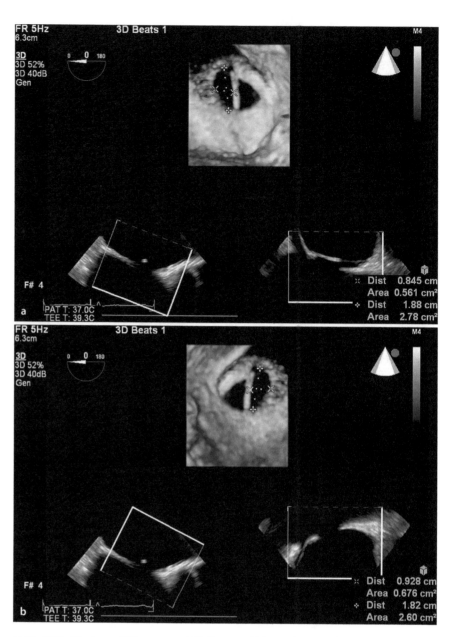

Fig. 9.13 The larger ASD measures 19*8.5 mm and is located in the left side from LA side **a** and is located in the right side from RA side and measures 18*9 mm **b**

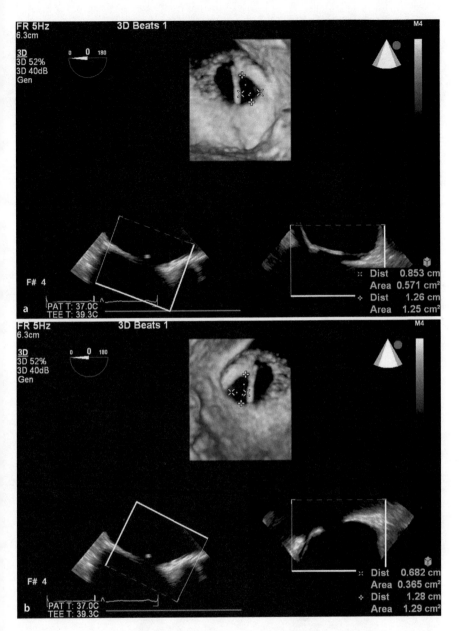

□ **Fig. 9.14**   The smaller ASD measures 13*8.5 mm and is located in the right side from LA side **a** and is located in left side from RA side and measures 13*7 mm from RA side **b**

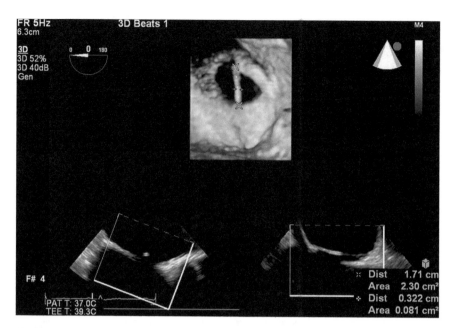

■ **Fig. 9.15**   The flap measures 3*17 mm from LA side

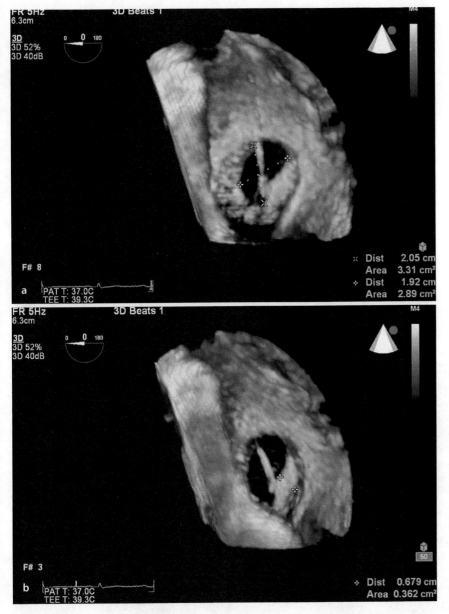

□ Fig. 9.16 Considering two ASDs together, they measure 21*19 mm from RA side **a**, distance between ASD and PFO measures 6.7 mm from RA side **b**

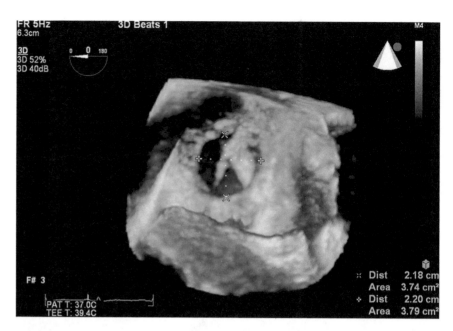

Fig. 9.17 Considering two ASDs and PFO, they measure 22*22 mm from LA side

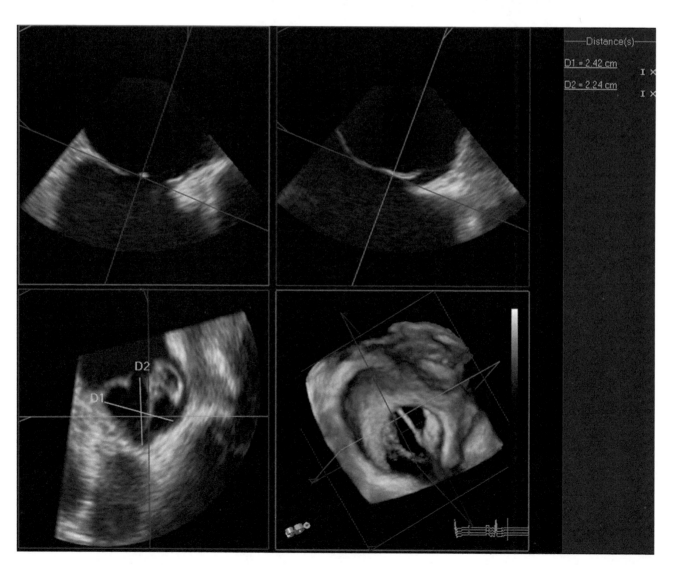

Fig. 9.18 Considering two ASDs together, ASD measures 22*24 mm with 3DQ

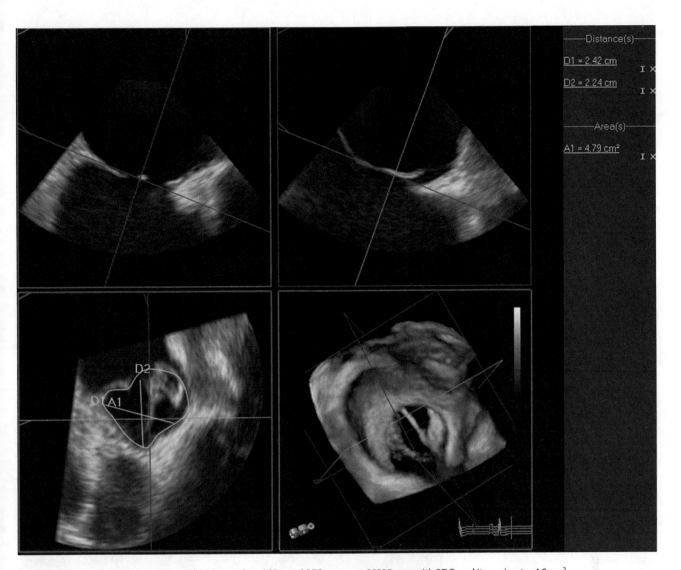

◘ **Fig. 9.19**   Considering two ASDs and PFO together, ASDs and PFO measure 22*25 mm with 3DQ and its perimeter 4.8 cm²

Diagnosis   Two ASDs ostium secundum which are separated by a flap and one PFO.

Comment   ASDs device closure.

Lesson   3D echo has changed our imagination from ASD flaps. We can see now easily that flap is a thin tissue within ASD.

9.7   Case 2: ASD Ostium Secundum with a Flap

A 38-year-old woman presented with dyspnea on exertion functional class II of recent exacerbation.

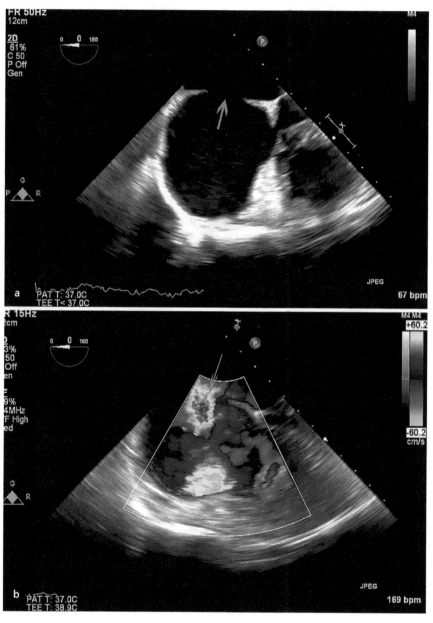

Fig. 9.20   ASD ostium secundum is seen in TEE 0° view by two-dimensional **a** and color Doppler study **b** (*arrows*)

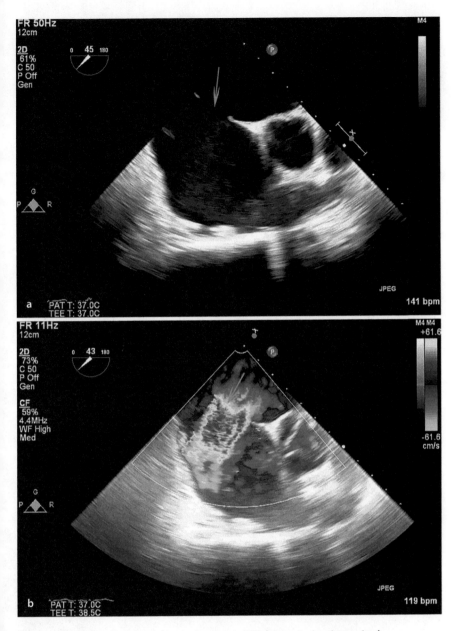

☐ **Fig. 9.21** ASD ostium secundum is also seen in TEE short-axis view (*arrows*) **a, b**

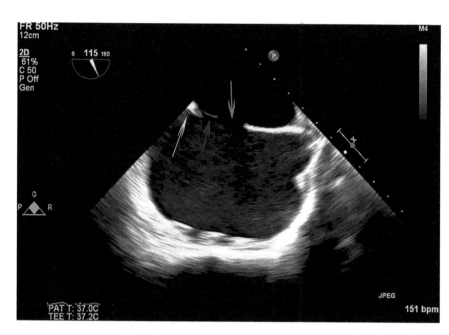

Fig. 9.22 ASD ostium secundum is also seen in TEE bicaval view (*arrow*). It is of notice that the rim of ASD to IVC has a thin part (*pink arrow*) and a thick part (*yellow arrow*)

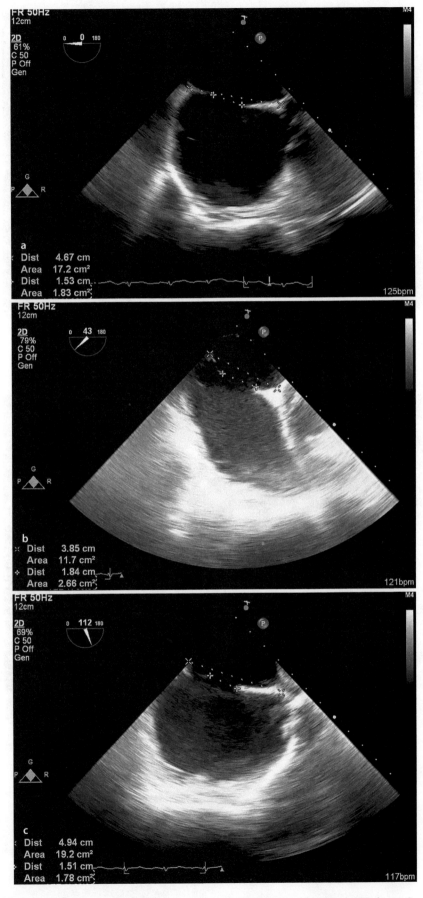

FR 50Hz
12cm

2D
61%
C 50
P Off
Gen

G

0 0 180

M4

P R

a
Dist   4.67 cm
Area   17.2 cm²
Dist   1.53 cm²
Area   1.83 cm²

125bpm

FR 50Hz
12cm

2D
79%
C 50
P Off
Gen

0 43 180

M4

G

P R

b
Dist   3.85 cm
Area   11.7 cm²
Dist   1.84 cm
Area   2.66 cm²

121bpm

FR 50Hz
12cm

2D
69%
C 50
P Off
Gen

0 112 180

M4

G

P R

c
Dist   4.94 cm
Area   19.2 cm²
Dist   1.51 cm
Area   1.78 cm²

117bpm

Fig. 9.23 The ratio of ASD/IAS measures 15/47 in TEE 0° view **a** and 18/39 in TEE short-axis view **b** and 15/49 in TEE bicaval view **c**

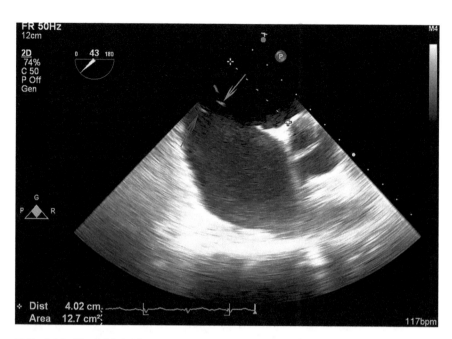

■ **Fig. 9.24** The atrial depth measures 40 mm in TEE short-axis view, it is of notice that a flap separates two ASDs from each other (*green arrow*), the eustachian valve is also evident in this view (*pink arrow*)

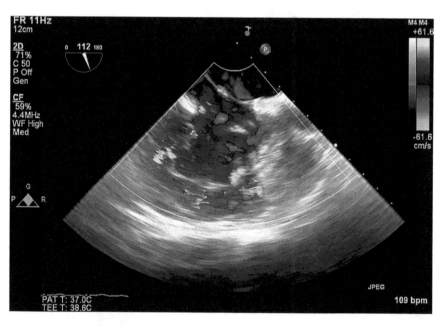

■ **Fig. 9.25** The ASD cannot be visualized in TEE bicaval view by some rotation

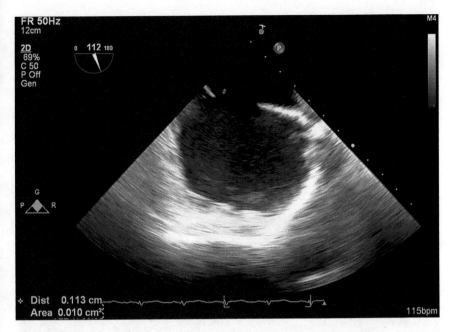

Fig. 9.26 The flap measures 1 mm in thickness in TEE bicaval view

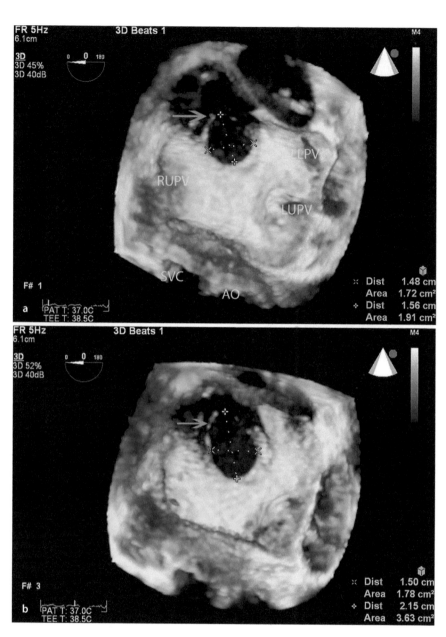

◘ Fig. 9.27 Two left pulmonary veins are fully visualized with 3D zoom from LA side, one right pulmonary vein (*upper*) is clear in the right side of the septum, ASD measures 16*15 mm in this view from LA side with direct measurement **a**, there is another ASD near the first one, they are separated by a flap (*arrows*) **a**, **b**, ASD measures 22*15 mm with some rotation of the image **b**. *SVC* superior vena cava, *AO* aorta, *LUPV* left upper pulmonary vein, *LLPV* left lower pulmonary vein, *RUPV* right upper pulmonary vein

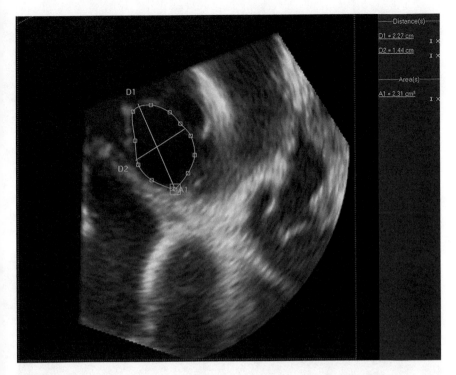

◻ Fig. 9.28 ASD measures 23*14 mm by 3DQ method, area is 23 mm²

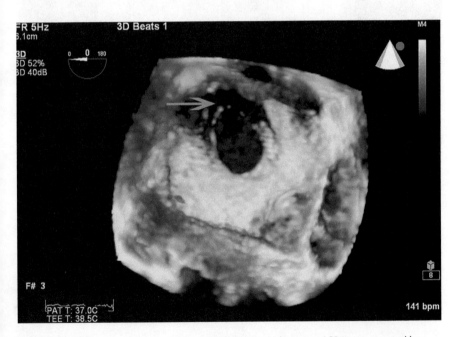

◻ Fig. 9.29 There is an ASD around the first ASD (*arrow*), these two ASDs are separated by a flap (3D zoom from LA side)

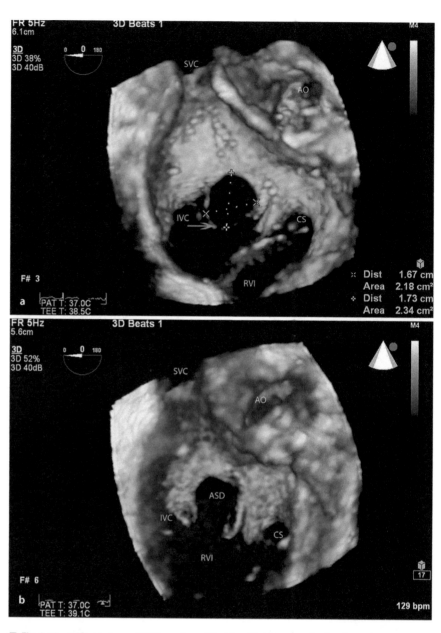

Fig. 9.30 ASD measures 17*17 mm from RA side with 3D zoom, the flap (*arrow*) separates the second ASD from IVC **a**, coronary sinus is fully visualized in this view **b**. *SVC* superior vena cava, *IVC* inferior vena cava, *AO* aorta, *RVI* right ventricular inflow tract

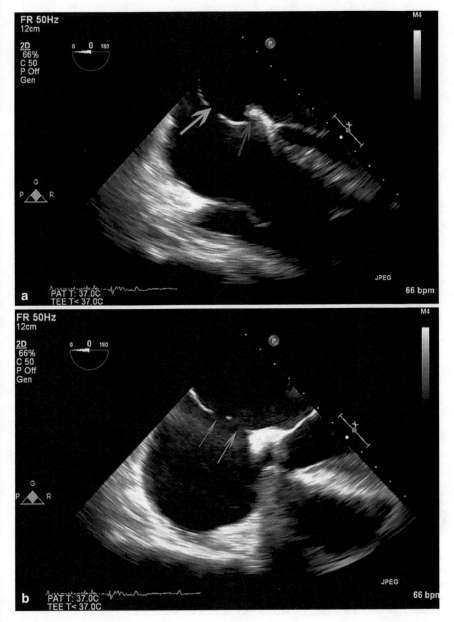

■ **Fig. 9.31** ASD from RA side (*arrow*) **a**, ASD and coronary sinus (*arrows*) (CS) with more rotation **b**

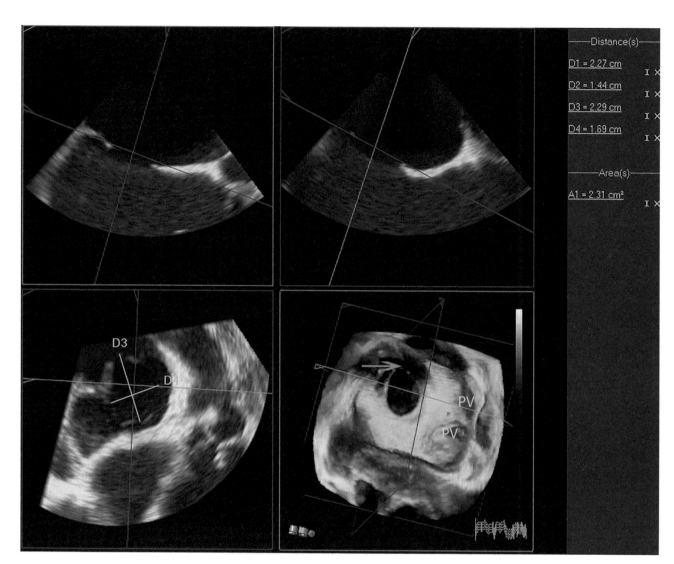

Fig. 9.32 3DQ measurement of ASD: (1) *Left upper quadrant of screen*: It looks at ASD from *green plane*, *red* and *blue* lines are placed vertical to each other, *blue* line at the margins of ASD and *red* line in the center of ASD, (2) *right upper quadrant of screen*: It looks at ASD from *red plane*, *green* and *blue* lines are placed vertical to each other, *blue* line at the margins of ASD and green line in the center of ASD, (3) *left lower quadrant of screen*: It looks at ASD from *blue plane*, *green* and *red* lines are placed vertical to each other in previous views, (4) *right lower quadrant of screen*: It is the 3D image of ASD, ASD measures 23*17 mm by 3DQ modality, pulmonary veins and the second ASD are fully visualized

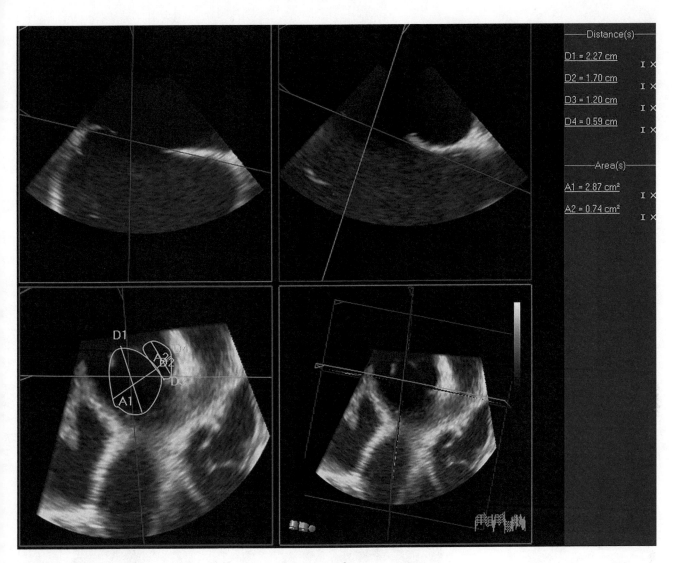

Fig. 9.33 The second ASD measures 12*6 mm and its surface is 0.7 cm²

Diagnosis   ASD ostium secundum with a flap. Maximum size of ASD is 18 mm by TEE two-dimensional echocardiography and 23 mm by TEE 3D echocardiography.

Comment   ASD Device closure.

Future aspects   Devices with more oval shape can be used for ASD device closure.

9.8   Case 3: ASD Ostium Secundum with Loose Posteroinferior Rims

A 35-year-old woman presented with dyspnea on exertion functional class II of 1 month exacerbation.

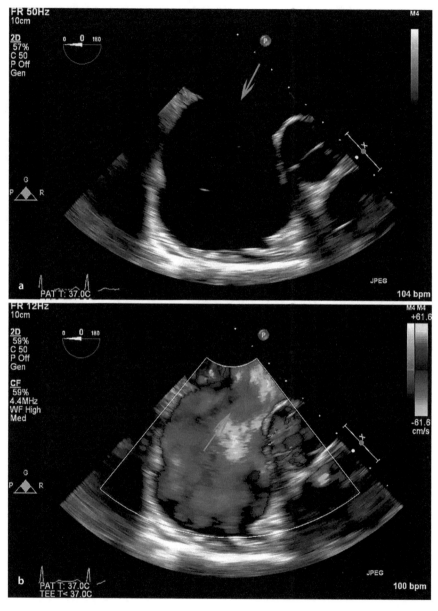

■ **Fig. 9.34** Large ASD ostium secundum is seen in TEE 0° view by two-dimensional (*arrow*) **a** and color Doppler study (*arrow*) **b**

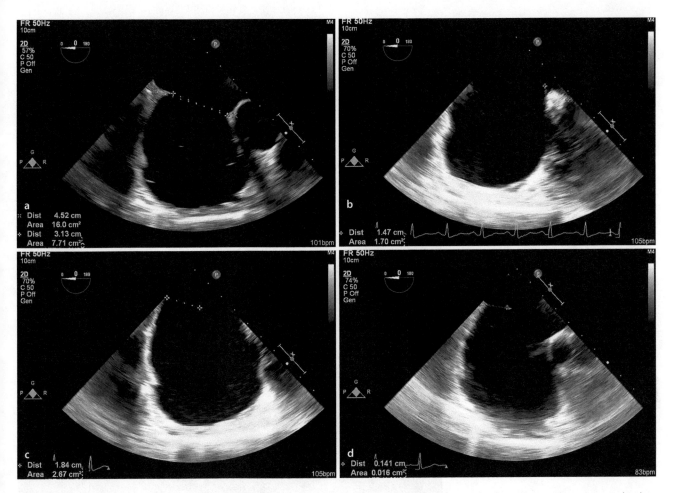

Fig. 9.35 ASD/IAS measures 31/45 mm in 0° view **a**, rim to mitral valve measures 15 mm **b** and posterior rim measures 18 mm **c**, posterior rim is very thin up to 1.4 mm **d**

9

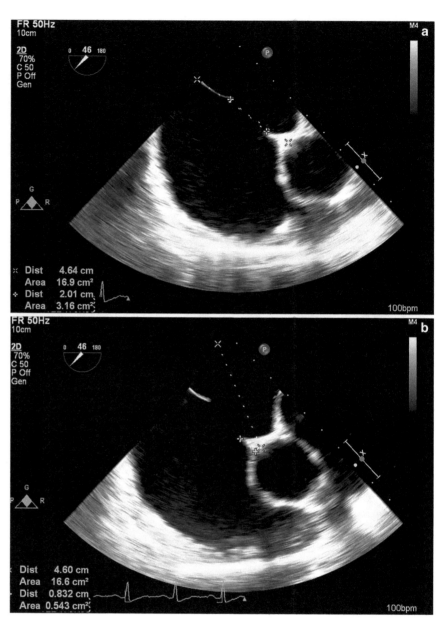

☐ **Fig. 9.36**   ASD/IAS measures 20/46 mm in 45° view **a**, rim to aortic valve measures 8 mm and atrial depth 46 mm **b**

9.8 · Case 3: ASD Ostium Secundum with Loose Posteroinferior Rims

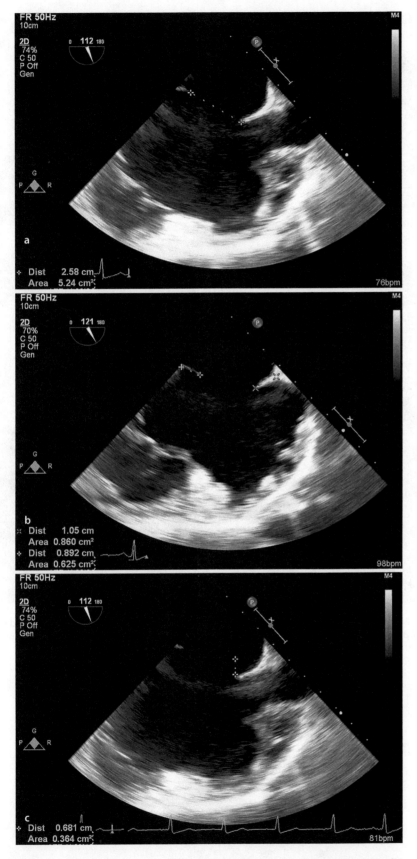

■ **Fig. 9.37** ASD measures 26 mm in TEE bicaval view **a**, rim to SVC measures 11 mm and rim to IVC 9 mm, respectively, in this view **b**, there is interatrial septal malalignment by this view about 6.8 mm **c**

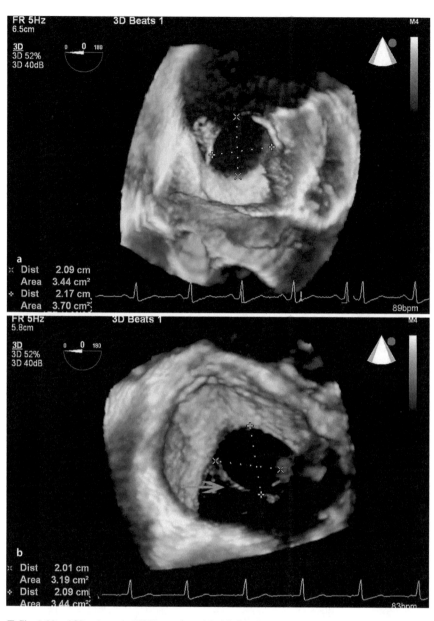

■ **Fig. 9.38** ASD measures 22*21 mm from LA side by 3D zoom **a** and 21*20 mm from RA side by direct measurement **b**. The hole which is seen in inferoposterior part of ASD is due to thin rim in this part (*arrow*)

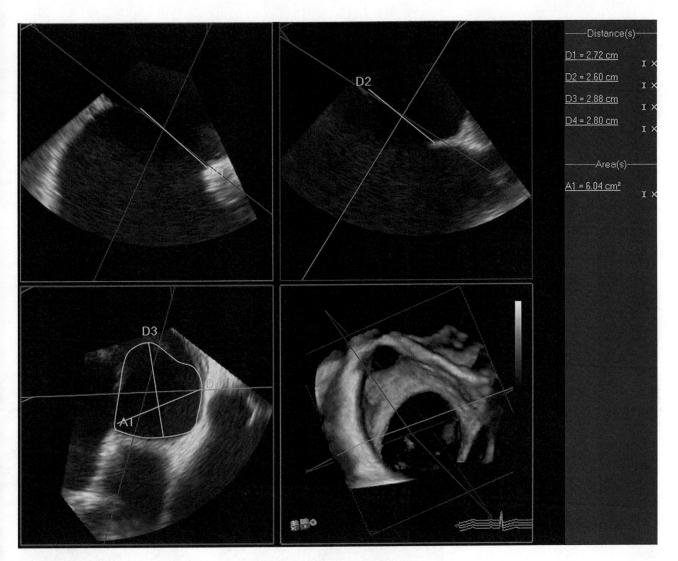

Distance(s)

D1 = 2.72 cm
D2 = 2.60 cm
D3 = 2.88 cm
D4 = 2.80 cm

Area(s)

A1 = 6.04 cm²

Fig. 9.39 Maximum size of ASD is 29 mm by 3DQ method

Diagnosis ASD ostium secundum type maximum size by 2D echo was 31 mm and by 3DQ was 29 mm with good rims but thin posteroinferior rim.

Comment Try for ASD device closure.

Lesson Thin rims cannot support device.

9.9   Case 4: ASD Ostium Secundum Near to SVC

An 18-year-old woman presented with dyspnea on exertion functional class II of recent exacerbation.

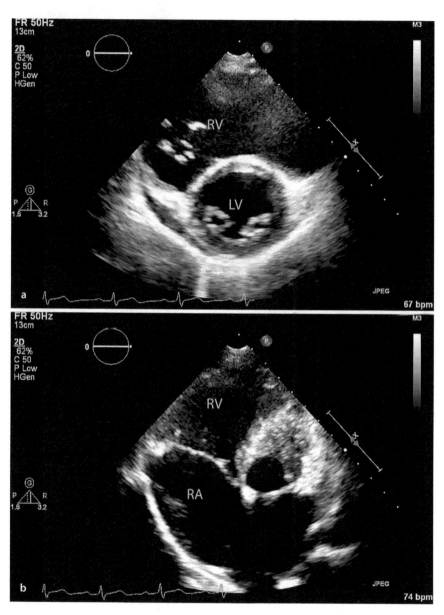

◻ **Fig. 9.40**   Severe RV dilation is evident in parasternal short-axis and apical four-chamber views **a**, **b**. *RA* right atrium, *RV* right ventricle, *LV* left ventricle

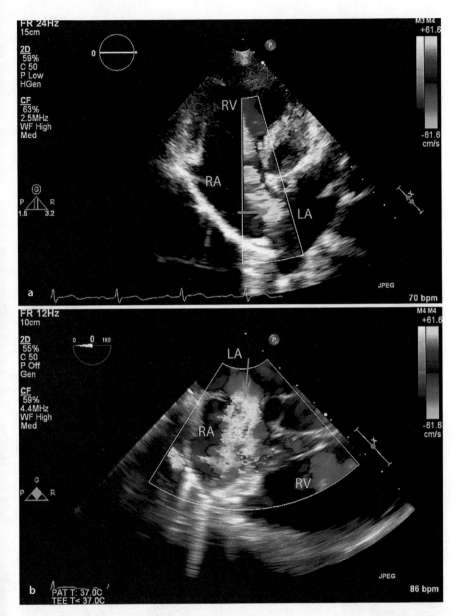

Fig. 9.41 ASD ostium secundum with left to right shunt (*arrows*) is evident in apical four-chamber and TEE 0° views **a**, **b**. *LA* left atrium, *RA* right atrium, *RV* right ventricle

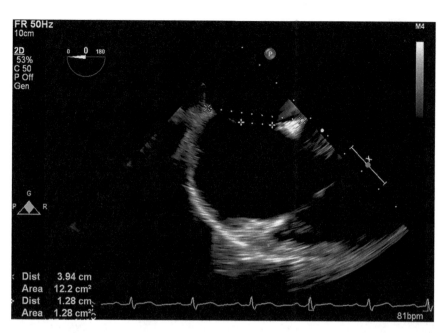

■ **Fig. 9.42**   ASD/IAS measures 13/39 in TEE 0° view

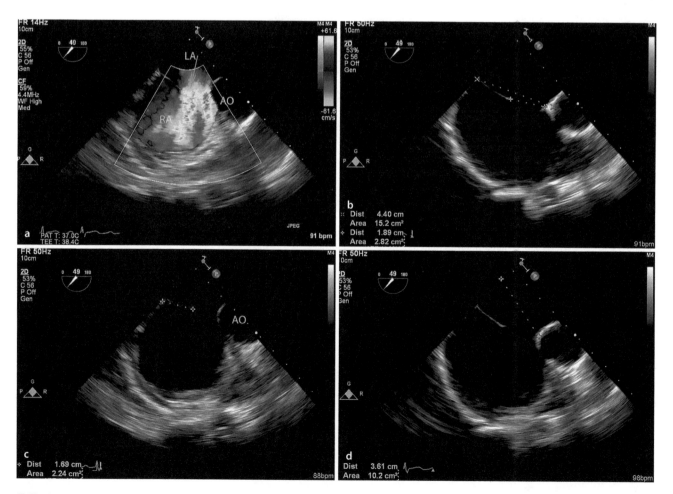

■ **Fig. 9.43**   ASD ostium secundum is also evident in TEE short-axis view (*arrow*) **a**, ASD/IAS measures 19/44 **b**, rim to aortic valve is deficient and opposite rim measures 17 mm **c** and atrial depth measures 36 mm **d**. *RA* right atrium, *LA* left atrium, *AO* aorta, *RV* right ventricle

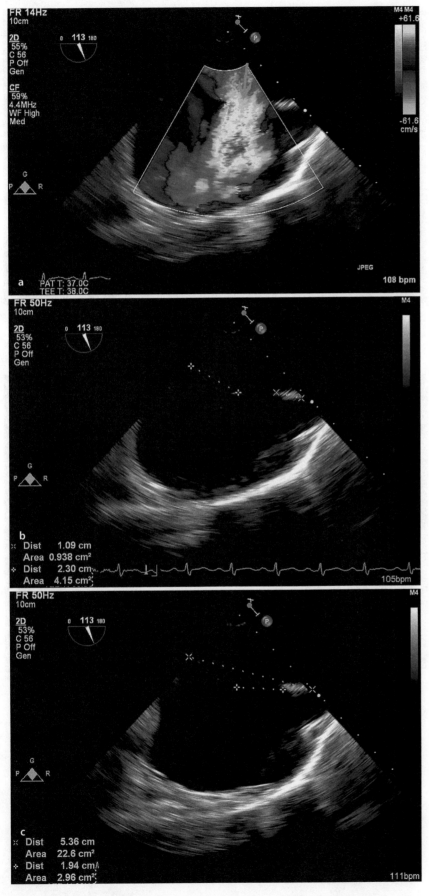

■ **Fig. 9.44** ASD is also evident in TEE bicaval view (*arrow*) **a**, rim to SVC and to IVC measures 23 and 11 mm, respectively **b**, ASD/IAS measures 19/54 mm **c**

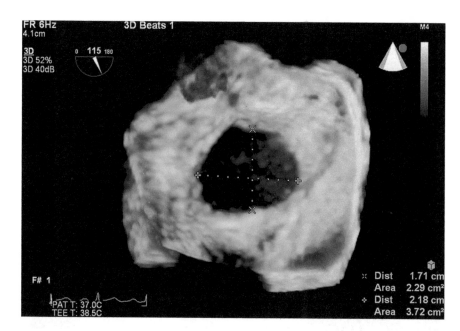

Fig. 9.45 ASD measures 22*17 mm from LA side by 3D zoom

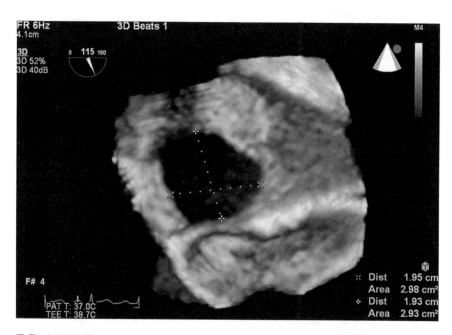

Fig. 9.46 ASD measures 20*19 mm from RA side by 3D zoom

9.9 · Case 4: ASD Ostium Secundum Near to SVC

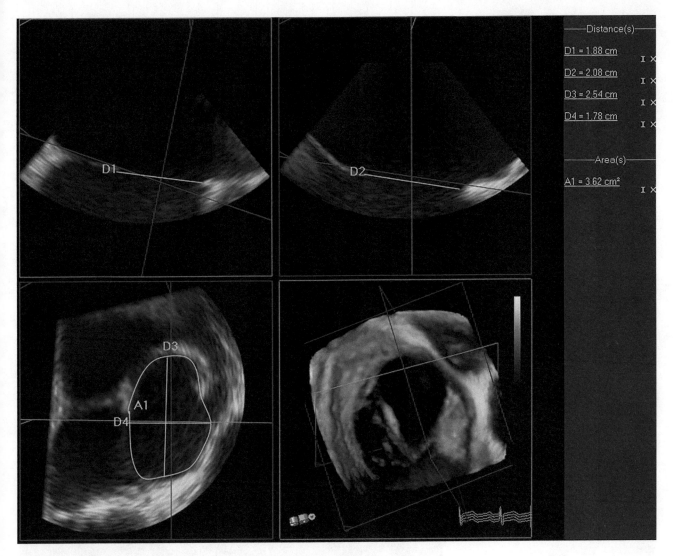

Fig. 9.47 ASD measures 19.1*25 mm by 3DQ method, area of ASD measures 36 mm²

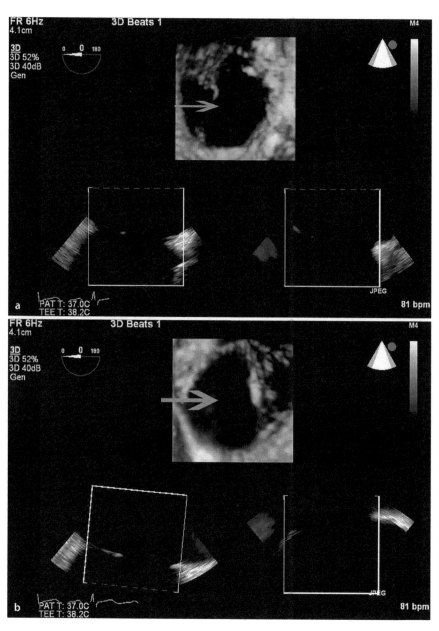

 ▪ **Fig. 9.48** I crop of ASD from LA **a** and RA **b** sides

Diagnosis   ASD ostium secundum with good rims and suitable size for ASD device closure.

Comment   ASD device closure.

This patient underwent ASD device closure, maximum size of ASD was 19 mm by TEE 2D and 25 mm by TEE 3D, balloon sizing of ASD measures 22 mm and final ASD device size was 24 mm.

9.10 Case 5: ASD Ostium Secundum with Partially Aneurysmal IAS

A 42-year-old woman presented with dyspnea on exertion functional class III.

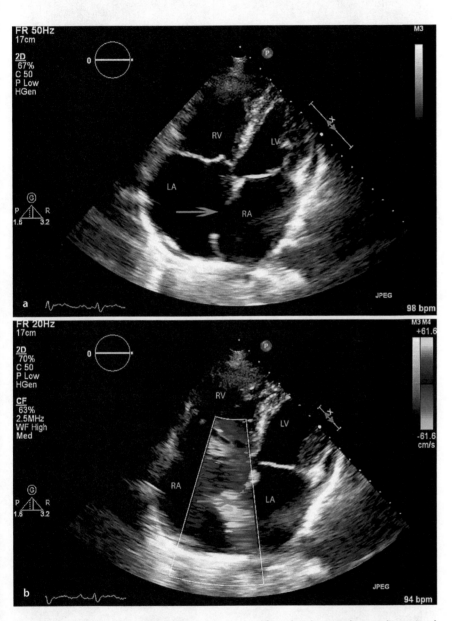

◧ **Fig. 9.49** ASD ostium secundum type is seen in apical four-chamber view by two-dimensional echocardiography **a** and color Doppler study (*arrows*) **b**, right ventricle is severely dilated. *LA* left atrium, *LV* left ventricle, *RA* right atrium, *RV* right ventricle

9

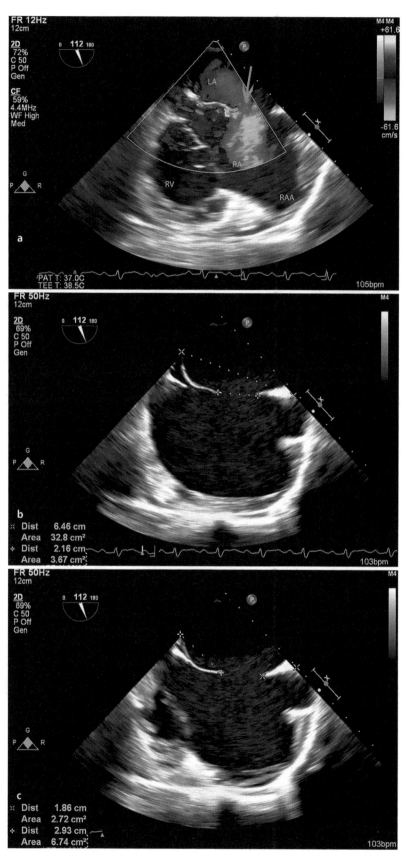

Fig. 9.50 The ASD ostium secundum is visualized in TEE bicaval view (*arrow*) **a**, ASD/IAS measures 22/65 mm in bicaval view **b**, rim to SVC measures 19 mm and rim to IVC measures 29 mm **c** in this view

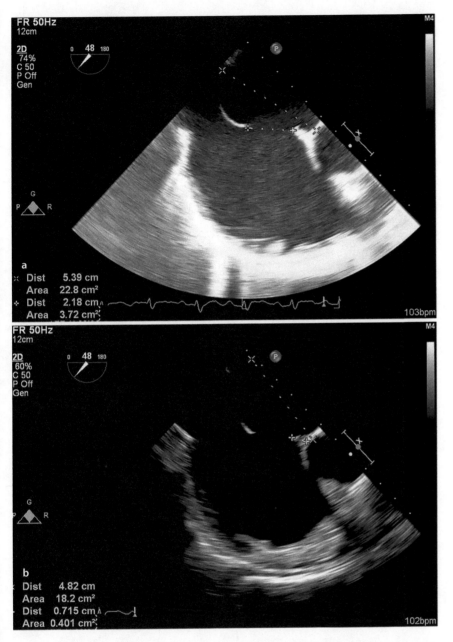

□ Fig. 9.51 ASD/IAS measures 22/54 mm in TEE short-axis view **a**, rim to aortic valve measures 7 mm and the opposite rim measures 30 mm in this view, atrial depth is 48 mm **b**

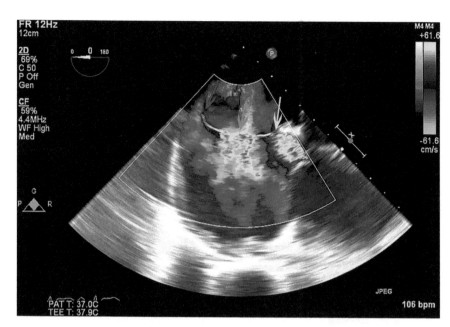

◻ Fig. 9.52   There is a large ASD ostium secundum in TEE 0° view (*green arrow*), there is another ASD in posterior part of IAS (*pink arrow*) and there is a small flow through PFO (*yellow arrow*)

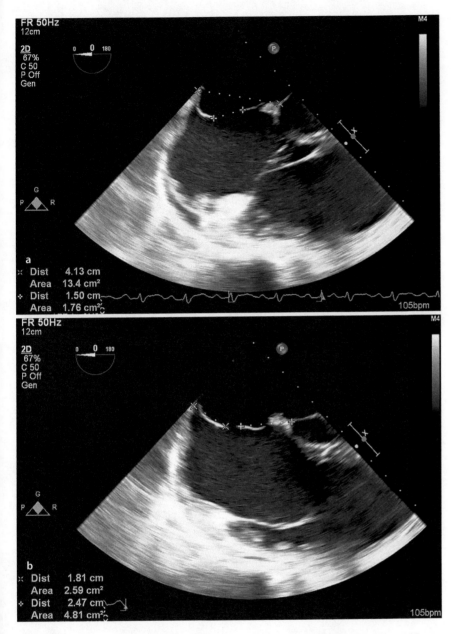

☐ **Fig. 9.53** ASD/IAS measures 15/41 mm in TEE 0° view **a**, rim to mitral valve measures 25 mm and posterior rim measures 18 mm **b** in this view

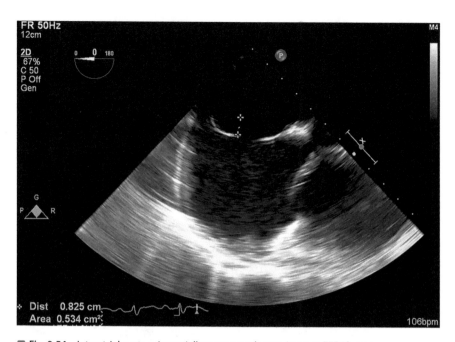

Fig. 9.54 Interatrial septum is partially aneurysmal up to 8 mm in TEE 0° view

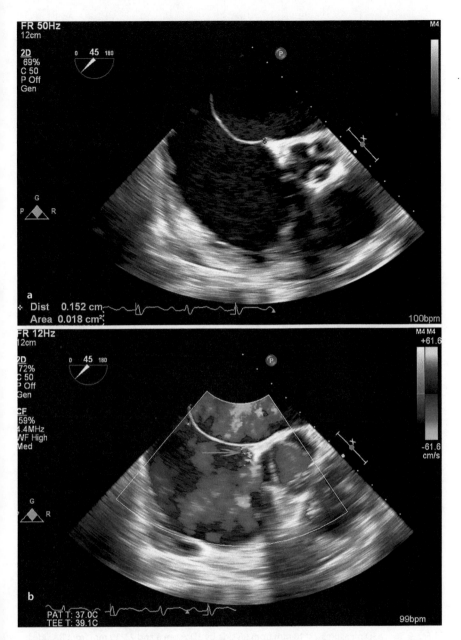

■ **Fig. 9.55** The distance between two layers of interatrial septum measures 1.5 mm in TEE short-axis view **a** and there is small flow across it (*arrow*) **b**

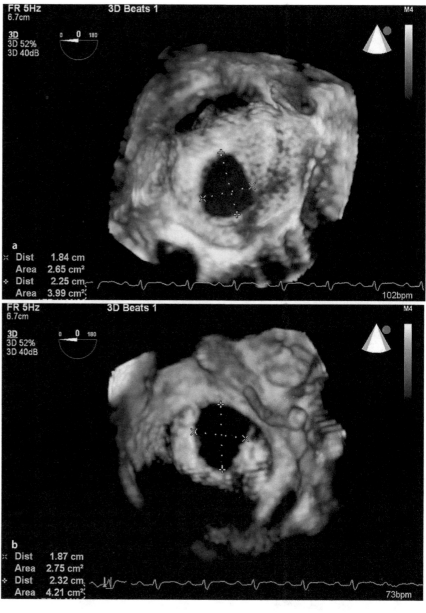

☐ **Fig. 9.56** ASD measures 23*18 mm from LA side by 3D zoom **a** and 23*19 mm from RA side **b**

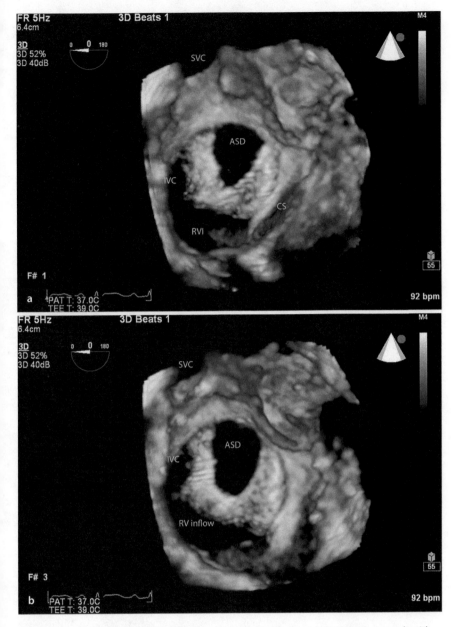

Fig. 9.57 Rims of ASD to SVC, RV inflow, CS, and IVC are adequate in this 4D view **a, b** with 3D zoom of interatrial septum from RA side. *SVC* superior vena cava, *IVC* inferior vena cava, *CS* coronary sinus, *RV inflow* right ventricular inflow

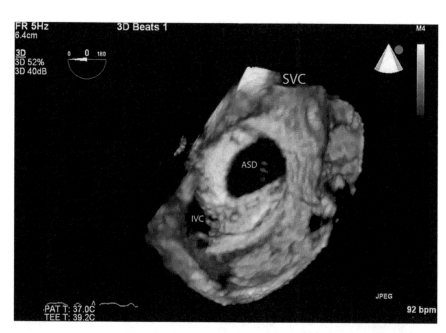

☐ **Fig. 9.58**   SVC and IVC and ASD in another aspect from RA side by 3D zoom. *SVC* superior vena cava, *IVC* inferior vena cava

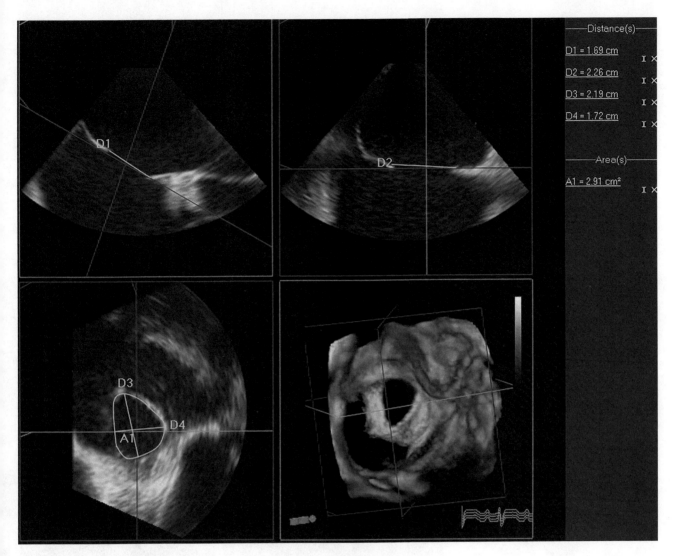

Distance(s)

D1 = 1.69 cm
D2 = 2.26 cm
D3 = 2.19 cm
D4 = 1.72 cm

Area(s)

A1 = 2.91 cm²

Fig. 9.59 By 3DQ method, maximum size of ASD is 23 mm and area measures 29 mm²

Diagnosis ASD ostium secundum with adequate rims to neighboring structures and maximum size of 23 mm, and second small ASD and PFO.

Comment ASD device closure for larger defect and follow-up for smaller defect and PFO.

9.11   Case 6: Small ASD and Elevated Pulmonary Arterial Systolic Pressure

A 33-year-old woman presented with multiple episodes of faint and one syncopal attack during recent years. Transthoracic echocardiography showed normal LV size and systolic function, normal RV size and systolic function, pulmonary arterial systolic pressure (PAPs) was equal to 40 mmHg (mildly elevated).

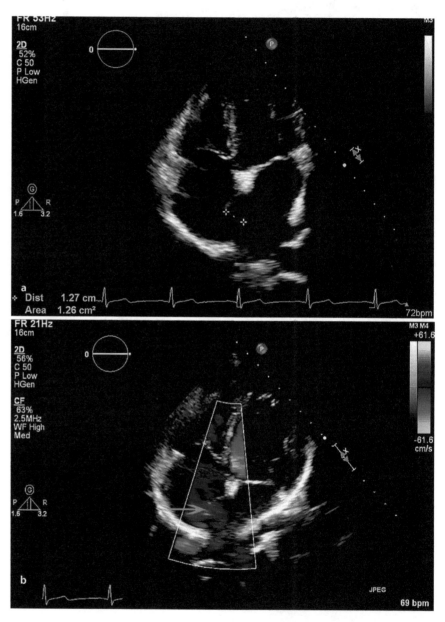

■ **Fig. 9.60**   Apical four-chamber view shows that IAS is aneurysmal up to 13 mm **a** and left to right shunt across IAS in favor of ASD ostium secundum (*arrow*) by color Doppler study **b**

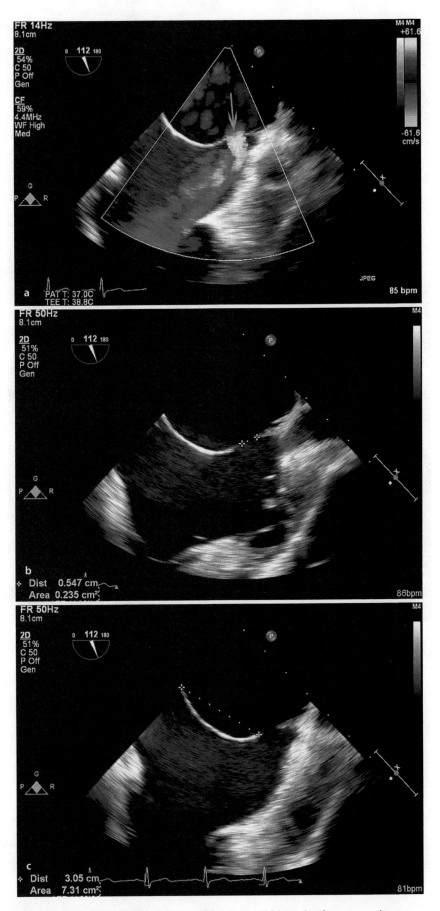

□ **Fig. 9.61** TEE bicaval view reveals a small flow across IAS (*arrow*) **a** close to superior vena cava (SVC), ASD measures 5.5 mm in size **b** and rim to IVC measures 31 mm **c**

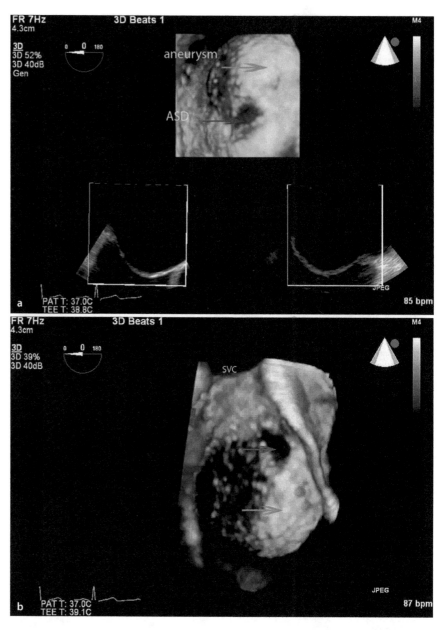

Fig. 9.62 Aneurysm of IAS (*green arrow*) is evident by 4D echo with 3D zoom from LA side **a** and RA side **b** , there is also a small ASD (*pink arrow*) between this aneurysm and SVC

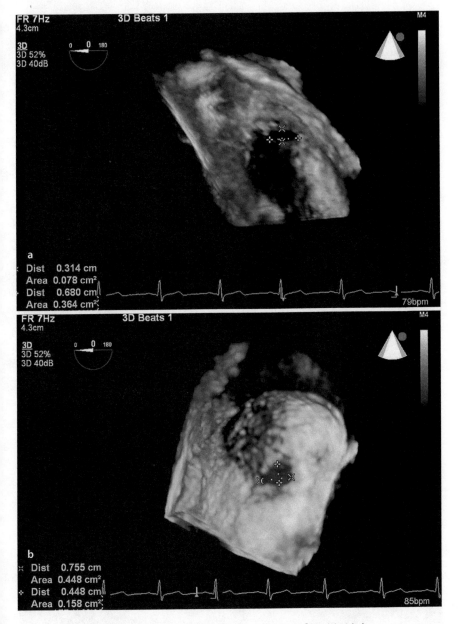

☐ **Fig. 9.63**   ASD measures 7*3 mm from RA side **a** and 5*8 mm from LA side **b**

Diagnosis   Small ASD ostium secundum with Qp/Qs = 1.2 and no RA and RV dilation but elevated PAPs.

Comment   The patient referred for ASD device closure.

9.12   Case 7: ASD Ostium Secundum

A 35-year-old woman presented with dyspnea on exertion of recent exacerbation.

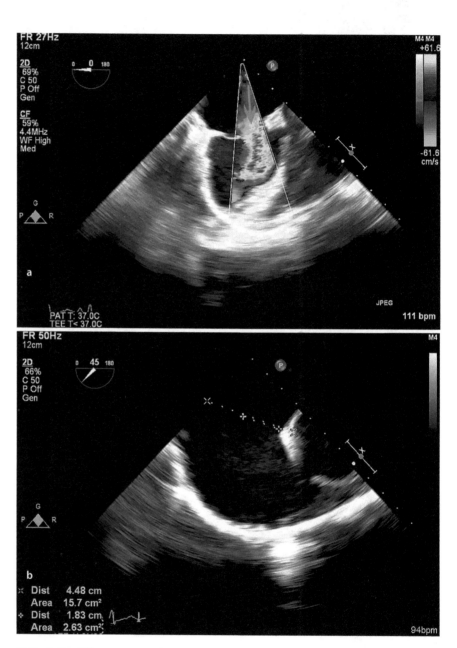

▫ **Fig. 9.64**   ASD ostium secundum is evident in TEE 0° view (*arrow*) **a**, ASD measures 18 mm in TEE short-axis view **b**

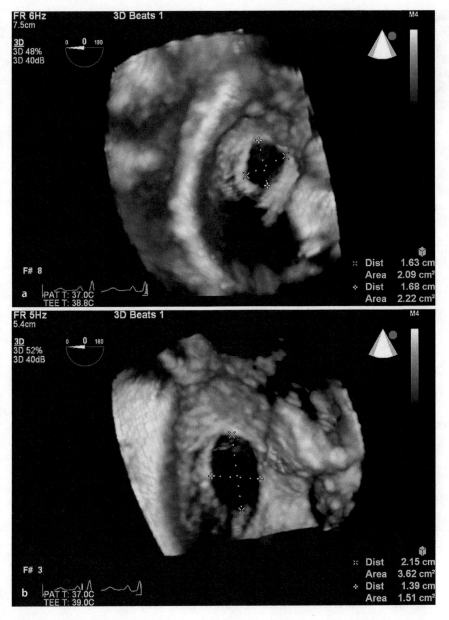

■ **Fig. 9.65**   ASD measures 17*16 mm from RA side **a** by 3D zoom and 22*14 mm from LA side by direct measurement **b**

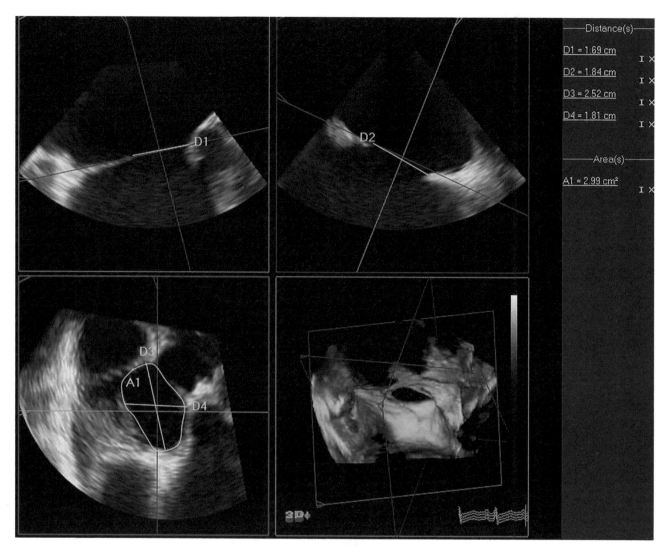

Distance(s)

D1 = 1.69 cm

D2 = 1.84 cm

D3 = 2.52 cm

D4 = 1.81 cm

Area(s)

A1 = 2.99 cm²

◻ Fig. 9.66   ASD measures 25*18 mm by 3DQ method and its area measures 3 cm²

Diagnosis   Large ASD ostium secundum with good rims.

Comment   The patient referred for ASD device closure.

Lesson   There is difference between the size of ASD obtained by direct measurement on 3D zoom from LA and RA sides and with 3DQ method. It is recommended to use 3DQ method for all measurements by 3D.

9.13   Case 8: Iatrogenic ASD Post-PTMC

A 55-year-old woman presented with dyspnea on exertion functional class II–III of recent duration. She was a known case of MS and underwent PTMC 18 years ago.

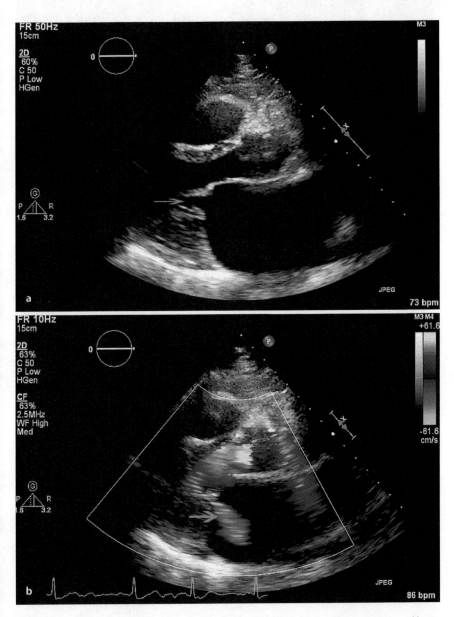

■ **Fig. 9.67**   Severe mitral stenosis (*arrow*) and mild MR (*arrow*) are evident by parasternal long-axis views **a**, **b**

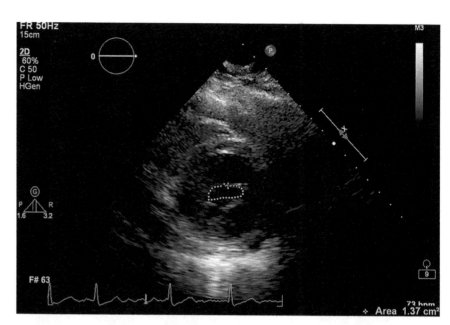

◨ **Fig. 9.68**   Mitral valve area measures 1.37 cm² by direct plannimetery by parasternal short-axis view

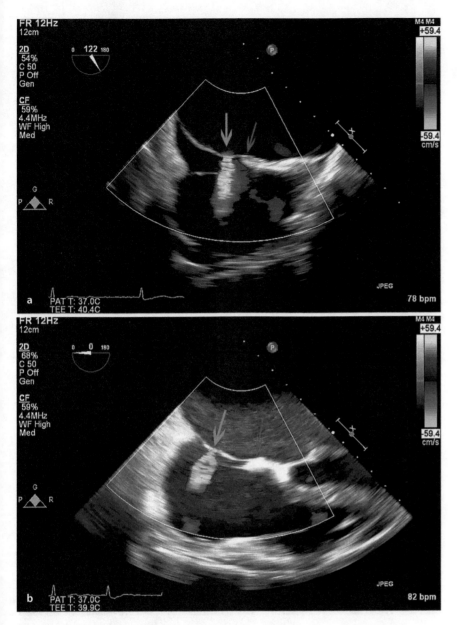

□ **Fig. 9.69** There is a turbulent flow across IAS in favor of iatrogenic ASD (*green arrow*) just above PFO site by TEE long-axis **a** and TEE 0° view **b**

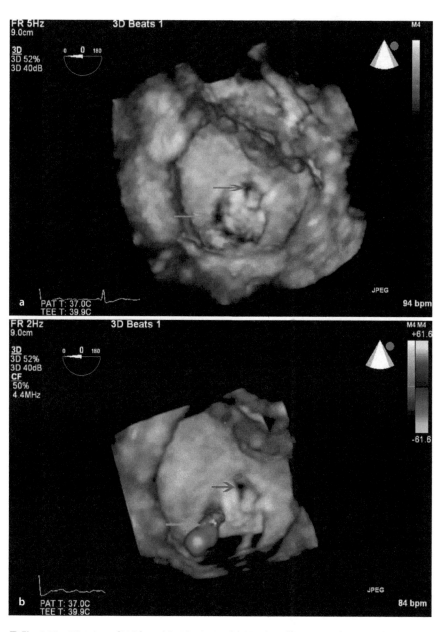

■ **Fig. 9.70**   3D zoom of IAS from RA side shows the PFO (*pink arrow*) and iatrogenic ASD (*green arrow*) (**a**, without color and **b**, with color Doppler study)

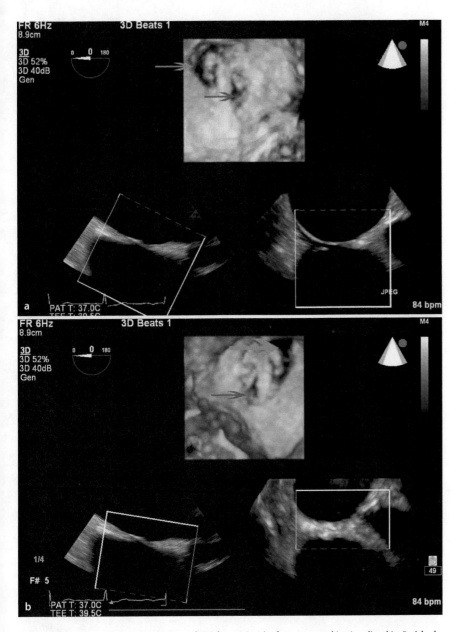

☐ **Fig. 9.71** 3D zoom reconstruction of IAS from LA side, foramen oval is visualized in 5 o'clock (*pink arrow*) **a** and iatrogenic ASD in 10 o'clock (*green arrow*) **a**, I crop from RA side shows foramen oval at 7 o'clock and iatrogenic ASD at 2 o'clock (just mirror image) **b**

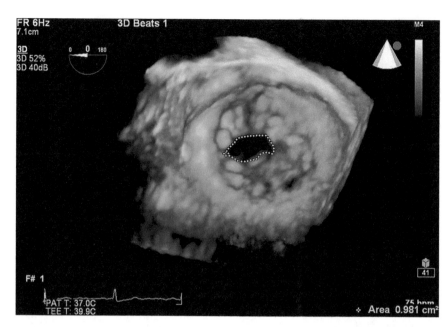

Fig. 9.72   Mitral valve area measures 0.98 cm² by direct plannimetery by 4D

9

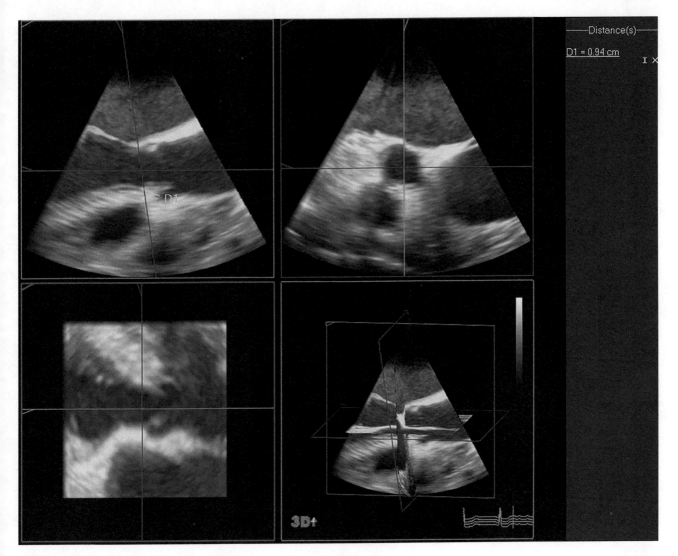

☐ **Fig. 9.73** Distance of RCA from aortic leaflets measures 9.4 mm by 3DQ method

Diagnosis Severe MS, mild MR, and spontaneous contrast grade III in LAA impending to fresh clot formation in LAA, iatrogenic ASD.

Comment Intensive anticoagulant therapy for 3 months and TEE after that.

Lesson Iatrogenic ASD is one of the complications of PTMC and occurs in near 10.5% of cases post-PTMC [8].

9.14   Case 9: Two ASDs Ostium Secundum and a Flap Within it

A 32-year-old woman presented with dyspnea on exertion functional class II. She was a known case of ASD (her diagnosis was made during pregnancy).

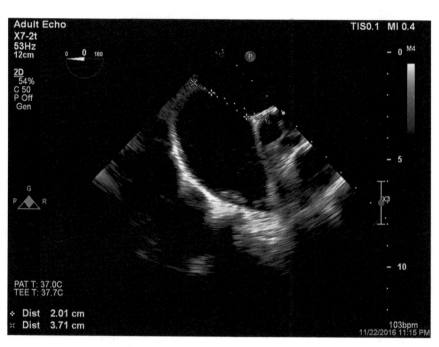

◘ Fig. 9.74   ASD ostium secundum about 20 mm in size is shown by TEE 0° view

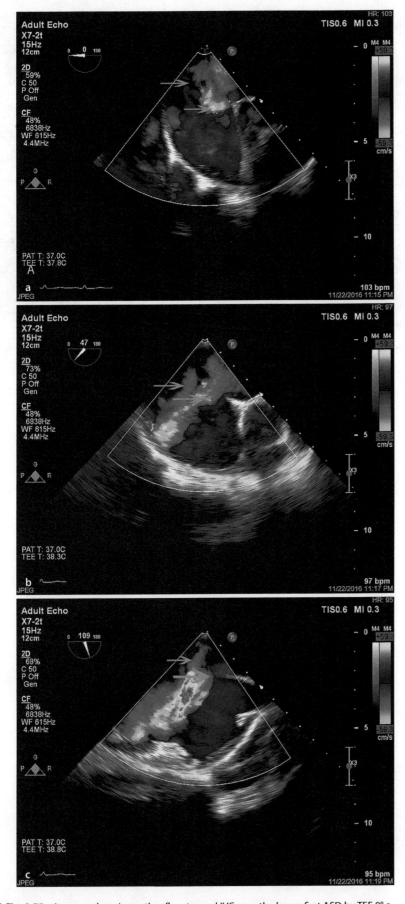

■ **Fig. 9.75** It seems there is another flow toward IVC near the larger first ASD by TEE 0° **a**, short-axis **b** and bicaval **c** views (*arrows*)

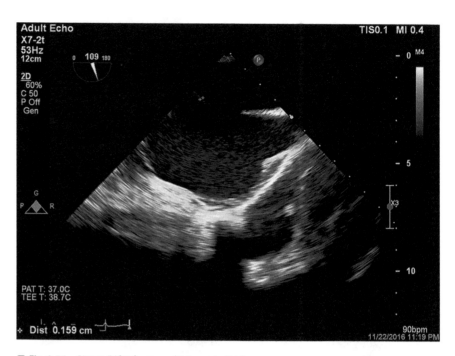

Fig. 9.76   Rim to IVC is loose and 1.6 mm in thickness

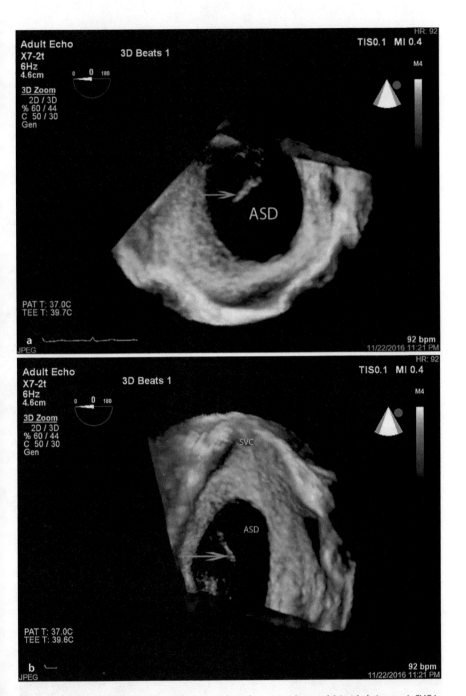

Fig. 9.77 There is a flap within ASD by 3D zoom from LA side **a** and RA side **b** (*arrows*), SVC is also visualized from RA side

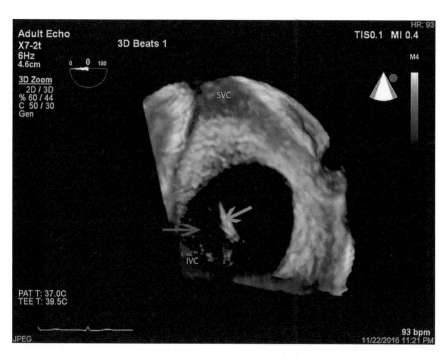

Fig. 9.78   This flap is toward IVC and there is loose tissue (*pink arrow*) between this flap (*green arrow*) and IVC

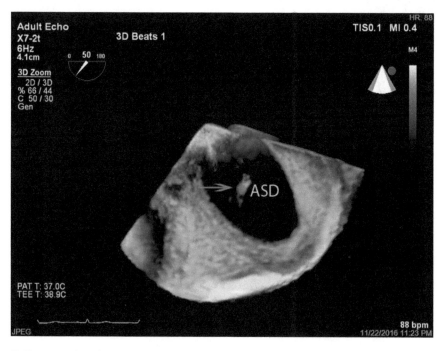

Fig. 9.79   Flap of ASD is also visualized by TEE 50° by 3D zoom from LA side (*arrow*)

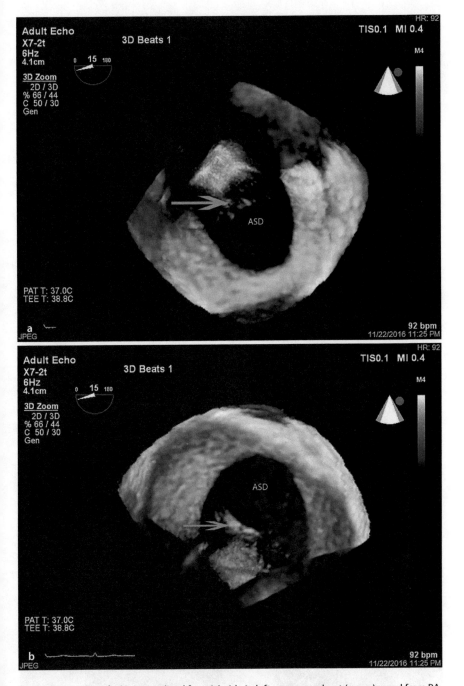

■ **Fig. 9.80** Flap of ASD is visualized from LA side in left upper quadrant (*arrow*) **a** and from RA side in left lower quadrant (*arrow*) **b**

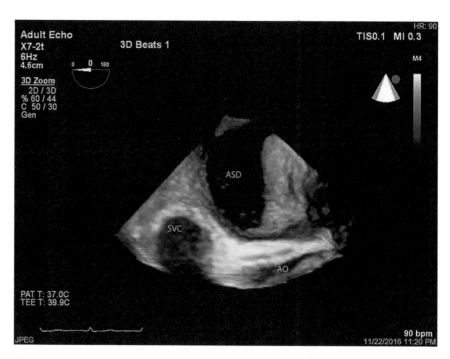

Fig. 9.81 Seeing ASD from LA side by 3D zoom, SVC and aorta are shown in the figure

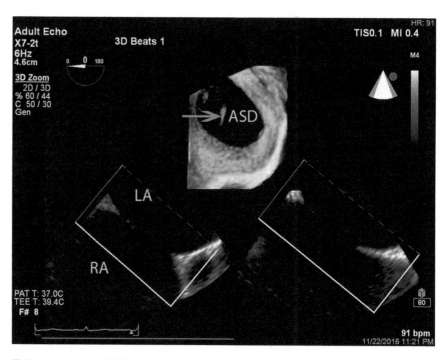

Fig. 9.82 I crop of ASD from LA side is showing the flap (*arrow*)

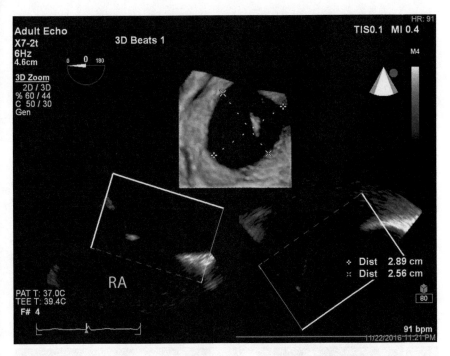

Fig. 9.83 I crop of ASD from RA side, ASD measures 29*26 mm by direct measurement

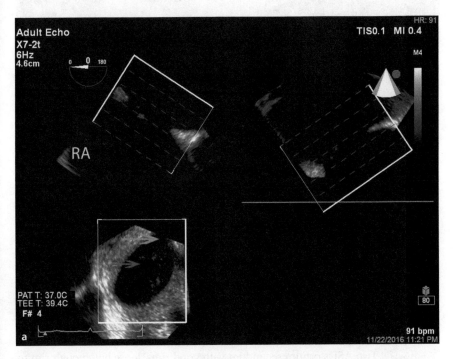

Fig. 9.84 I slice of ASD from RA side to LA side **a–c**, ASD measures 29*31 mm by direct measurement **b**, loose tissue around ASD is marked by green flash and the second ASD is marked by pink flash **a, c**. It is of notice that ASD is in right upper quadrant from right atrial I crop **a** and in left upper quadrant from left atrial I crop **c**, (mirror image)

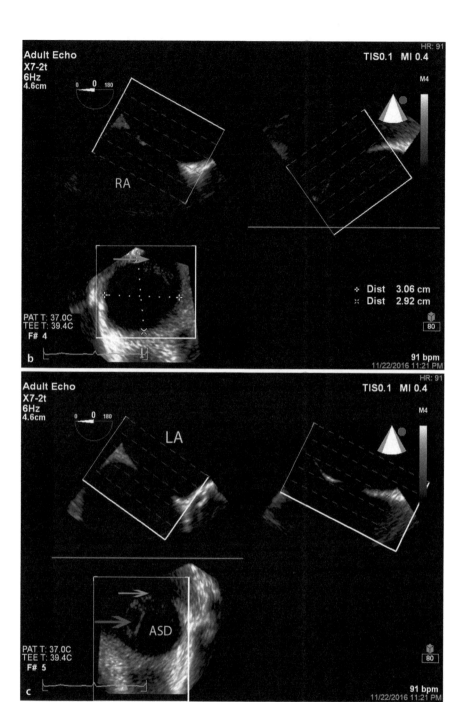

Fig. 9.84 (continued)

Diagnosis   Two ASDs ostium secundum with good rims, loose but enough rim to IVC and a flap which separates two ASDs.

Comment   The patient referred for ASD device closure.

9.15 Case 10: ASD with Isenmenger Syndrome

A 17-year-old man presented with dyspnea on exertion functional class III. Physical examination revealed loud P2 and systolic ejection murmur at pulmonic area. ECG revealed tall R in right precordial leads.

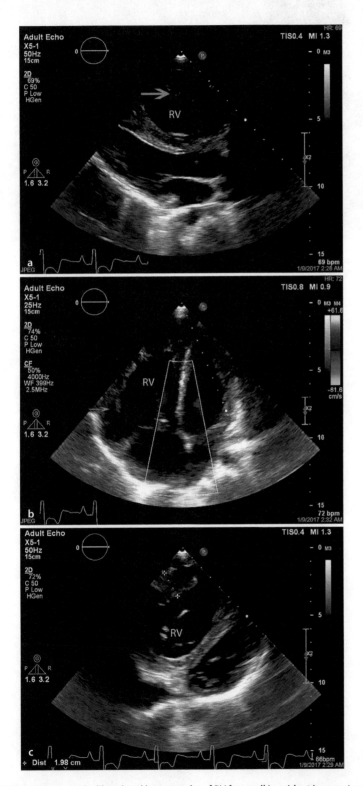

☐ **Fig. 9.85** RV is severely dilated and hypertrophy of RV free wall is evident in parasternal long-axis view (*arrows*) **a** and apical four-chamber view **b**, RV free wall measures 20 mm in apical four-chamber view **c**

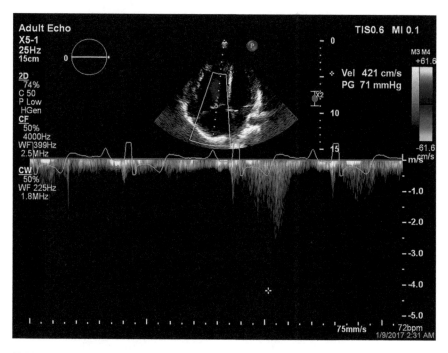

☐ Fig. 9.86   TRG measures 71 mmHg

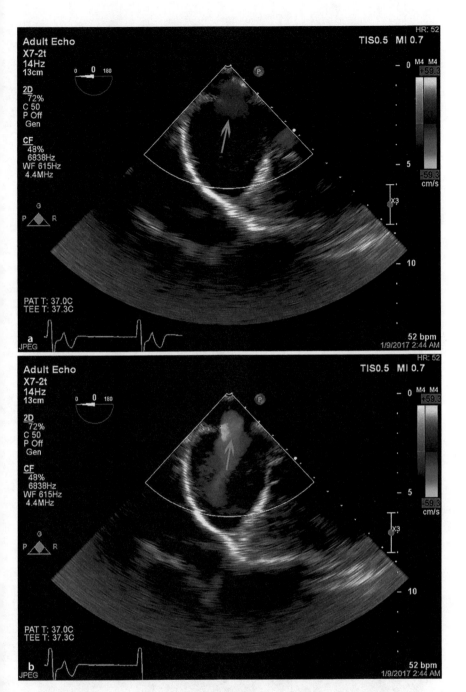

Fig. 9.87 There is bidirectional flow across ASD (*arrows*) in TEE 0° view **a, b**

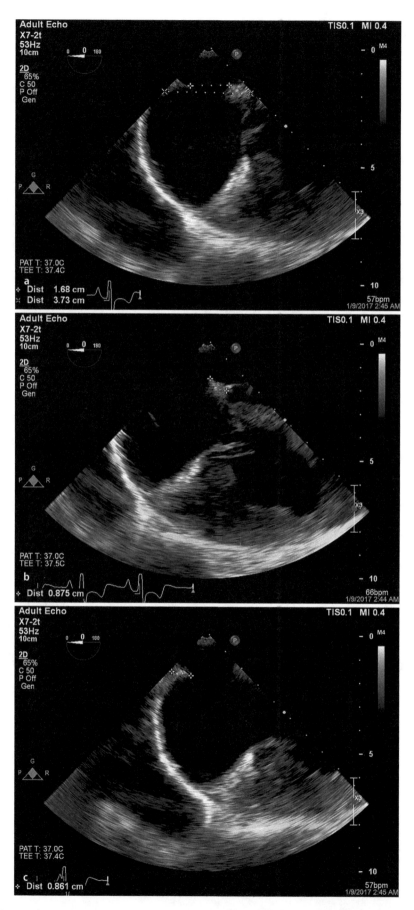

Fig. 9.88 ASD/IAS measures 17/37 mm in 0° view **a**, rim to mitral valve measures 9 mm **b** and posterior rim measures 9 mm in this view **c**

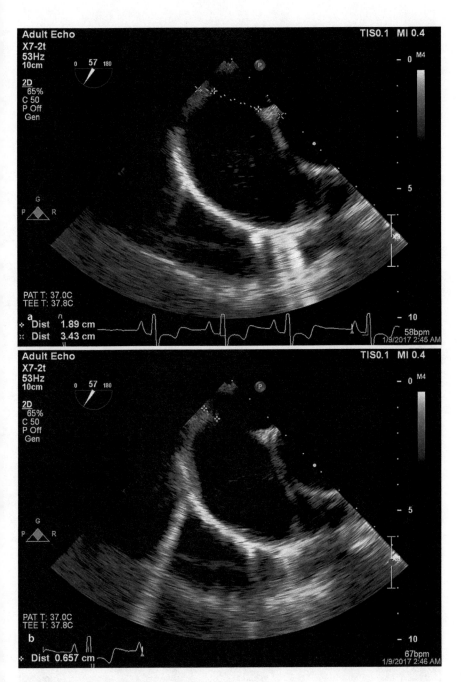

Fig. 9.89 ASD/IAS measures 19/34 mm in TEE short-axis view **a**, posterior rim measures 6.5 mm in this view **b**

9

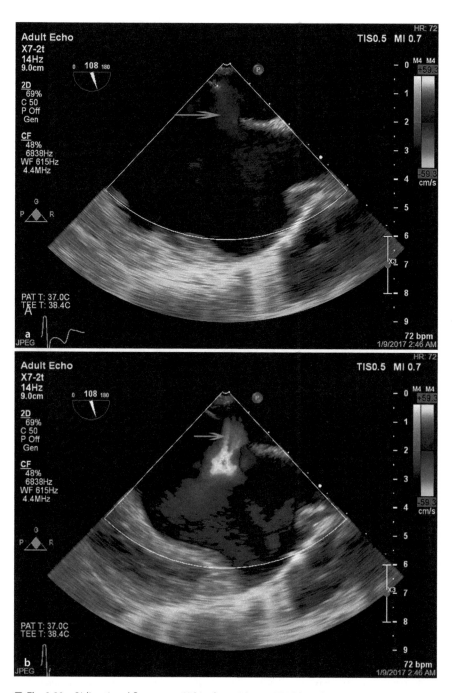

■ **Fig. 9.90** Bidirectional flow across IAS is also evident in TEE bicaval view (*arrows*) (**a, b**)

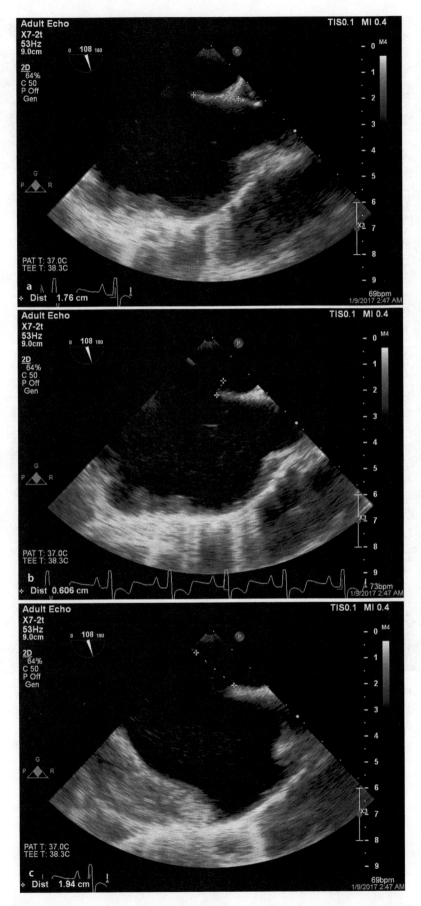

☐ **Fig. 9.91**   Rim to SVC measures 18 mm in TEE bicaval view **a**, there is also interatrial septal malalignment 6 mm **b**, and ASD measures 19 mm in this view **c**

9

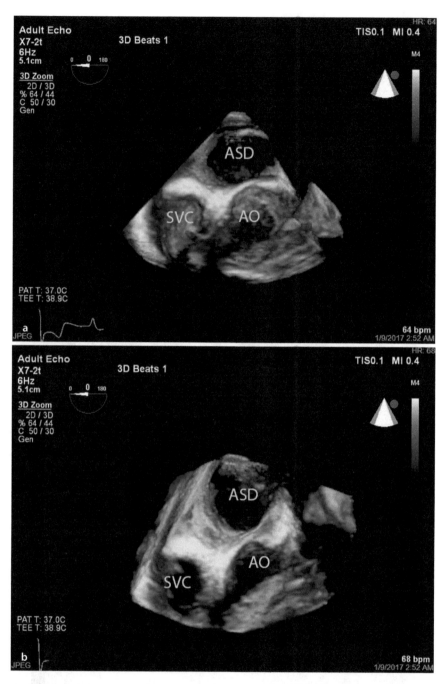

☐ **Fig. 9.92**   ASD is demonstrated in TEE 0° view by 3D zoom from LA side, SVC and aorta are visible in this view **a, b**

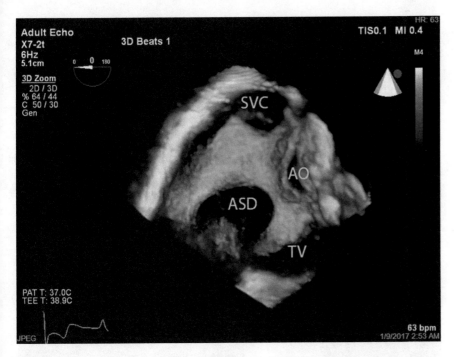

◻ Fig. 9.93   ASD from RA side in TEE 0° view by 3D zoom. SVC, aorta, and TV are visible in this view

Diagnosis   ASDPH. Qp/Qs = 1.
   PVR was 7 unit, after 10 min of O2:
   PAPs decreased to 60 mmHg
   PAPm reached from 30 to 25 mmHg
   but PVR reached to 6 and is until above 5.

Comment   Medical therapy and follow-up.

Lesson   Pulmonary vasoreactivity is defined as more than 10 mmHg reduction in PAPm or the absolute figure for PAPm reached to 40 mmHg [9].

9.16   Case 11: Sinus Venosus ASD with PAPVC

A 55-year-old man with a history of dyspnea on exertion, palpitation, and easy fatigability and in physical examination he had normal sinus rhythm and a systolic murmur grade III/VI on left sternal border.

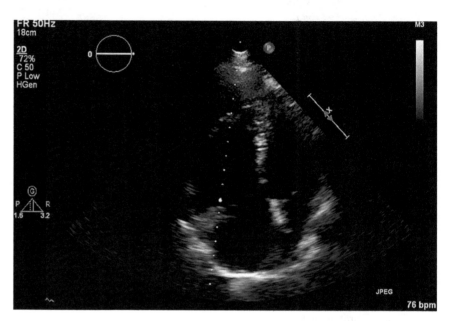

◻ **Fig. 9.94**   Apical four-chamber view shows severe right ventricular dilation with normal right systolic function

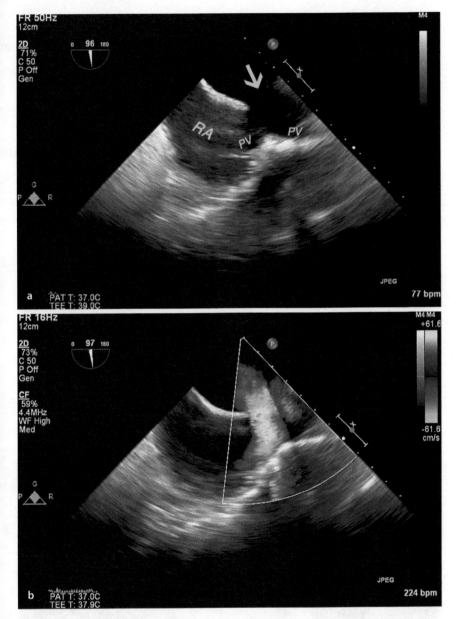

◼ Fig. 9.95 Mid esophageal bicaval view depicts a defect above to superior vena cava in favor of sinus venosus type atrial septal defect (**a**, *arrow*) and connection between SVC and both atrium is visible clearly **b** and also this view shows two pulmonary veins connection to SVC **a**

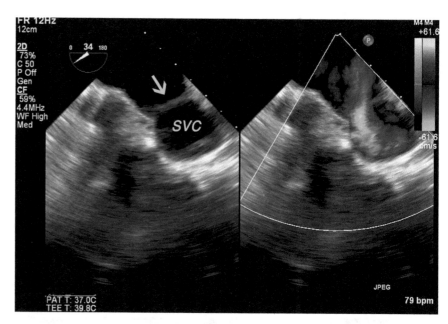

■ **Fig. 9.96**   Upper esophageal 34° view shows superior vena cava (*arrow*) is not round and there is a defect on it in favor of connection of SVC to the left atrium

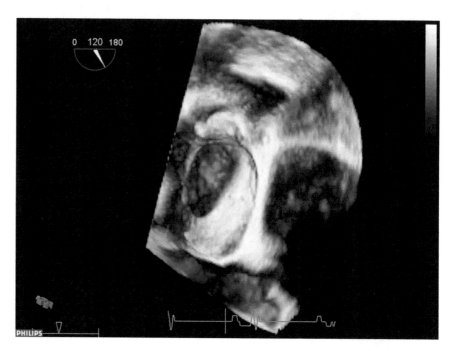

■ **Fig. 9.97**   3D zoom view acquisition of bicaval view shows oval shape atrial septal defect

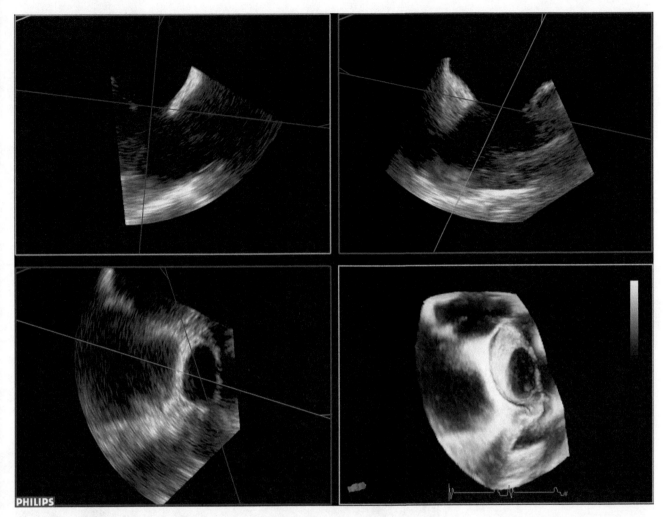

☐ **Fig. 9.98** 3D dataset in a patient with sinus venosus atrial septal defect, right lower shows enface view of ASD from the left atrial side and it shows clearly shape, area, and diameter of ASD, the top two planes represent two orthogonal 2D cross-sectional views (*green* and *red* planes) perpendicular to the interatrial septum

Diagnosis Sinus venosus ASD with partial anomalous pulmonary vein drainage.

Lesson Surgical closure of atrial septal defect and correction of abnormal pulmonary veins is recommended.

9.17 Case 12: Sinus Venosus ASD, PAPVC, and Moderate Valvaular PS

A 45-year-old man presented with dyspnea on exertion (functional class II). Physical examination revealed a load S2, systolic murmur in pulmonic area, and fixed splitting of S2.

Transthoracic echocardiography revealed right ventricular dilation and right ventricular hypertrophy.

Transesophageal echocardiography was done for evaluation of the cause of right ventricular dilation.

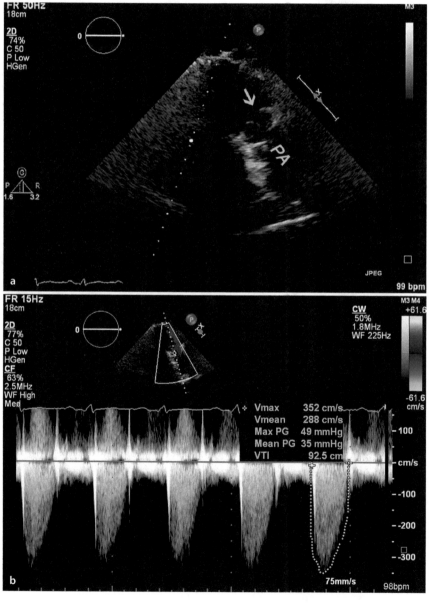

■ **Fig. 9.99** Parasternal long-axis view with probe tilting to medial side shows thick pulmonary valve (*arrow*, **a**) and color Doppler flow study across pulmonary valve depicts maximum peak gradient equal to 48 mmHg and mean gradient about mmHg **b** in favor of moderate pulmonary stenosis

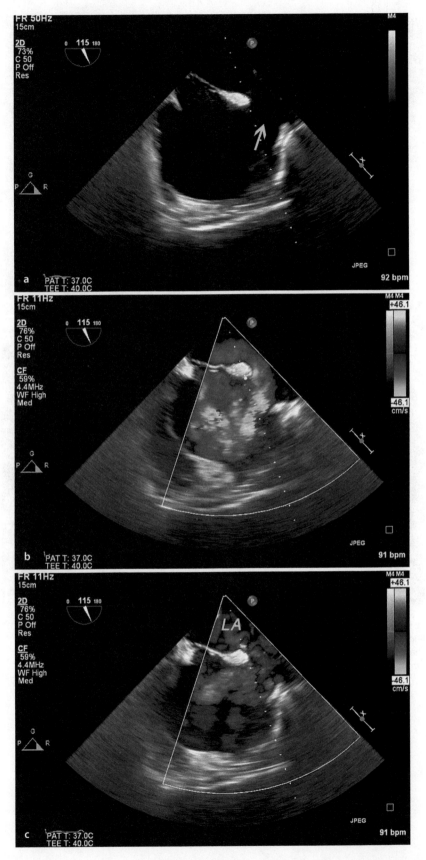

◨ **Fig. 9.100**   Mid esophageal bicaval view demonstrates an atrial septal defect (ASD) sinus venosus type (*arrow*) below the superior vena cava (SVC) **a** and the SVC is attached to left atrium and right atrium simultaneously with bidirectional shunt **b, c**

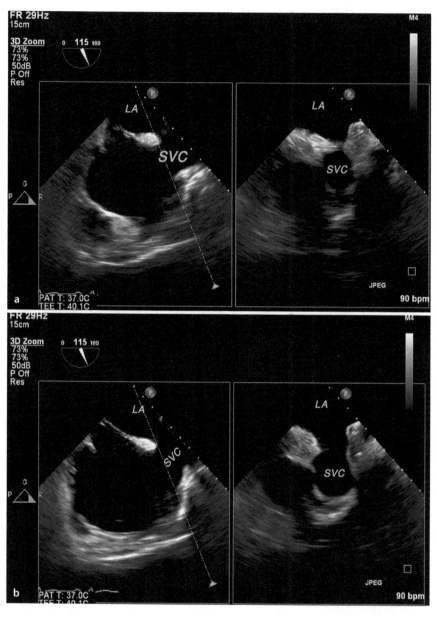

Fig. 9.101 X plane bicaval view shows clearly defect of superior vena cava, at first X plain line is passed from left atrium, interatrial septum and superior vena cava **a**, SVC is seen round shape in orthogonal view and then X plane line is moved to the site of atrial septal defect (**b**, *arrow*) and depicts connection of SVC to left atrium and defect of superior vena cava (*arrow*)

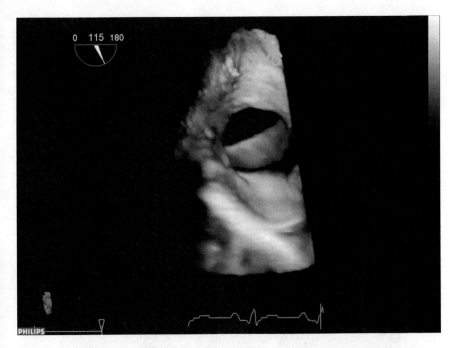

◼ **Fig. 9.102** 3D zoom view shows large round shape sinus venosus atrial septal defect

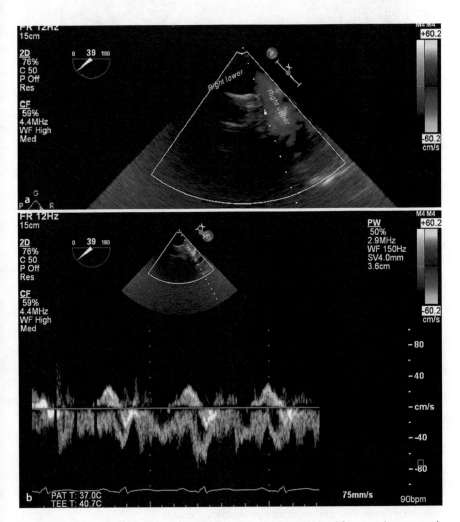

◼ **Fig. 9.103** Upper esophageal short-axis view shows abnormal blood flow in right upper pulmonary vein (*blue*, **a**) and color Doppler flow reveals reversal flow in right upper pulmonary vein **b** (in normal condition flow is visible red color and flow is seen above base line)

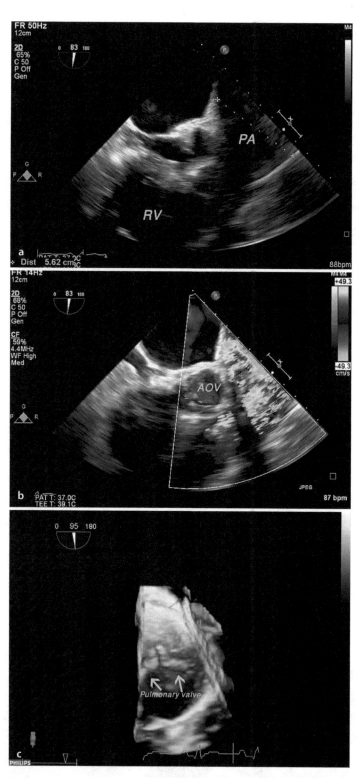

Fig. 9.104 Mid esophageal 80° view demonstrates dilated pulmonary artery up to 56 mm **a** and turbulent flow in it in favor of pulmonary stenosis **b** and 3D view depicts thick pulmonary leaflets (**c**, *arrow*)

Diagnosis   Sinus venosus ASD with anomalous connection between the right lower pulmonary vein SVC and moderate pulmonary stenosis.

Comment   The patient was referred for surgery.

9.18 Patent Foramen Ovalis

In fetal circulation, blood flow is toward LA from RA via fossa ovalis. Pulmonary veins transfer only 5–10% of flow in fetus, due to this fact that the lungs are inactive in fetal life. The remaining flow of left atrium and left ventricle passes through IAS (fossa ovalis) and membrane of vieuscence which is a marker of LA in fetus is just in above portion of IAS in LA in the path of flow.

After birth, the lungs will be activated with the first cry, then patent foramen ovalis (PFO) will be closed physiologic within 48 h after birth. In up to ¼ of population, the foramen ovale is not anatomically closed until adulthood.

Most PFO remains asymptomatic, if the patient is symptomatic despite aspirin or warfarin, PFO device closure should be considered. Large PFO with aneurysm of interatrial septum can more benefit from PFO device closure.

There are two classifications for PFO: (1) Anatomic and (2) Physiologic.

In anatomic classification, PFO is considered as small when distance of two layers is less than 2 mm, moderate size when distance of two layers is between 2 and 4 mm, and large when distance of two layers is more than 4 mm.

In physiologic classification, the number of bubbles passed through IAS is the criteria for classification, PFO is considered as small when <9 bubbles passed through IAS, moderate size when between 10 and 20 bubbles passed through IAS, and large when >20 bubbles passed through IAS [10].

Although, there are some clinical cases that PFO is small from anatomic point of view but moderate from physiologic point of view or vice-versa. Besides, there are some cases which there is PFO flow at rest but no bubble passage with contrast and valsalva maneuver.

IAS aneurysm is an aneurysm more than 10–15 mm by echocardiography [10].

9.19   Case 13: Aneurysm of Interatrial Septum and PFO

A 47-year-old woman presented with dyspnea on exertion functional class II. Transthoracic echocardiography revealed moderate mitral stenosis and moderate mitral regurgitation.

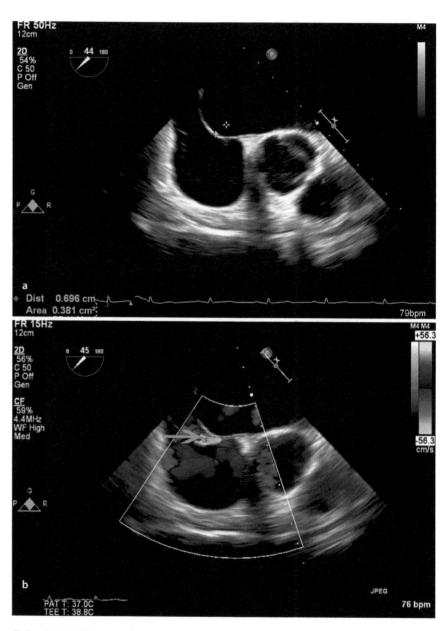

Fig. 9.105   IAS is partially aneurysmal up to 7 mm by TEE short-axis view **a**, left to right shunt is seen by color Doppler study in this view (*arrow*) **b**

9.19 · Case 13: Aneurysm of Interatrial Septum and PFO

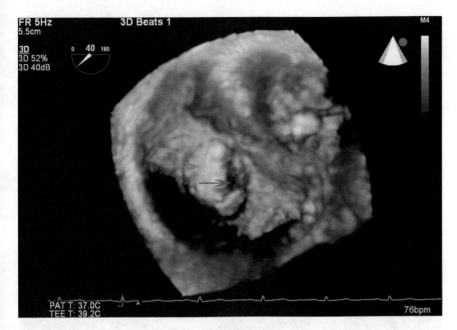

Fig. 9.106 Aneurysm (*green arrow*) of IAS and PFO (*pink arrow*) is seen from RA side by 3D echocardiography 3D zoom in TEE short-axis view

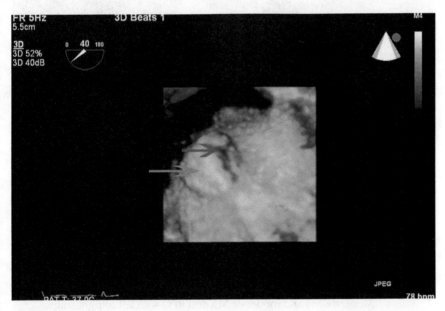

Fig. 9.107 Aneurysm (*green arrow*) of IAS and PFO (*pink arrow*) is seen from LA side by 3D echocardiography

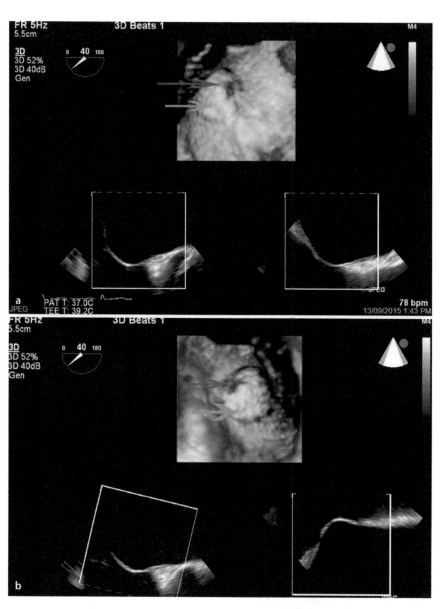

■ **Fig. 9.108** I crop of IAS shows aneurysm and bulging of IAS from LA toward RA (*green arrows*) (**a**, from LA side and **b**, from RA side), PFO is seen from LA side in 2 o'clock **a** and from RA side in 10 o'clock (*pink arrows*) **b**

Diagnosis   Moderate MS and moderate MR and PFO with left to right shunt.

Comment   medical treatment and follow-up.

9.20   Case 14: AMVL Cleft and ASD

A 33-year-old man with history of recent onset dyspnea with functional class II and in physical examination he had pan systolic murmur in mitral area and fix splitting of S2.

Transthoracic echocardiography showed mild left ventricular dilation and sub-optimal left ventricular function.

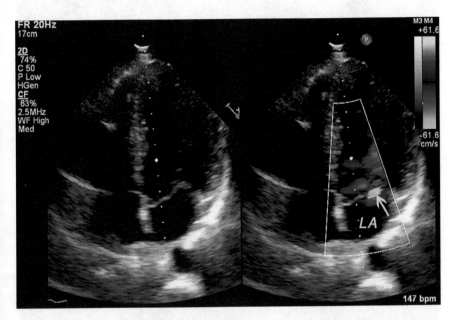

◻ **Fig. 9.109**   Apical four-chamber view shows moderate mitral regurgitation (*arrow*) which is not compatible with pan systolic murmur in physical examination. *LA* left atrium

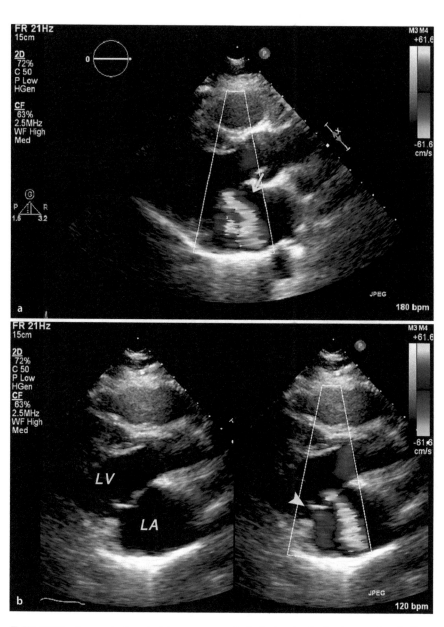

■ **Fig. 9.110** Long-axis view depicts more amount of mitral regurgitation (*arrow*, **a**) and off axis of long-axis view shows this jet of mitral regurgitation is not from coaptation site (*arrow head*) and it is from mid belly of anterior mitral leaflet **b**. *LA* left atrium, *LV* left ventricle

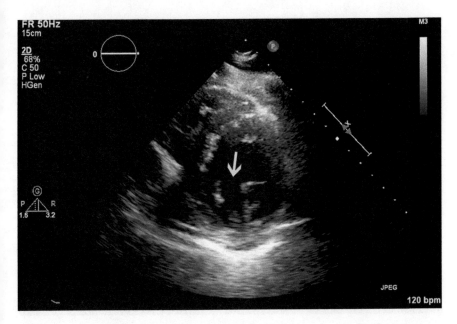

Fig. 9.111 Parasternal short-axis view depicts defect in the anterior mitral leaflet (*arrow*) indicative for mitral cleft

Transesophageal echocardiography was performed for more evaluation of mitral valve and rolled out of associated common anomaly such as ventricular septal defect and primum type atrial septal defect. There was not evidence of ventricular septal defect and primum type atrial septal defect.

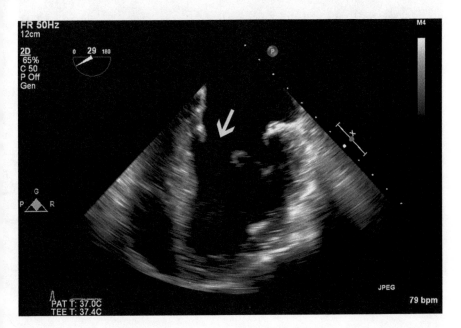

Fig. 9.112 Mid esophageal 29° view shows a large defect (*arrow*) in anterior mitral leaflet. *LA* left atrium, *LV* left ventricle

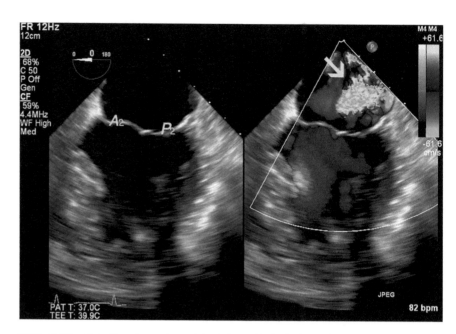

◘ Fig. 9.113 Color Doppler study at mid esophageal 0° in the level of A2, P2 shows a turbulent flow in left atrium with swirling to lateral wall of left atrium (*arrow*), in favor of severe mitral regurgitation, but mitral regurgitation doesn't origin from mitral valve coaptation

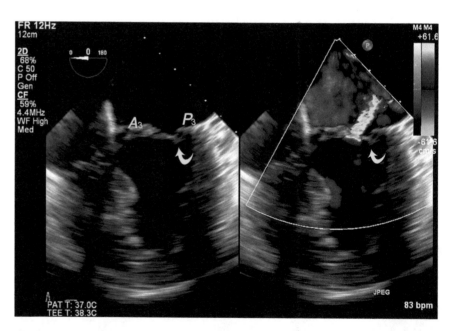

◘ Fig. 9.114 Mid esophageal 0° with deep insertion of probe shows A3, P3 scallops and depicts that the origin of mitral regurgitation is in this level and also reveals that it is in different site from coaptation point (*curved arrow*) in favor of pathology is in the level of A3 scallop

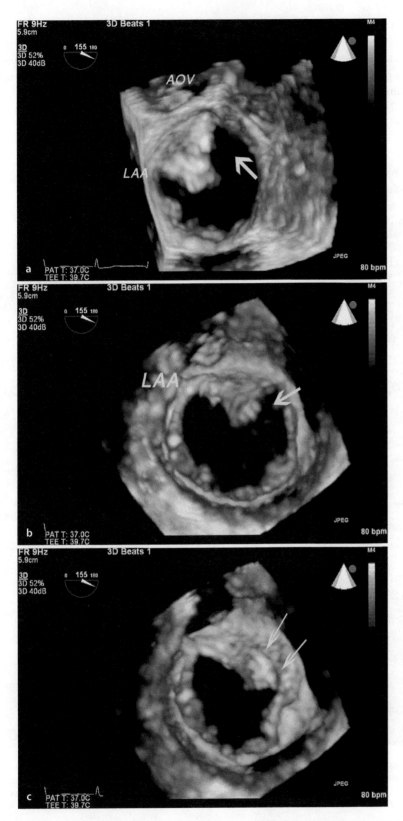

■ Fig. 9.115   3D zoom view of mitral leaflets shows a large cleft in the level of A3 (a, atrial side and b ventricular side, c during systole). *AOV* aortic valve, *LAA* left atrial appendage

Recommendation   With respect to severity of mitral regurgitation and decrease left ventricular function and enlarged size of left ventricle, the patient referred for MV repair.

9.21   Case 15: Cleft of MV

A 34-year-old lady who had undergone common AV canal surgery several years ego presented with dyspnea on exertion (functional class II–III) and in physical examination a pan systolic murmur is heard in the mitral area.

Transthoracic echocardiography showed normal left ventricular function and size.

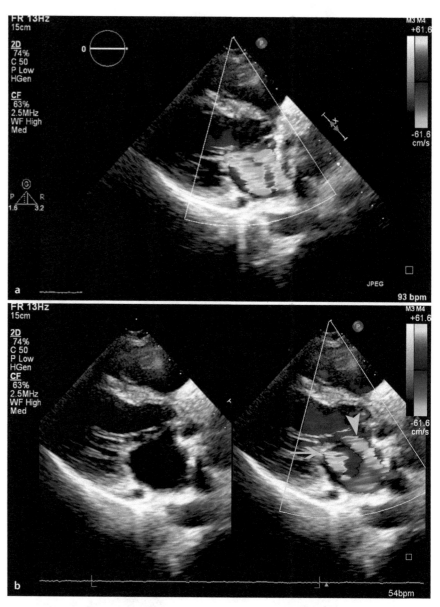

☐ **Fig. 9.116** Parasternal long-axis view shows significant mitral regurgitation **a** and off axis parasternal long axis demonstrates two sites of mitral regurgitation **b** one of them originates from coaptation point (*arrow*) and another originates from mid belly of anterior mitral leaflet (*head arrow*)

9.21 · Case 15: Cleft of MV

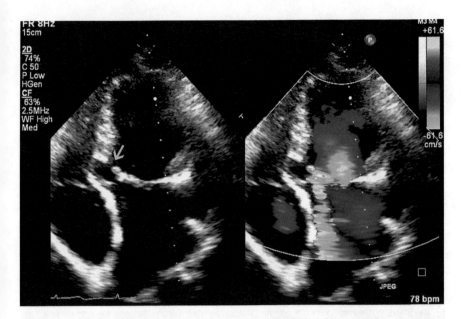

☐ **Fig. 9.117** Apical four-chamber view depicts a site of defect (*arrow*) in anterior mitral leaflet in favor of failing mitral valve repair

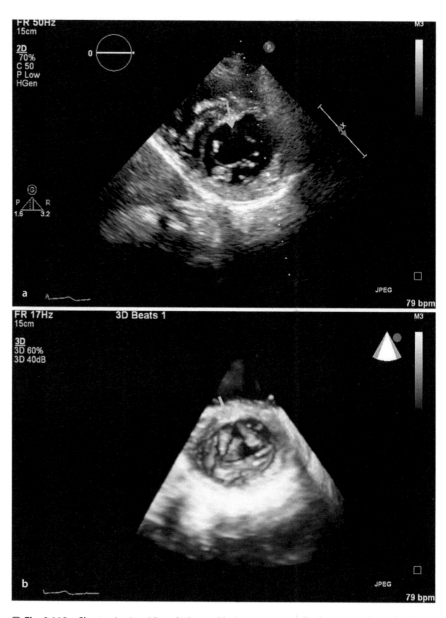

Fig. 9.118 Short-axis view 2D and 3D **a** and **b** demonstrate cleft of anterior of mitral valve (*arrow*) and mitral valve seems tricuspid

Transesophageal echocardiography was performed for evaluation definite cause and severity of mitral regurgitation

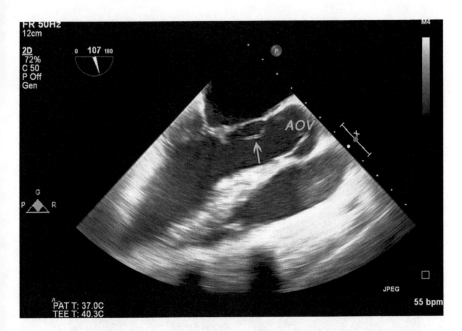

☐ **Fig. 9.119**　Mid esophageal long-axis view depicts a linear hyper echo density in left ventricular outflow tract (*arrow*) that it attaches to anterior mitral leaflet indicative for pericardial patched rupture of previous repaired anterior mitral leaflet cleft

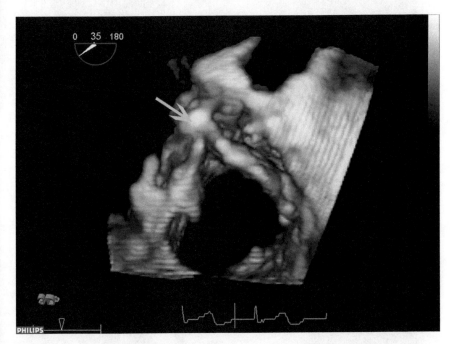

☐ **Fig. 9.120**　3D zoom view of mitral valve demonstrates a large defect in A2 scallop that it extends up to annulus (*arrow*)

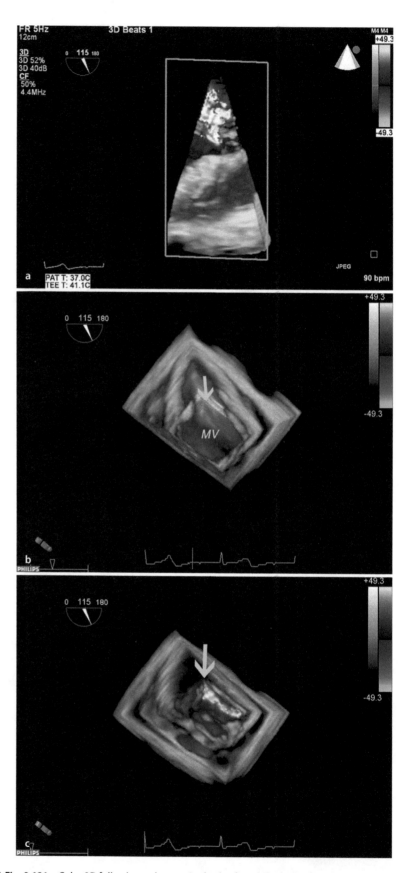

Fig. 9.121 Color 3D full volume shows mitral valve from left atrial side **a** and origination site of mitral regurgitation from anterior mitral cleft during systole (**b**, **c**, *arrow*) and mitral regurgitation volume is measured about 70 cm³ (doesn't show)

Diagnosis   Failed repair of mitral valve cleft with severe mitral regurgitation.

Recommendation   Patient was sent for mitral valve surgery and redo repair.

References

1. Baumgartner H, Bonhoeffer P, De Groot NM, de Haan F, Deanfield JE, Galie N, et al. ESC guidelines for the management of grown-up congenital heart disease (new version 2010). Eur Heart J. 2010;31(23):2915–57.
2. Rojas CA, El-Sherief A, Medina HM, Chung JH, Choy G, Ghoshhajra BB, et al. Embryology and developmental defects of the interatrial septum. AJR Am J Roentgenol. 2010;195(5):1100–4.
3. Sadeghian H, Savand-Roomi Z. Echocardiographic atlas of adult congenital heart disease. 1st ed. Cham: Springer International Publishing; 2015. 517p
4. Hajizeinali A, Sadeghian H, Rezvanfard M, Alidoosti M, Zoroufian A, Volman MA. A comparison between size of the occluder device and two-dimensional transoesophageal echocardiographic sizing of the ostium secundum atrial septal defect. Cardiovasc J Afr. 2013;24(5):161–4.
5. Sadeghian H, Hajizeinali A, Eslami B, Lotfi-Tokaldany M, Sheikh Fathollahi M, Sahebjam M, Hakki E, Zoroufian A, Kassaian SE, Alidoosti M. Measurement of atrial septal defect size: a comparative study between transesophageal echocardiography and balloon occlusive diameter method. J Tehran Univ Heart Center. 2010;5(2):74–7.
6. Abdel-Massih T, Dulac Y, Taktak A, Aggoun Y, Massabuau P, Elbaz M, et al. Assessment of atrial septal defect size with 3D-transesophageal echocardiography: comparison with balloon method. Echocardiography. 2005;22(2):121–7.
7. Galie N, Humbert M, Vachiery JL, Gibbs S, Lang I, Torbicki A, et al. 2015 ESC/ERS guidelines for the diagnosis and treatment of pulmonary hypertension: the joint task force for the diagnosis and treatment of pulmonary hypertension of the European Society of Cardiology (ESC) and the European Respiratory Society (ERS), endorsed by Association for European Pediatric and Congenital Cardiology (AEPC), International Society for Heart and Lung Transplantation (ISHLT). Eur Heart J. 2016;37(1):67–119.
8. Ali LA, Riaz R, Hussain M. Percutaneous transmitral commissurotomy. Prof Med J. 2016; 23(1):104–13.
9. Mclaughlin VV, Sadeghi HM. Pulmonary hypertension. In: Mann DL, Zipes ZD, Libby P, Bonow RO, Braunwald E, editors. Braunwald's heart disease. 2. 10th ed. Philadelphia, PA: Elsevier Saunders; 2015. p. 1682–702.
10. Carroll JD, Saver JL, Thaler DE, Smalling RW, Berry S, MacDonald LA, et al. Closure of patent foramen ovale versus medical therapy after cryptogenic stroke. N Engl J Med. 2013; 368(12):1092–100.

VSD, PDA, Coarctation of Aorta, Subvalvular AS

Videos can be found in the electronic supplementary material in the online version of the chapter.
On http://springerlink.com enter the DOI number given on the bottom of the chapter opening page.
Scroll down to the Supplementary material tab and click on the respective videos link.

© Springer International Publishing AG 2017
H. Sadeghian, Z. Savand-Roomi, *3D Echocardiography of Structural Heart Disease*,
DOI 10.1007/978-3-319-54039-9_10

10.1 VSD

Ventricular septal defect (VSD) is one of the most common congenital heart diseases. In fetal life, there may be muscular or perimembranous VSD in septum, most of them are closed until birth or in early life or until puberty.

There are five types of VSD:
1. Perimembranous,
2. Muscular,
3. Outlet or doubly committed,
4. Inlet VSD,
5. Malalignment VSD [1].

Perimembranous VSD are near aortic valve, doubly committed are near pulmonary valve, muscular are in different sites of interventricular septum, inlet VSDs are most often associated by other congenital heart disease, and malalignment VSDs are associated by anomalies like Tetralogy of Fallot.

There are also VSDs complicated myocardial infarction or sometimes as a complication post-surgery of hypertrophic cardiomyopathy.

10.2 Case 1: Perimembranous VSD

An 18-year-old girl referred for echocardiography due to dyspnea on exertion functional class II–III. She was a known case of VSD and was under follow-up from childhood. Physical examination revealed holosystolic murmur at lower sternal border.

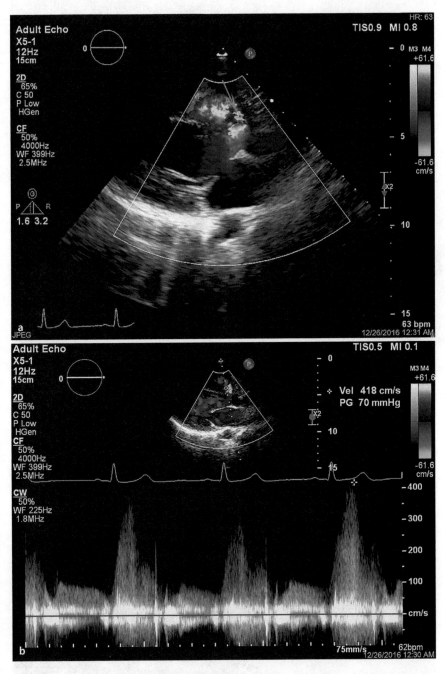

■ **Fig. 10.1** Systolic turbulent flow across IVS in favor of perimembranous VSD (*arrow*) **a**, peak gradient across IVS measures 70 mmHg **b**

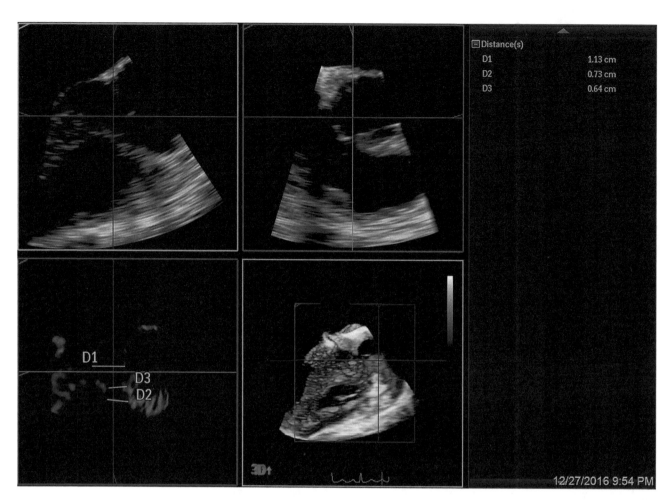

❑ **Fig. 10.2**   VSD measures 11 mm in LV side and 7 mm in RV side by 3DQ 3D zoom

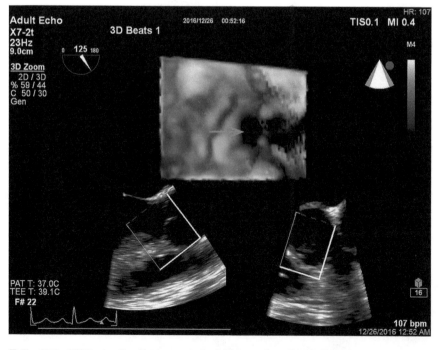

❑ **Fig. 10.3**   VSD is visualized by I crop method, 3D zoom from LV side (*arrow*)

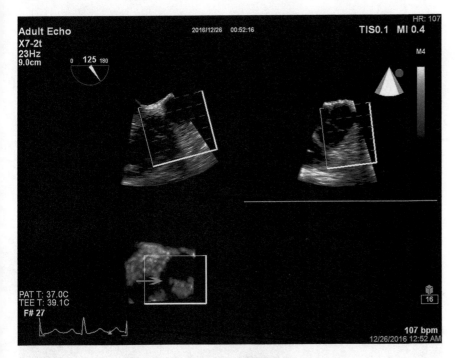

■ **Fig. 10.4** VSD is shown by l slice method, 3D zoom from LV side (*arrow*)

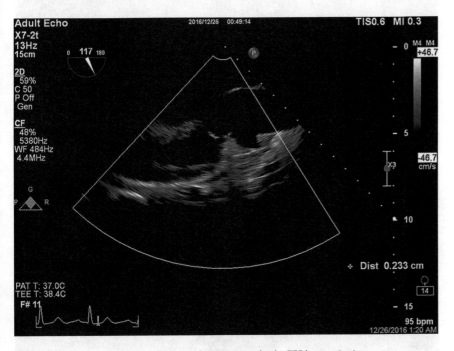

■ **Fig. 10.5** Rim of VSD measures 2 mm from aortic valve by TEE long-axis view

Diagnosis Perimembranous VSD with small aortic rim, normal LV size, PG across VSD = 70 mmHg, Qp/Qs = 1.2, PAPs = 37 mmHg.

Comment The patient referred for cardiac catheterism and surgery.

Lesson Although left to right shunt is not significant but the patient was symptomatic and mildly elevated PAPs. Due to small aortic rim via TEE and nearly no rim by 3D echocardiography, percutaneous VSD closure is not suitable.

10.3 Case 2: Residual VSD Post-Surgery

A 25-year-old man referred for echocardiography. He was a known case of VSD and underwent surgery at 14, at his follow-up echocardiography, there was a residual VSD. And one time after his surgery, he developed infective endocarditis and treated completely with full medical treatment.

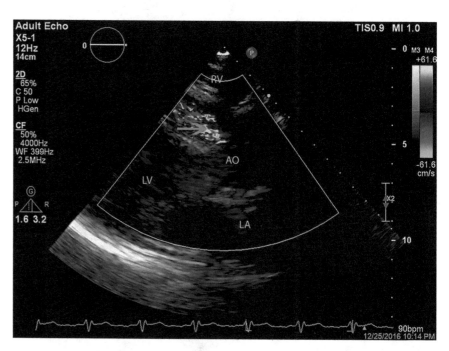

☐ **Fig. 10.6** Systolic turbulent flow across IVS in favor of residual perimembranous VSD (*arrow*). *LA* left atrium, *LV* left ventricle, *AO* aorta, *RV* right ventricle

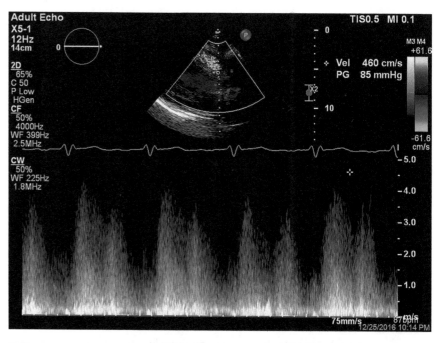

☐ **Fig. 10.7** Peak gradient across VSD is 85 mmHg but the flow is also diastolic

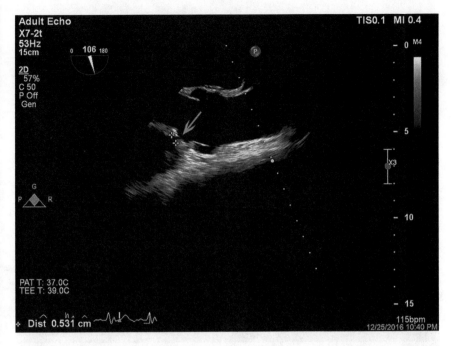

Fig. 10.8 TEE long-axis view shows the residual VSD (*arrow*) and it measures 5.3 mm in RV side

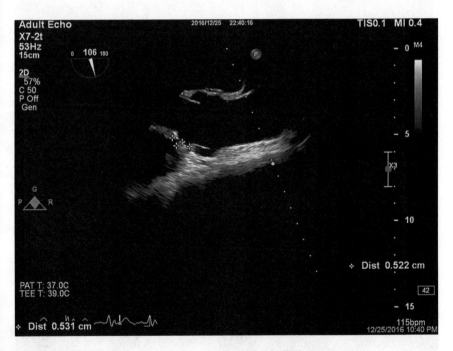

Fig. 10.9 Rim of VSD to aortic valve measures 5.2 mm in TEE long-axis view

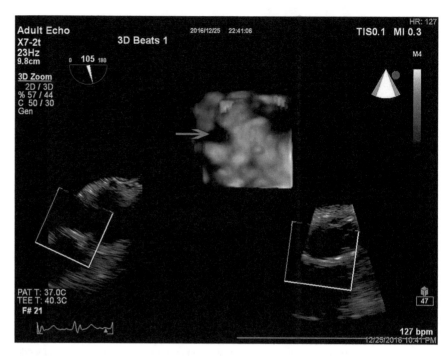

☐ **Fig. 10.10** VSD is visualized by I crop from LV side by 3D zoom (*arrow*)

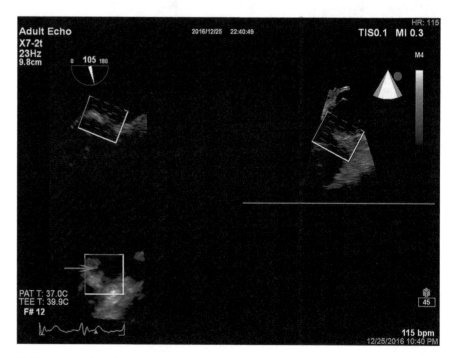

☐ **Fig. 10.11** VSD is determined by I slice from LV side by 3D zoom (*arrow*)

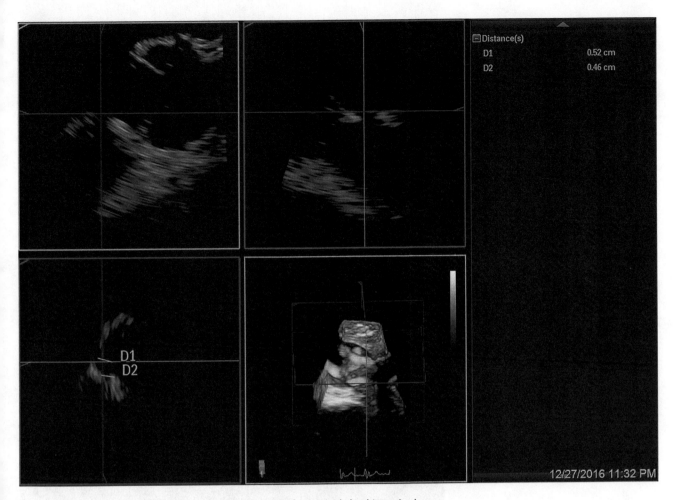

Distance(s)	
D1	0.52 cm
D2	0.46 cm

12/27/2016 11:32 PM

Fig. 10.12 VSD measures 5.2 from LV side by 3DQ and 4.7 from RV side by this method

Diagnosis   Small residual VSD post-surgery with Qp/Qs = 2.2, mild LV dilation, PAPs = 40 mmHg, good rim of VSD to aortic valve.

Comment   The patient referred for VSD device closure.

10.4   Case 3: VSD Post-Surgery HOCM

A 45-year-old woman referred for echocardiography after septal myectomy for HOCM and MVR. She developed CVA after surgery in recovery.

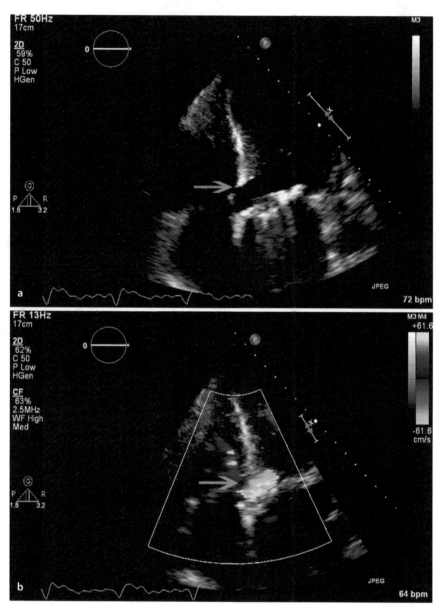

Fig. 10.13   Apical four-chamber view shows VSD (*arrow*) **a**, there is a turbulent flow across this VSD in systole (*arrow*) **b**

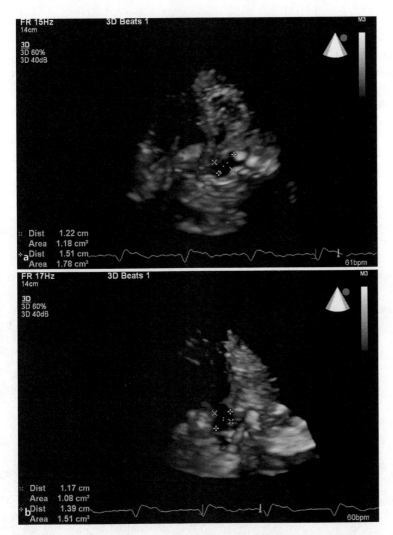

☐ **Fig. 10.14** This VSD measures 15*12 mm from LV side **a** and 12*14 mm from RV side **b** with 3D zoom

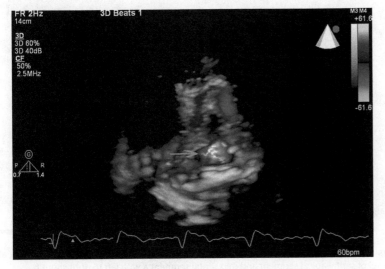

☐ **Fig. 10.15** 3D zoom echocardiography with color flow study reveals flow across VSD from LV side (*arrow*)

Diagnosis   VSD post-surgery myectomy and MVR.

Comment   If symptomatic, VSD device closure.

10.5   Case 4: Post-Myocardial Infarction VSD

A 62-year-old woman with a history of new recent acute anterior myocardial infarction and primary PCI on LAD. She presented 3 days after PCI with new onset chest pain and dyspnea and a new harsh systolic murmur at left sternal border and her electrocardiogram revealed new RBBB. She was referred to our echocardiography laboratory for evaluation of the cause of systolic murmur.

Transthoracic echocardiography showed regional wall motion abnormality in LAD territory.

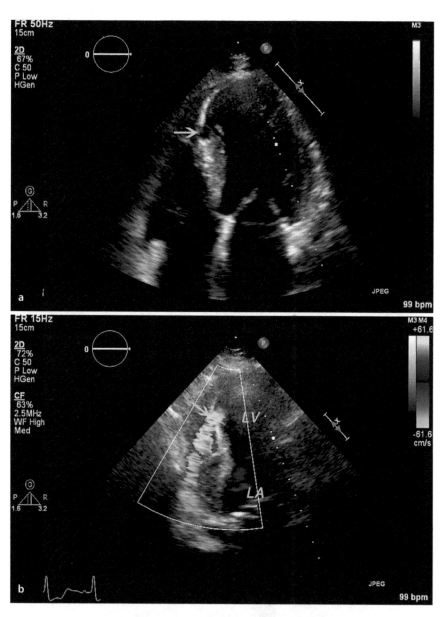

☐ **Fig. 10.16**   Apical four-chamber view shows a tunnel shape muscular VSD near to apex at the level of septal apical segment and mid septal segment **a** with left to right shunt **b**

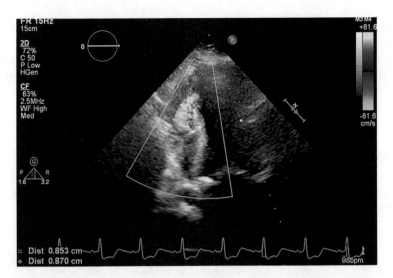

☐ **Fig. 10.17** The size of ventricular septal defect at the left ventricular aspect is measured 8 mm and at right ventricular side is measured 9 mm

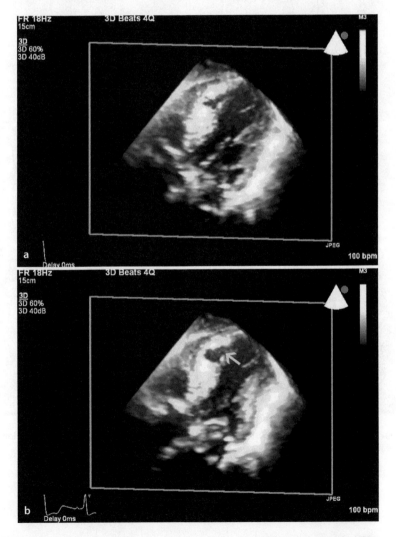

☐ **Fig. 10.18** 3D full volume four-chamber view depicts a narrow tunnel muscular VSD **a** and septal crop demonstrates the size of muscular VSD is larger than first looking **b** in favor of bundle branch damage occurs with extension of VSD along with interventricular septum

Diagnosis   Post-myocardial infarction ventricular septal defect.

10.6   Case 5: PDA

A 31-year-old man presented with dyspnea on exertion functional class II. Physical examination showed a continuous murmur at the left second intercostal space. Electrocardiography was normal.

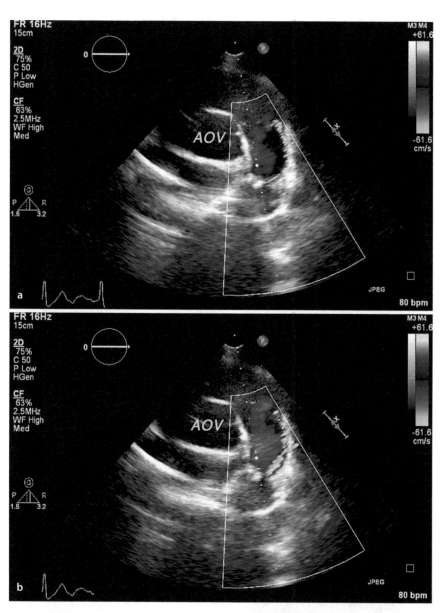

☐ **Fig. 10.19**   The parasternal short-axis view depicts a turbulent systolic **a** and diastolic flow **b** in the pulmonary artery, in favor of a patent ductus arteriosus (PDA). *AOV* aortic valve

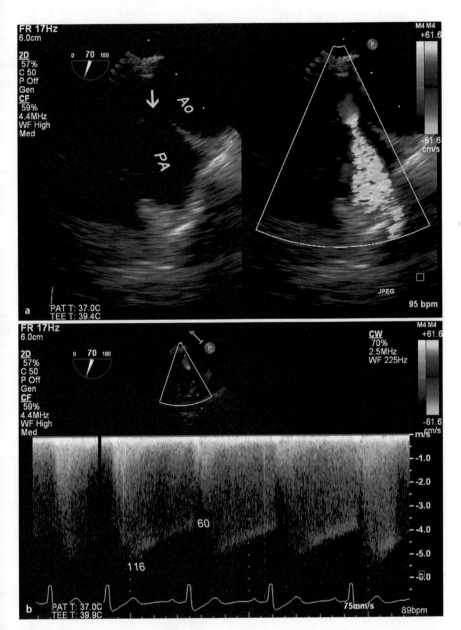

Fig. 10.20 Transesophageal echocardiography (70°), about 28 cm from dental arcade, shows the turbulent flow across descending aorta toward the pulmonary artery (*arrow*) **a**, the continuous Doppler study shows that the peak systolic and diastolic gradients are 116 and 64 mmHg, respectively **b**. *AO* aorta, *PA* pulmonary artery

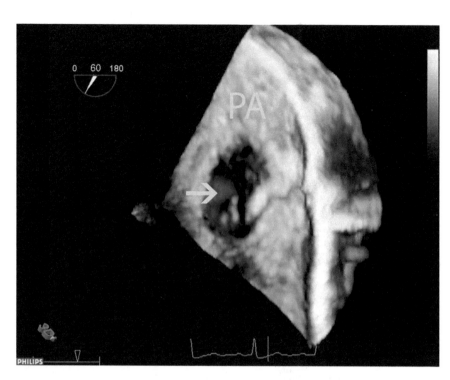

□ **Fig. 10.21**   In upper esophageal view 60° 3D zoom acquisition of pulmonary artery shows patent ductus arteriosus (PDA) enface view (*arrow*) from pulmonary artery side

Diagnosis   PDA.

Comment   The patient referred for PDA device closure.

10.7   Case 6: Subaortic Aortic Stenosis Membranous Type

A 35-year-old man presented with history of dyspnea on exertion and frequent episodes of palpitation. Physical examination revealed a diastolic murmur (grade III/VI) in the aortic area. Echocardiography demonstrated mild LV dilation and suboptimal LV systolic function as well as mild concentric left ventricular hypertrophy.

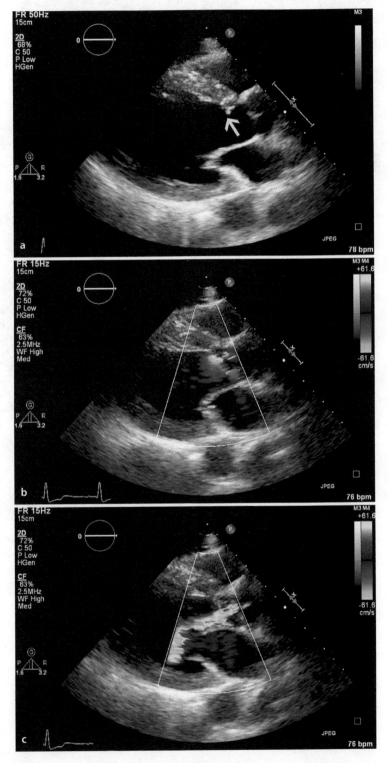

■ **Fig. 10.22** The long-axis view shows a subaortic membrane below the aortic valve which is attached to the interventricular septum (*arrow*, **a**) without systolic turbulancy in this area, in favor of non-significant stenosis of subaortic web **b**, a severe diastolic flow originates from aortic valve suggestive for severe aortic regurgitation **c**

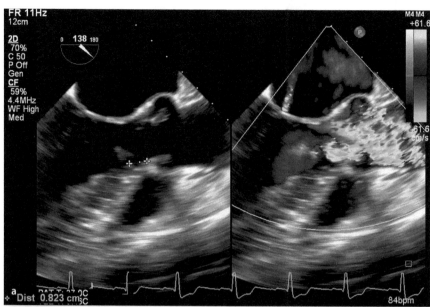

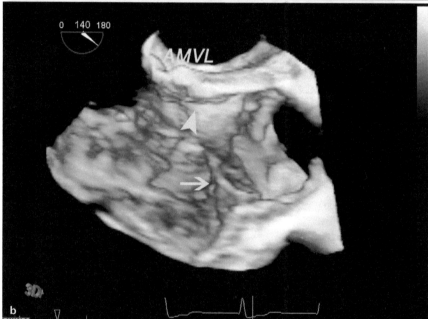

Fig. 10.23 Transesophageal echo (TEE) long-axis view depicts this membrane, this membrane is about 8 mm away from the aortic valve **a** and there is no attachment to anterior mitral leaflet in 3D long-axis view by 3D zoom (*arrowhead*, **b**). *AMVL* anterior mitral leaflet

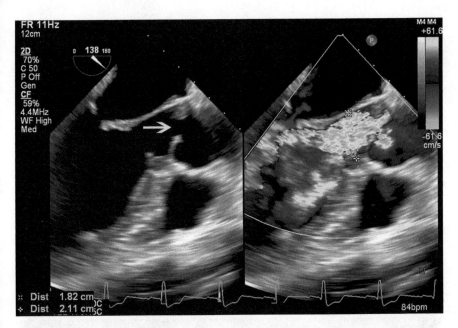

☐ **Fig. 10.24** Transesophageal echo (TEE) long-axis view shows severe AI due to malcoaptation of aortic leaflets in diastolic time (*arrow, left*) and it reveals width of AI/LVOT more than 60% (18/21, right **b**)

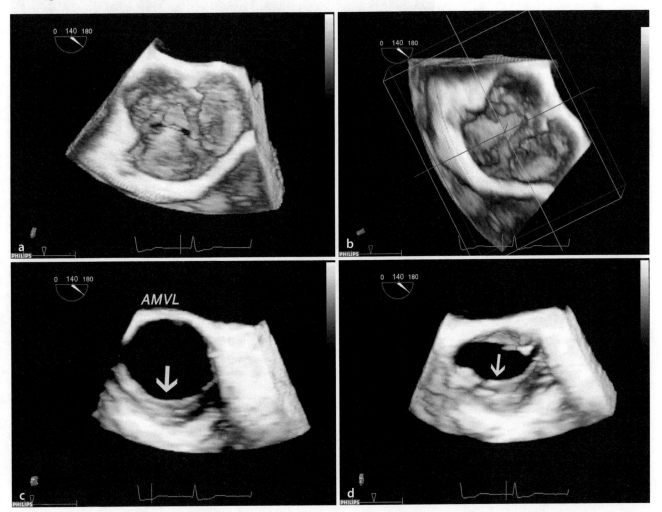

☐ **Fig. 10.25** Transesophageal 3D zoom short-axis enface view of aortic valve shows malcoaptation and restricted leaflets with thick borders in favor of chronic damage of leaflets due to subvalvular membrane **a** and after cropping along the red axis **b**, aortic leaflets are eliminated and subvalvular membrane's attachment to interventricular septum is apparent (*arrow*) without any attachment to anterior mitral leaflet **c, d**

Diagnosis The patient was diagnosed with severe aortic regurgitation and noncircular type subvalvular aortic membrane.

Comment AVR and resection of subvalvular membrane was recommended. Although subvalvular membrane had non-significant stenosis, resection of membrane is recommend for preventing of hemodynamic effect on prosthetic valve function.

Lesson:
1. RT 3D TEE of aortic valve provides detail morphologic information about leaflets, borders, coaptation of leaflets, mechanism of aortic regurgitation, and vena contracta's shape, size, and location.
2. After cropping along red axis view left ventricular out flow visualized clearly and revealed circular and noncircular subaortic membrane and this clue is very important for surgeon and successful operation.
3. This view is for another patient with circular type subaortic membrane stenosis.

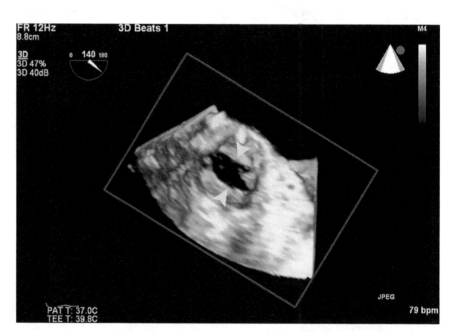

◘ Fig. 10.26 Crop of aortic valve leaflets reveals circular type of subaortic membrane which it has interventricular septal attachment and attachment to anterior mitral leaflet (*arrowheads*)

10.8   Case 7: Coarctation of Aorta

A 22-year-old man with history of hypertension referred for echocardiography. Physical examination showed hypertension and equal pulses in upper extremities but lower extremities pulses were weak.

Transthoracic echocardiography revealed normal left ventricular size and function and heart valves.

Transesophageal echocardiography was done for future evaluation of aortic arch.

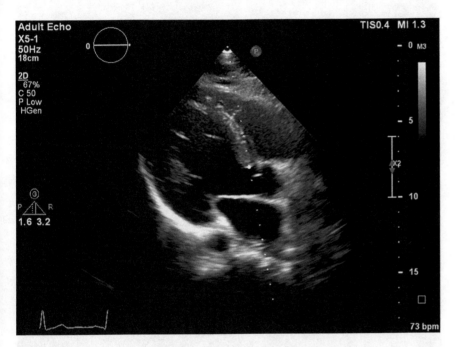

◻ Fig. 10.27   Parasternal long-axis view shows mild left ventricular hypertrophy

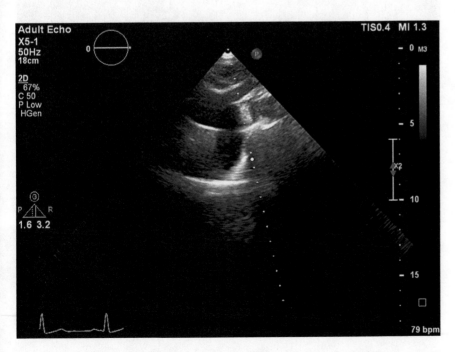

◻ Fig. 10.28   Suprasternal long-axis view reveals normal aortic arch at first looking

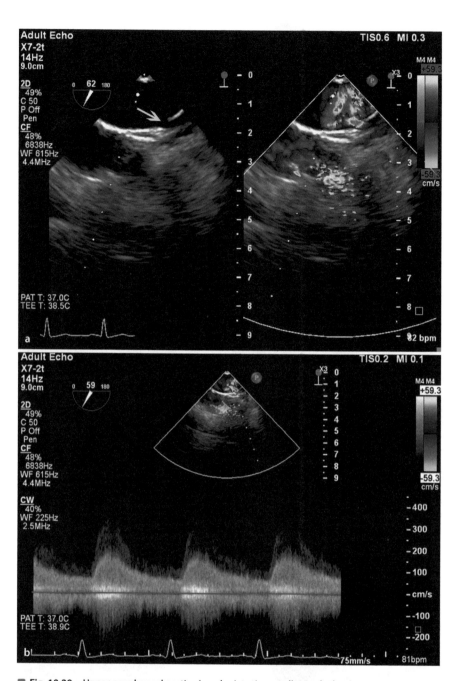

◘ Fig. 10.29 Upper esophageal aortic view depicts tiny small vessels that it connects to aorta **a** with continuous flow with systolic accentuation **b** in favor of collaterals

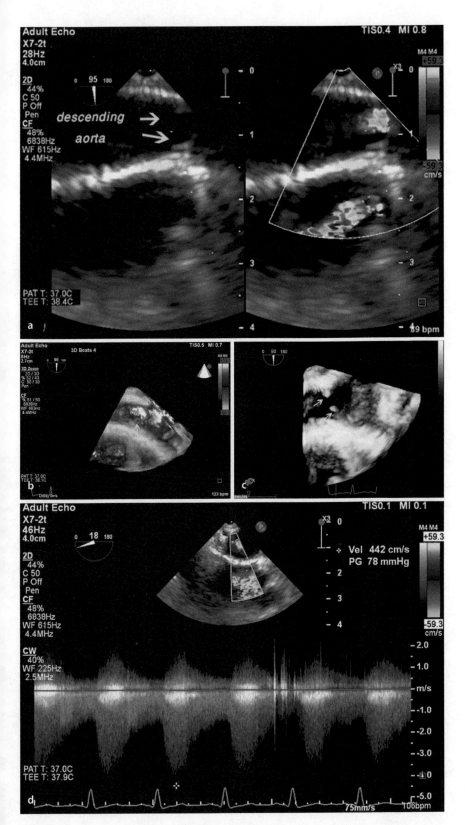

Fig. 10.30 Pull back of probe in upper esophageal view demonstrates a significant narrowing in aorta with turbulency at this site **a–c** and gradient across narrowing is measured 76 mmHg and the flow has antegrade diastolic component in favor of coarctation of aorta **d**

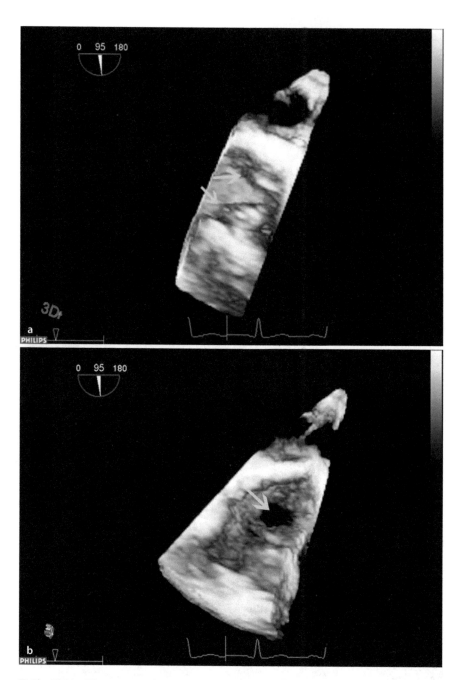

☐ **Fig. 10.31**   3D zoom view demonstrates very nice circular shape of coarctation of aorta **a, b**

Diagnosis   Coarctation of aorta with long distance from subclavian artery.

Recommendation   Patient was sent for coarctation stenting.

10.9   Case 8: Subaortic Web

A young age lady with a history of frequent transient ischemic attack that she is referred for evaluation cardiac source of emboli, physical examination was normal.

All transthoracic data was normal, transesophageal echocardiography was done for evaluation cardiac source of emboli.

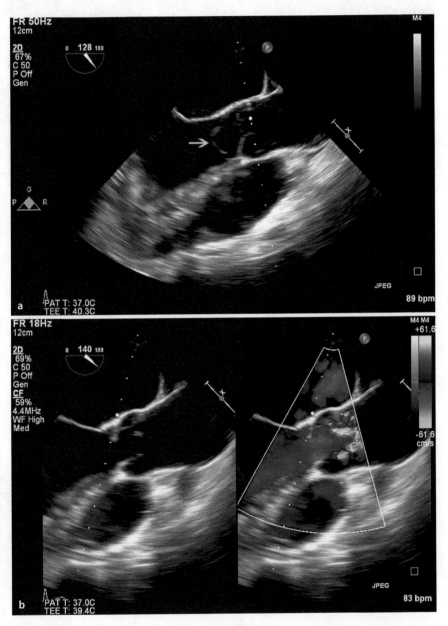

☐ **Fig. 10.32**   Mid esophageal long-axis view depicts a long membrane in left ventricular out flow tract (**a**, *arrow*) without any interaction with aortic valve function **b**

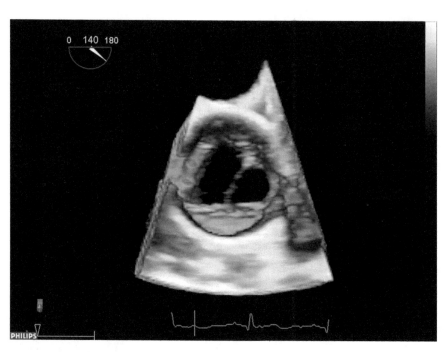

☐ **Fig. 10.33**   3D zoom view of aortic valve demonstrates this membrane is attached to right coronary cusp and left coronary cusp

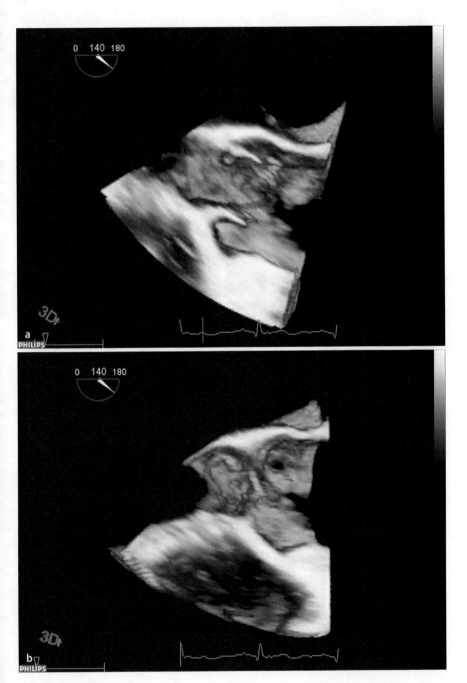

Fig. 10.34 Parasternal long-axis 3D zoom view shows that this membrane is hyper mobile and protrudes to aortic sinus during systolic time **a** and retracts to left ventricular out flow during diastolic time **b**

Diagnosis A membrane below aortic valve without stenosis.

Recommendation Due to the presence of PFO, the patient referred for PFO device closure and follow-up for subaortic web.

Reference

1. Sadeghian H, Zahra S-R. Echocardiographic atlas of adult congenital heart disease. Cham: Springer; 2015.

Cardiac Mass

Videos can be found in the electronic supplementary material in the online version of the chapter.
On http://springerlink.com enter the DOI number given on the bottom of the chapter opening page.
Scroll down to the Supplementary material tab and click on the respective videos link.

© Springer International Publishing AG 2017
H. Sadeghian, Z. Savand-Roomi, *3D Echocardiography of Structural Heart Disease*,
DOI 10.1007/978-3-319-54039-9_11

For differentiation cardiac masses, it is essential to consider the underlying disease, the cardiac chamber involved, and hyper or hypovascularity of the mass.

LA masses are clot or myxoma, if the patient has mitral stenosis, the probability of clot is increased. Cardiac myxoma is usually single and often is located in LA and is attached to IAS with a stalk. Thrombosis is often originated from LAA or is attached to LA roof.

The cardiac masses in LV are clot or cardiac tumors like rhabdomyoma. The clots are often associated by hypokinesia or akinesia of surrounding wall.

The masses in RA and RV are most likely thrombosis with systemic origin like tumors and hypercoagulable state.

Multiple masses are most likely metastasis, hyper or hypovascularity can help differentiation benign lesions from malignant tumor. Hypervascularity is in favor of malignancy.

11.1   Case 1: LAA Clot in DCM Patient

A young man with history of paroxysmal nocturnal dyspnea and orthopnea from 2 months ago following a common cold developped atrial fibrillation rhythm. Physical examination showed S3. He was candidate for cardio-version so he was sent for transesophageal echocardiography and rolled out of left atrial appendage clot.

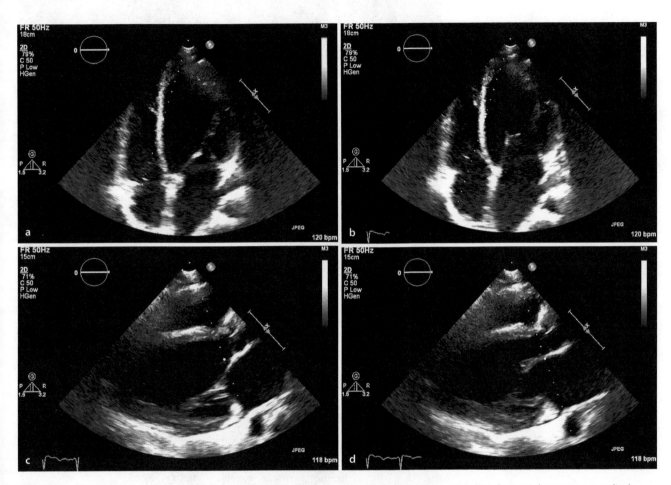

▫ **Fig. 11.1**   Apical four-chamber (**a**, systole and **b**, diastole) and long-axis view (**c**, systolic time and **d**, diastolic time) show severe systolic dysfunction and global hypokinesia indicative for myocarditis

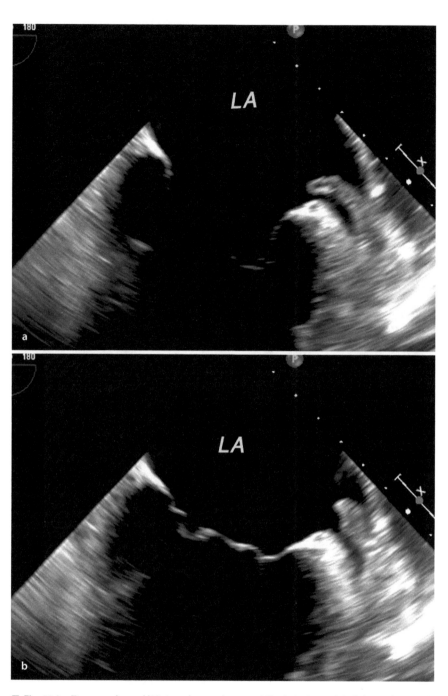

□ **Fig. 11.2**   Transesophageal l0° view shows a large mobile thrombus **a, b** in left atrial append-age (*arrow*)

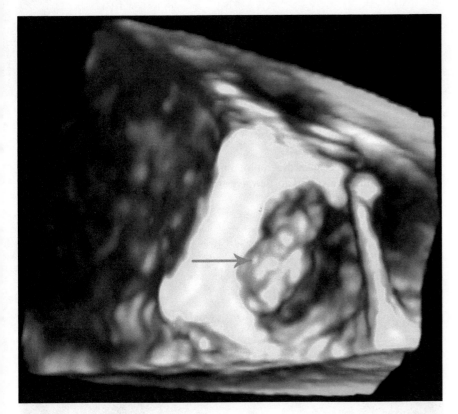

◘ Fig. 11.3   3D zoom view of left atrial appendage from left atrial view shows the clot in LAA which protrudes to left atrium

With respect to large left atrial appendage clot, cardio-version could not be possible so only appropriate anticoagulation therapy and heart rate control recommended.

11.2   Case 2: LA and LAA Clot Due to MS

A 45-year-old women who presented with dyspnea on exertion functional class IV and abdominal pain and cholecystitis was referred by surgeon for pre-operation evaluation.

In physical examination she had a diastolic murmur in mitral area grade III/VI and a systolic murmur in aortic area.

Transthoracic echocardiography showed normal left ventricular systolic function and severe mitral stenosis.

Transesophageal echocardiography was performed for evaluation of mass and exact size of mitral valve and aortic valve area.

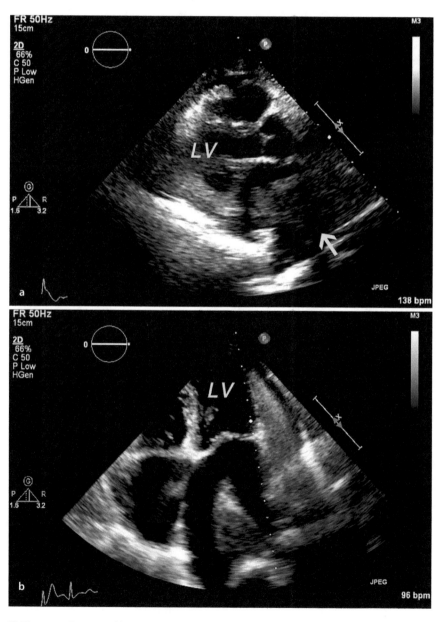

☐ **Fig. 11.4**   Parasternal long-axis view shows a large echo dense haziness in left atrium which filled more than 2/3 of LA **a** and apical four-chamber view shows that this lesion originated from roof of left atrium **b**

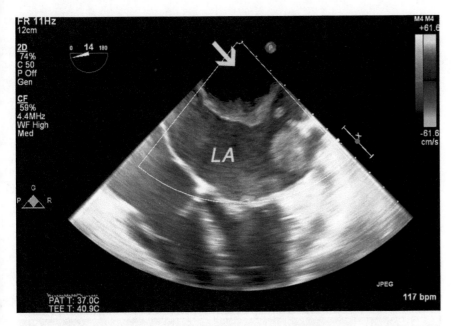

☐ **Fig. 11.5** Transesophageal echo 14° view shows a large mass in left atrium with some necrosis in it (*arrow*) in favor of clot formation in left atrium due to mitral stenosis

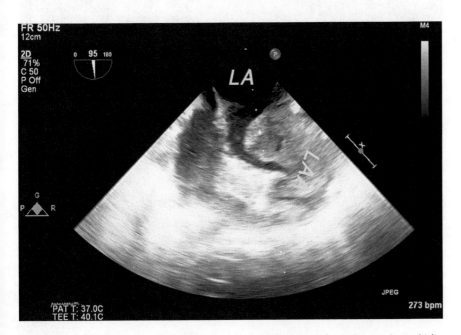

☐ **Fig. 11.6** Transesophageal short-axis view shows a large clot in left atrial appendage which filled whole left atrial appendage and extends to left atrium

11

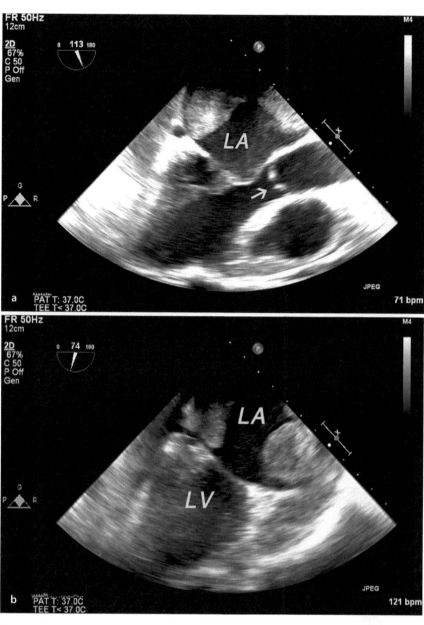

◘ Fig. 11.7 Long-axis **a** and short-axis **b** transesophageal views reveal that left atrial clot extends from one side to other side of left atrium and also long-axis view reveals that aortic valve is thick and dome (*arrow*) **a** and aortic valve area measures 1, 2 cm² (didn't show) indicative for moderate AS

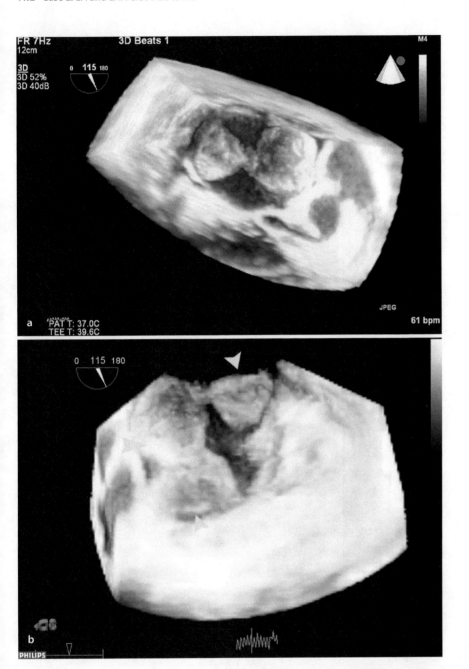

Fig. 11.8 Live 3D echo shows left atrial clot from the left atrial view which is dumbbell shape **a** and by some rotation in Z axis, extension of clot is better visualized than 2D views (*arrow heads*, **b**)

Diagnosis Severe mitral stenosis, moderate valvular aortic stenosis, and very large clot in left atrium and left atrial appendage with some necrosis within it.

The patient was sent to operation room for MVR and AVR and removal of left atrium and left atrial appendage clot and left atrial appendage closure.

11.3   Case 3: LA Myxoma

A 55-year-old woman with history of recurrent TIA was referred to our echo-lab for evaluation of cardiac cause of emboli. In physical examination she had normal S1 and S2 and faint diastolic and systolic murmur in mitral area.

Transthoracic echocardiography revealed normal left ventricular size and systolic function.

Transesophageal echocardiography was performed for more depiction of mass.

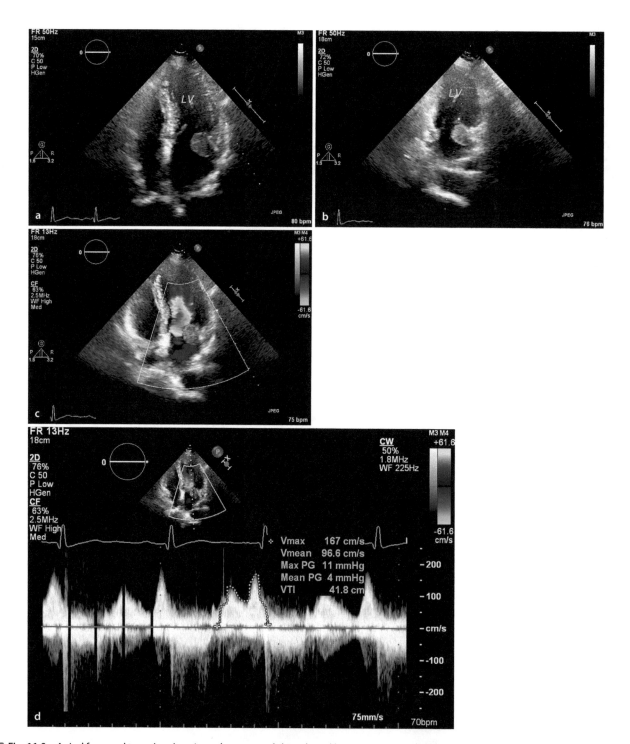

■ **Fig. 11.9**   Apical four- and two-chamber views show a round shape broad base mass attached to posterior mitral leaflet and left atrial wall **a, b**, color Doppler study reveals mild diastolic turbulency across mitral valve **c**, peak and mean gradient across mitral valve are 11 and 4 mmHg, respectively (mildly increased) **d**

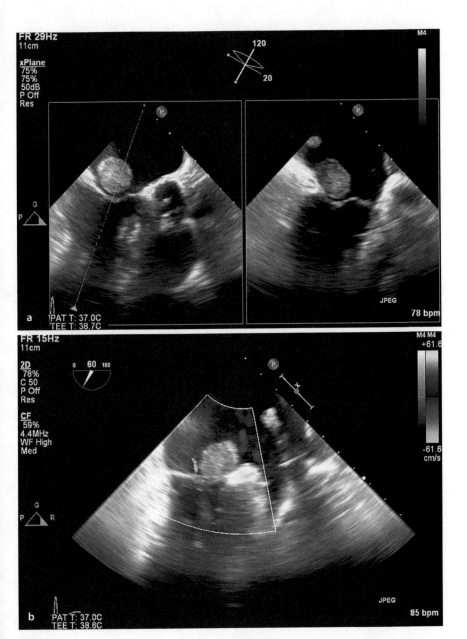

Fig. 11.10 Transesophageal echocardiography X plain two-chamber view shows that the left atrial mass doesn't have any attachment to posterior mitral leaflet **a** and it induces trivial mitral regurgitation **b**

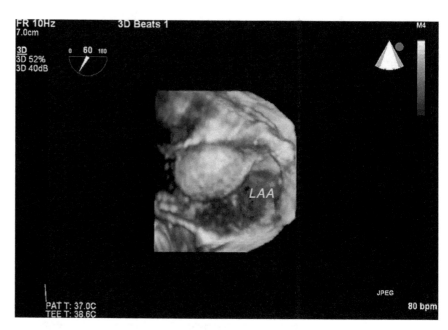

☐ **Fig. 11.11** 3D zoom view shows clearly that the mass does not originate from left atrial appendage and completely is separate from posterior mitral leaflet, 3D zoom view acquisition was performed in transesophageal two-chamber view from left atrial side

This mass seems unusual type of left atrial myxoma.

With respect to the patient had neurological evidence of recurrent TIA, the patient was sent for mass resection and after resection, pathology confirmed benign vascular tumor.

11.4   Case 4: LA Myxoma with Severe MR

A 65-year-old man presented with history of dyspnea on exertion functional class III. In physical examination he had systolic murmur in mitral area, he was referred to our echo-lab for evaluation of the cause of dyspnea.

Transthoracic echocardiography showed normal left ventricular size and systolic function.

Usually left atrial myxoma attached to the PFO (patent foramen oval) site and by TTE parasternal long-axis view it could be seen.

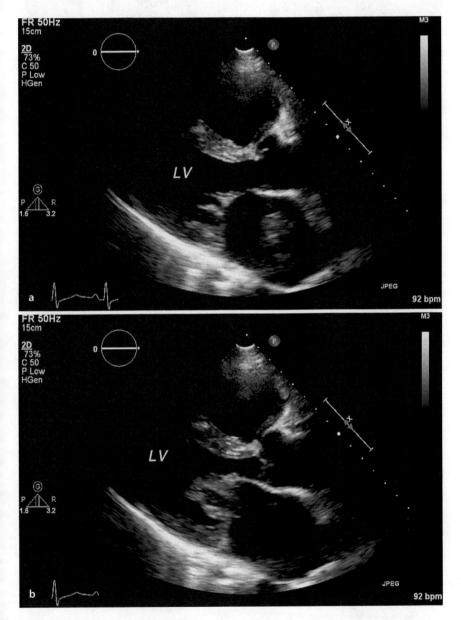

☐ **Fig. 11.12**   Long-axis views **a**, **b** show large hyper-mobile mass in left atrium which protrudes to the left ventricle in diastolic time **b**. *LV* left ventricle

11

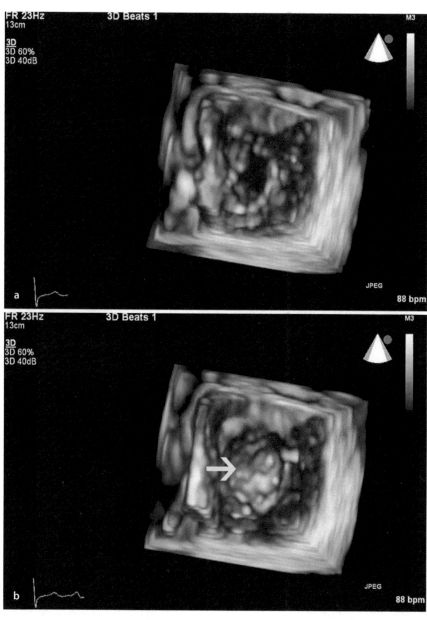

■ **Fig. 11.13**   3D zoom short-axis views **a**, **b** of mitral valve from left ventricular side show clearly protrusion of this mass into left ventricle during diastolic time (*arrow*) **b**

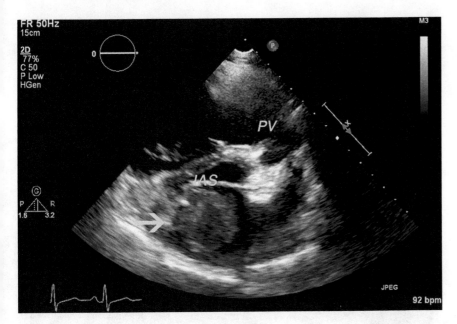

■ **Fig. 11.14**   Parasternal short-axis view depicts attachment of this mass (*arrow*) to the inter-atrial septum. *IAS* interatrial septum, *PV* pulmonary valve

11

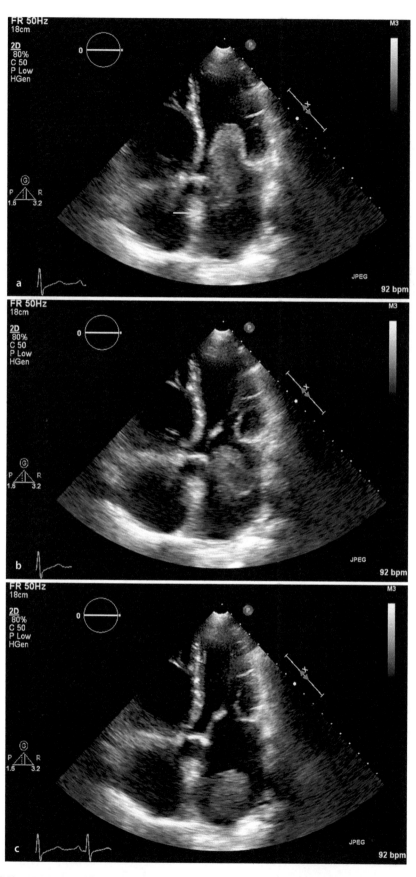

Fig. 11.15 Apical four-chamber views confirm the attachment of this mass to interatrial septum (*arrow*, **a**) but the location of this mass is different between views **b**, **c** and it differs according to cardiac cycle and so it seems more mobile than a usual type of myxoma

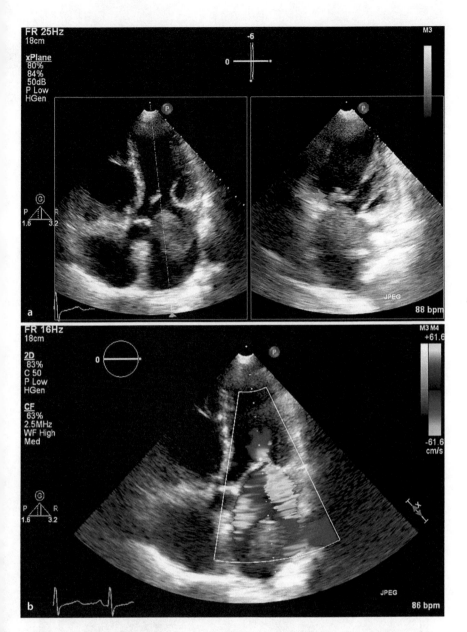

□ **Fig. 11.16** Apical four-chamber view by X plane mode shows mitral valve leaflets are thick (**a**, *arrow*) with severe mitral regurgitation **b**

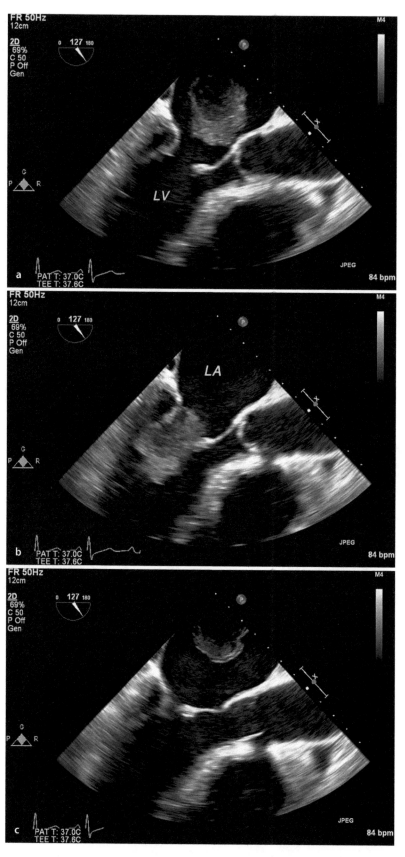

■ **Fig. 11.17** Transesophageal long-axis view depicts a large lobulated mass indicative for myxoma but the mobility of mass is more than usual, in early diastole it is in mid LA **a**, in late diastole, it protrudes into left ventricle **b** and in systole, it is located in roof of left atrium (**c**) and mitral leaflets seem thick and restricted and short due to recurrent mass injury **a**, **c**. *LV* left ventricle

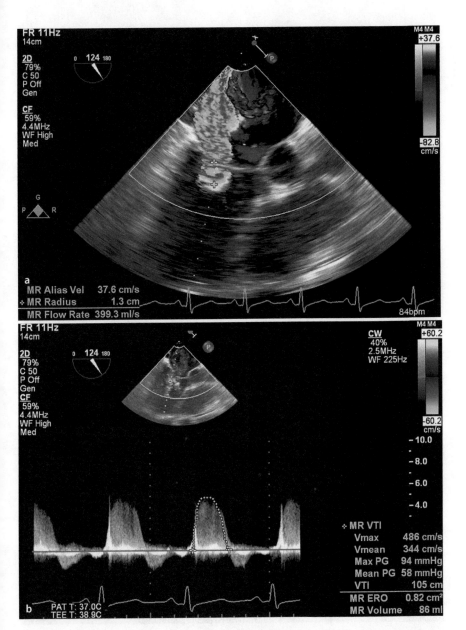

Fig. 11.18 Severe mitral regurgitation with mitral regurgitation volume more than 80 mL by PISA represents for severe MR **a**, **b**, for measuring MR volume by PISA, first, the velocity of aliasing of MR is reduced between 35 and 45 cm/s (37.6 in this case) at atrial level, then the radius of MR PISA is measured (13 mm in this case) **a**, then VTI of MR is traced (105 cm in this case) with peak velocity of 4.86 m/s **b** and finally MR volume is calculated

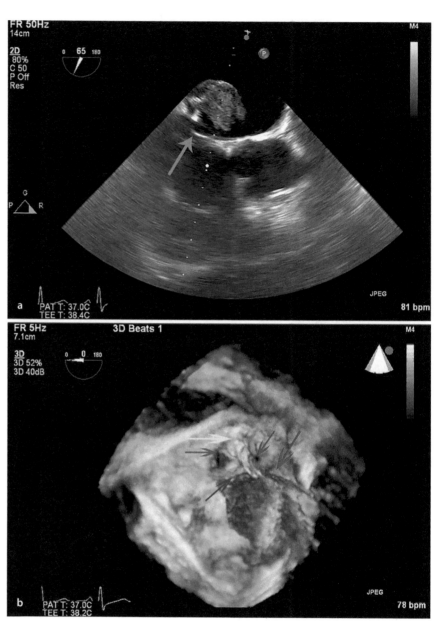

◘ Fig. 11.19 Transesophageal short-axis view reveals that the site of the mass attachment is not exactly at the site of fossa ovalis (*arrow*) **a** and 3D zoom of interatrial septum from LA side **b** shows tumor's whole extension and shape and surface structure, the mass extends up to the Fossa ovalis (*green arrow*), right lower pulmonary vein is also visualized in this view (*pink arrow*), the stalk of the mass is also seen in this view (*yellow arrow*)

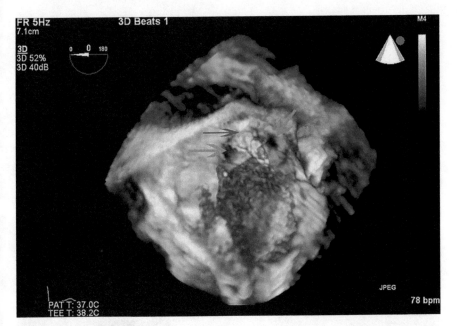

☐ **Fig. 11.20**   3D zoom view in 0° shows the site of myxoma attachment between the right pulmonary veins (*green arrows*), the stalk of attachment of this tumor is also well visualized in this view (*pink arrow*)

11.5 Case 5: Small Size Pulmonary Thromboemboli with Large RA Mass

A 25-year-old woman with history of abdominoplasty 1 week ago, who presented with atypical chest pain without dyspnea with normal blood pressure who was referred to our echocardiography laboratory for echocardiography. In physical examination a faint systolic murmur in left sternal border was heard.

Transthoracic echocardiography was performed: left and right ventricular sizes and function were normal and a large mass in right atrium was detected, transesophageal echocardiography was performed for evaluation of pulmonary artery and mass such as renal carcinoma and tumor metastasis.

Pulmonary artery is dilated but it was not any clot in it.

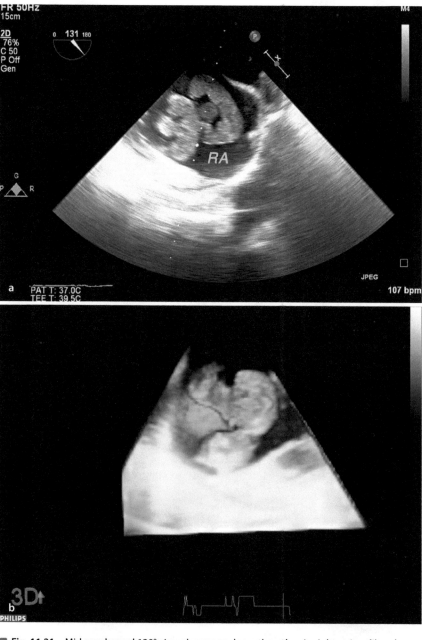

Fig. 11.21   Mid esophageal 130° view shows very large thrombus in right atrium like a long worm **a**, **b** in favor of a large clot in right atrium

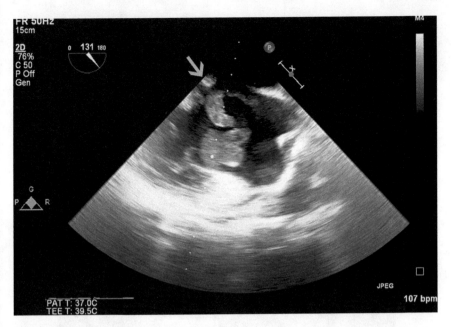

Fig. 11.22 Mid esophageal long-axis view depicts a thrombus in inferior vena cava (*arrow*) that protrudes to right atrium

Diagnosis   A large thrombus in right atrium impending to pulmonary emboli.

Recommendation   According to guideline 2014 of pulmonary emboli, negative predictive valve of echocardiography is 40–50% so a negative result cannot exclude pulmonary emboli, due to this fact that only moderate and large size pulmonary thromboemboli can be diagnosed by echocardiography. Pulmonary CT angiography was performed and it showed some small clot in left pulmonary artery, color Doppler sonography of both lower extremities did not show any deep vein thrombosis.

The patient had not any evidence of massive pulmonary emboli and she was stable but she was impending to massive pulmonary emboli, size of right atrial thrombus was too large and fibrinolytic therapy could induce multiple pulmonary emboli and on the other hand she had history of surgery 1 week ago, we preferred sending patient to the operation room and clot removal was performed and size of clot was reported 22 cm.

11.6   Case 6: LAA Thrombosis

A 65-year-old man with a history of stroke and left sided paralysis was sent to our echocardiography laboratory for evaluation of the cause of stroke. In physical examination he had irregular beats in favor of atrial fibrillation rhythms without significant murmur.

Transthoracic echocardiography revealed a large left atrium and a mass on the left atrium and normal valves.

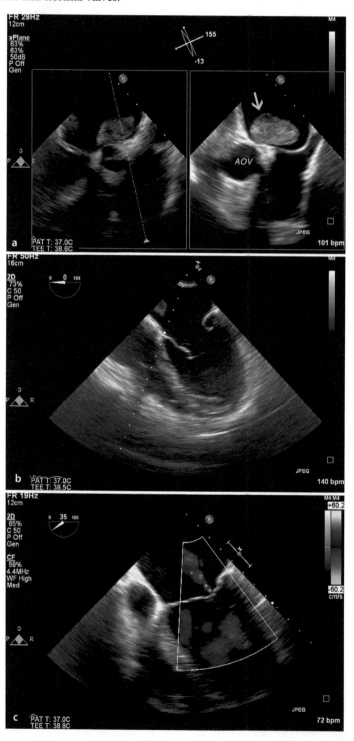

◘ Fig. 11.23   Mid esophageal X plane view depicts a left atrial mass (**a**, *arrow*) with attachment to anterosuperior part of interatrial septum near to aortic valve and far from mitral valve and without protrusion to mitral valve during diastolic time **b** and there is not any interaction to mitral valve function **c**

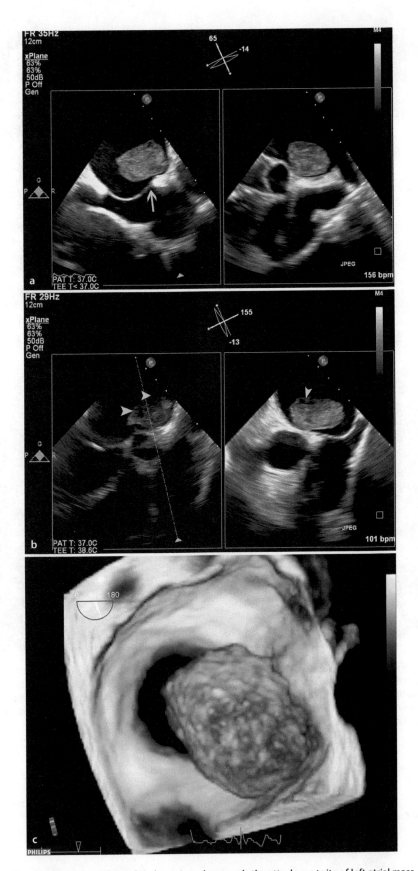

◻ Fig. 11.24 Mid esophageal X plane view also reveals the attachment site of left atrial mass is not in usual site of LA myxoma and doesn't have stalk **a** (LA myxoma usually attaches to PFO site, *arrow*) and there is some vacuolization in mass (*head arrows*, **b**) in favor of mass necrosis and 3D zoom view demonstrates heterogeneous appearance of mass **c** suggestive for left atrial thrombus

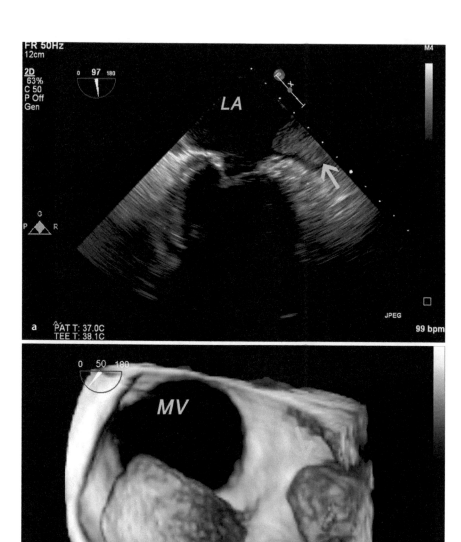

◻ Fig. 11.25 Mid esophageal view **a** and 3D zoom view **b** depict a large mass in left atrial appendage (*arrow*) that it protrudes to left atrium, the first mass might be considered as to be a myxoma, however, with detection of second mass growing out of the LA appendage and presence of other criteria of thrombus such as appearance of mass and necrosis in it and attachment (without stalk) in superior part of interatrial septum, both masses are most likely thrombi

Diagnosis   Large LA and LAA thrombus due to atrial fibrillation rhythm.

Recommendation   The patient was sent to operation room for LA and LAA removal clot and maze procedure during operation.

11.7   Case 7: RA Clots

A 55-year-old man presented by dyspnea on exertion functional class IV. He was a known case of coronary artery disease and low ejection fraction (LVEF = 20%) and severe ischemic mitral regurgitation.

TEE was performed for more evaluation of ischemic MR.

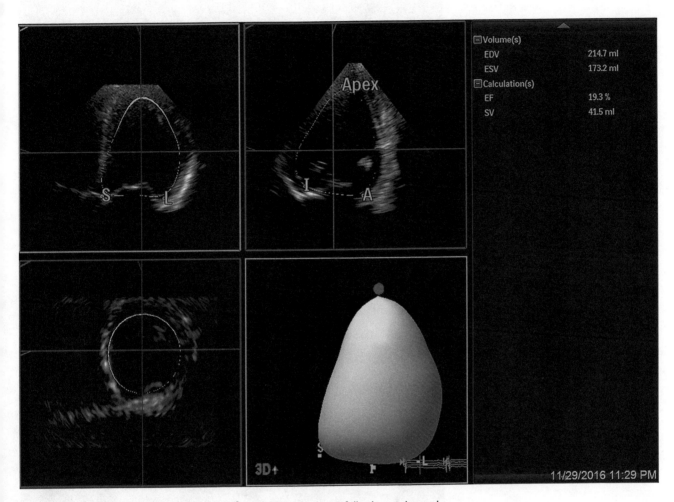

Fig. 11.26   LVEDV = 215 cm³, LVESV = 173 cm³, and LVEF = 19% by 3D full volume advanced

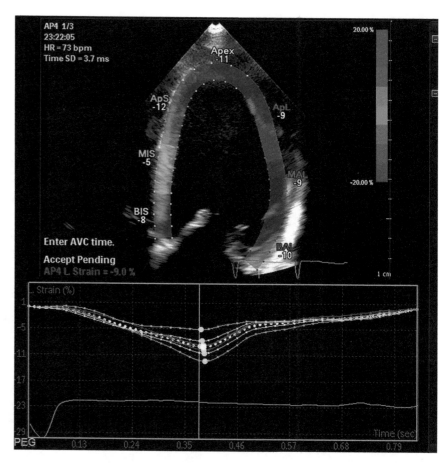

 Fig. 11.27 Longitudinal strain measures −9% in apical four-chamber view

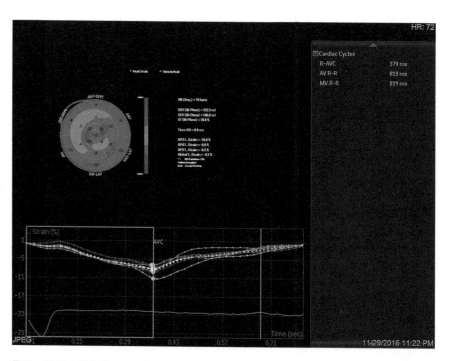

 Fig. 11.28 Global longitudinal strain measures −9%

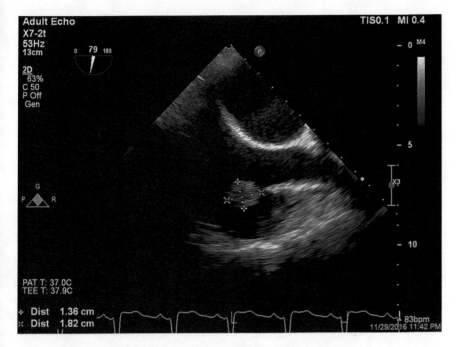

☐ **Fig. 11.29** There is a mobile mass 18*14 mm in right atrium

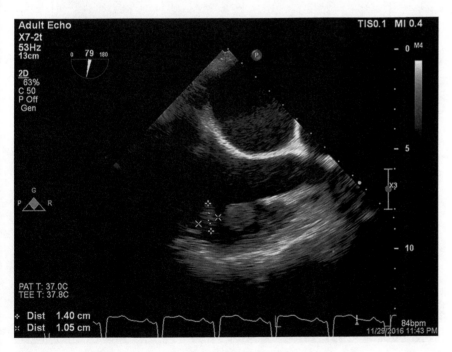

☐ **Fig. 11.30** There is another mass 14*11 mm in right atrium

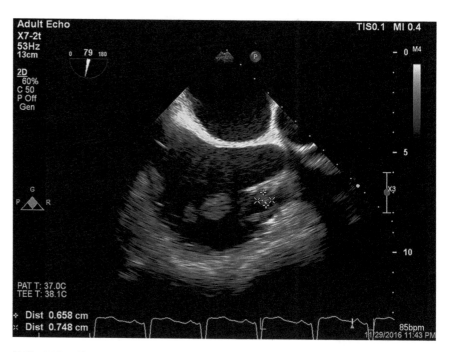

Fig. 11.31   There is third mass 7.5*6.5 mm in right atrial appendage

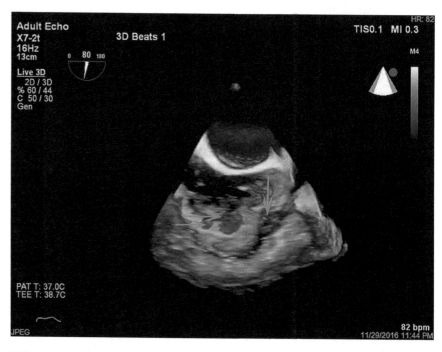

Fig. 11.32   There are three masses in right atrium by live 3D (*arrows*)

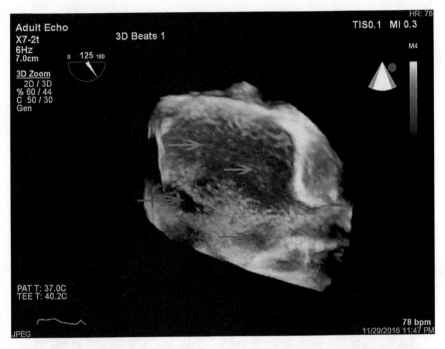

◘ Fig. 11.33 Pulmonary veins are visualized by 3D zoom of interatrial septum (*arrows*), due to reversal flow in pulmonary vein because of severe mitral regurgitation, two right pulmonary veins are empty of flow (*pink arrows*)

11

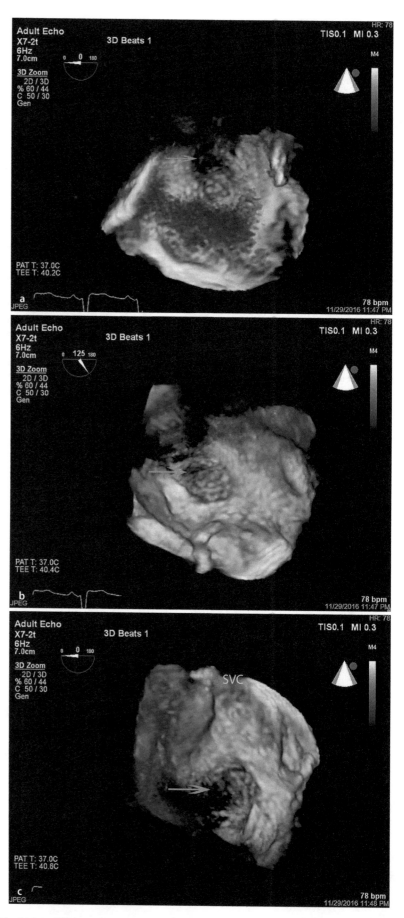

◘ **Fig. 11.34**   PFO is evident by 3D zoom from LA sides (0° and 125°, **a, b**) and by 3D zoom from RA side of interatrial septum **c** (*arrows*)

Diagnosis   Severe ischemic mitral regurgitation, LVEF = 20%, severe LV dilation, three RA clots, and PFO.

Comment   The patient referred for urgent surgery (MV repair + CABG + removal of RA clots + PFO closure).

Lesson:
1. Due to PFO, thrombolysis is dangerous for RA clots. Because that the clots may pass through PFO and cause systemic emboli, so urgent surgery was recommended.
2. Stress echocardiography is class I of indication for assessment of viability for secondary functional mitral regurgitation according to ACC/AHA guidelines [1].
3. Mitral valve surgery is class IIa in severe functional MR if CABG is needed according to both American and European guidelines [1, 2].
4. In this patient, stress echocardiography was not performed due to RA clots.
5. Global longitudinal LV strain in normal population is between −15.9% and 22.1% [3]. In this patient global longitudinal LV strain is severely reduced (−9%).

11.8   Case 8: LA Myxoma

A 42-year-old man presented by dyspnea on exertion functional class I.

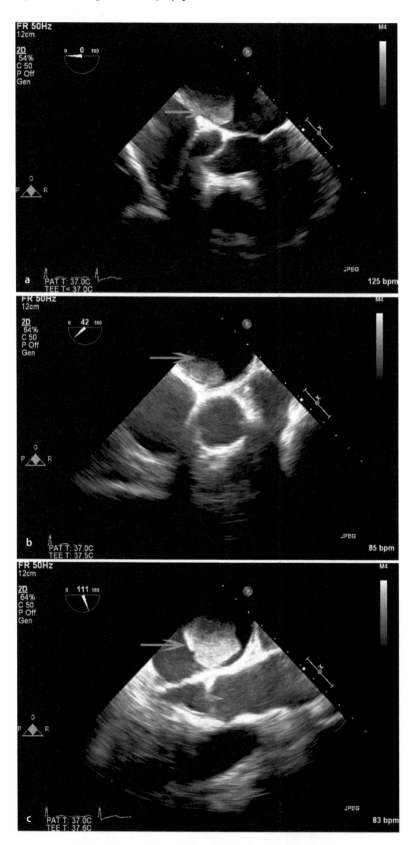

☐ **Fig. 11.35**   A large mass is seen in LA in TEE 0° **a**, short-axis **b** and long-axis I views (*arrows*) **c**

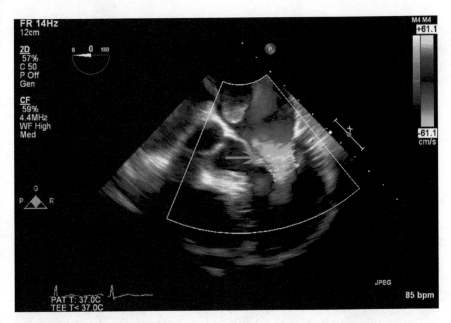

◻ Fig. 11.36 This mass is hypovascular and no obstructive effect on mitral valve by TEE 0°
view (*arrow*)

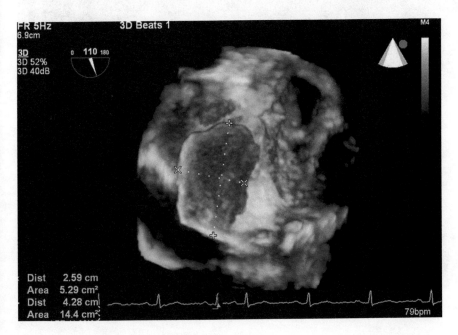

◻ Fig. 11.37 This mass measures 43*26 mm by 3D zoom

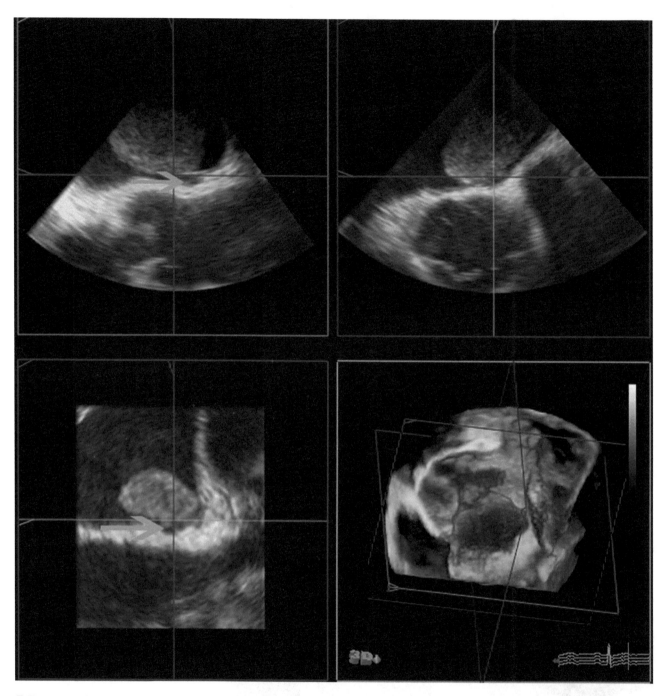

Fig. 11.38   This mass is attached to IAS by a small stalk (*arrows*) viewed by 3DQ

Diagnosis   A hypovascular mass in LA most probably myxoma without obstructive effect on other structures.

Comment   Surgery.

11.9   Case 9: Cardiac Hydatic Cyst

A 29-year-old man presented by atypical chest pain of recent duration.

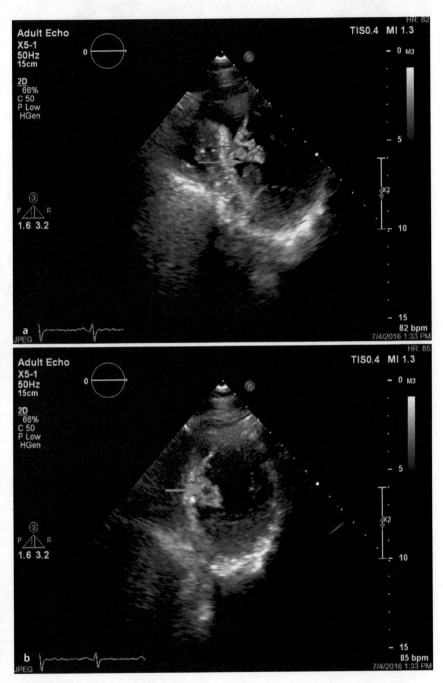

◘ **Fig. 11.39**   Septal apical and inferoapical are akinetic with a mass attached to these walls (*green arrow*) (**a**, modified apical), there is a hole in this mass (*pink arrow*) (**b**, short-axis)

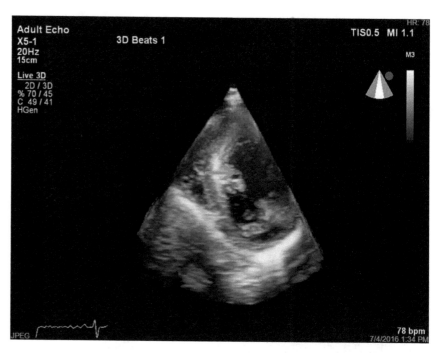

□ **Fig. 11.40** Live 3D fully shows this mass with a hole within it (*arrow*)

Diagnosis   Cardiac Hydatic cyst. Coronary angiography was normal and the cause for akinesia in septal apical and inferoapical was the pressure effect of the cyst.

Comment   The patient referred for cardiac surgery and the cyst completely removed and after that, echocardiography revealed no cyst.

References

1. Nishimura RA, Otto CM, Bonow RO, Carabello BA, Erwin 3rd JP, Guyton RA, et al. 2014 AHA/ACC guideline for the management of patients with valvular heart disease: a report of the American College of Cardiology/American Heart Association task force on practice guidelines. J Am Coll Cardiol. 2014;63(22):e57–185.
2. Joint Task Force on the Management of Valvular Heart Disease of the European Society of Cardiac, European Association for Cardio-Thoracic Surgery, Vahanian A, Alfieri O, Andreotti F, Antunes MJ, et al. Guidelines on the management of valvular heart disease (version 2012). Eur Heart J. 2012;33(19):2451–96.
3. Yingchoncharoen T, Agarwal S, Popovic ZB, Marwick TH. Normal ranges of left ventricular strain: a meta-analysis. J Am Soc Echocardiogr. 2013;26(2):185–91.

Intervention in Structural Heart Disease

Videos can be found in the electronic supplementary material in the online version of the chapter.
On http://springerlink.com enter the DOI number given on the bottom of the chapter opening page.
Scroll down to the Supplementary material tab and click on the respective videos link.

© Springer International Publishing AG 2017
H. Sadeghian, Z. Savand-Roomi, *3D Echocardiography of Structural Heart Disease*,
DOI 10.1007/978-3-319-54039-9_12

12.1   Case 1: ASD Device Closure

A 55-year-old woman presented by dyspnea on exertion functional class II–III of recent exacerbation.

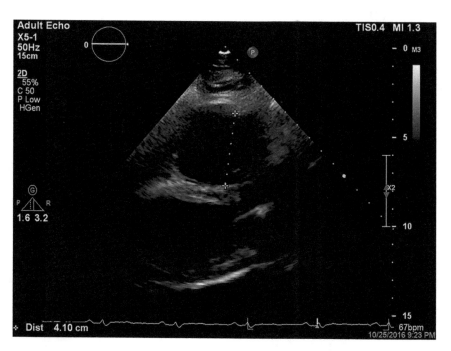

☐ **Fig. 12.1**   Right ventricle is dilated in parasternal long-axis view, right ventricle measures 41 mm in this view

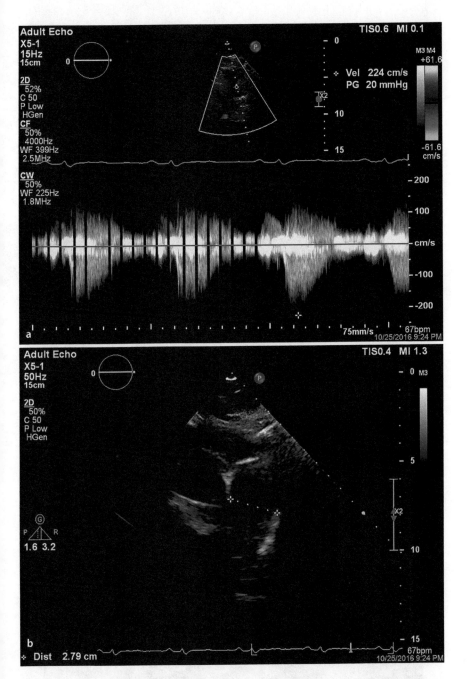

◻ Fig. 12.2 Peak gradient across pulmonary valve is 20 mmHg in parasternal short-axis view **a**, pulmonary artery measures 28 mm in this view **b**

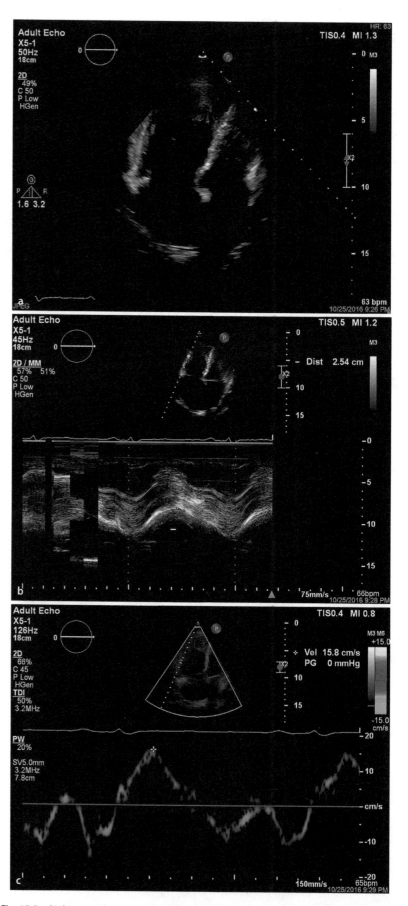

Fig. 12.3   Right ventricle is severely dilated in apical four-chamber view **a**, TAPSE measures 25 mm in this view **b**, RV Sm measures 16 cm/s in this apical four-chamber view **c**

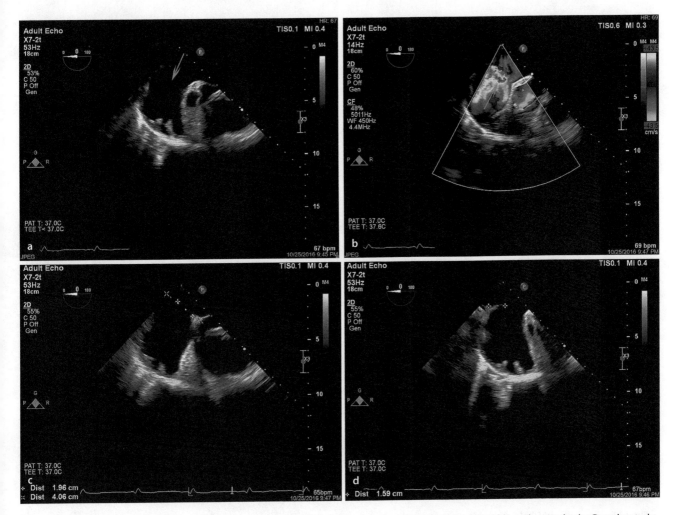

◻ Fig. 12.4 The defect of interatrial septum is evident by TEE 0° view (*arrows*) by two-dimensional echocardiography **a** and color Doppler study **b**, ASD/IAS measures 20/41 mm in this view **c** and posterior rim measures 16 mm in this view **d**

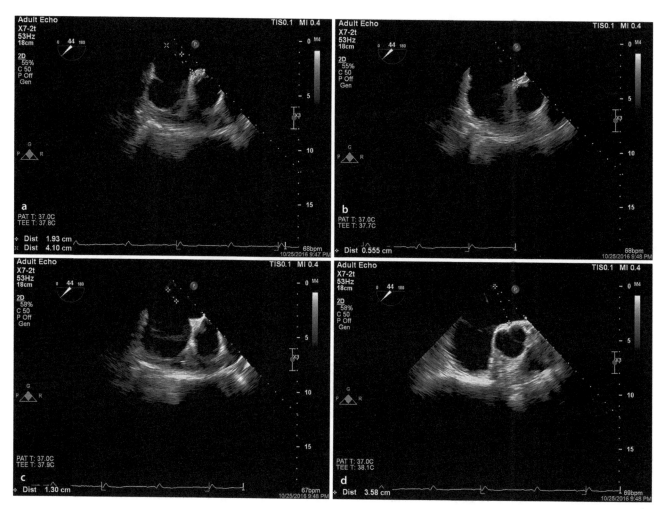

☐ **Fig. 12.5**   The ratio of ASD/IAS measures 19/41 mm in TEE short-axis view **a**, the rim to aortic valve measures 5.5 mm **b** and the opposite rim measures 13 mm **c** in this view, atrial depth measures 36 mm **d**

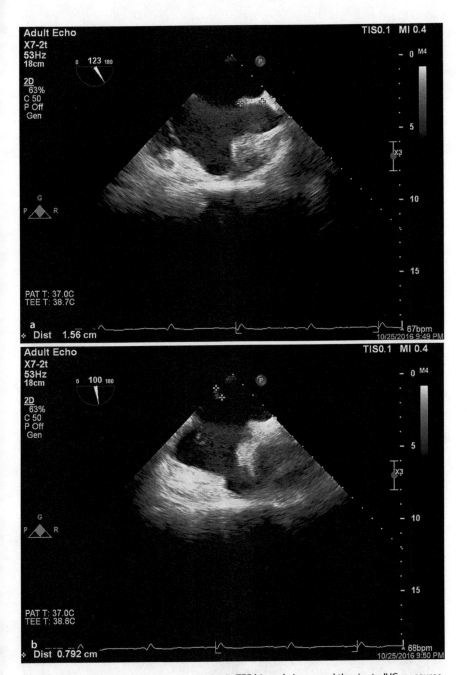

■ **Fig. 12.6**   The rim to SVC measures 16 mm in TEE bicaval view **a** and the rim to IVC measures 8 mm in this view **b**

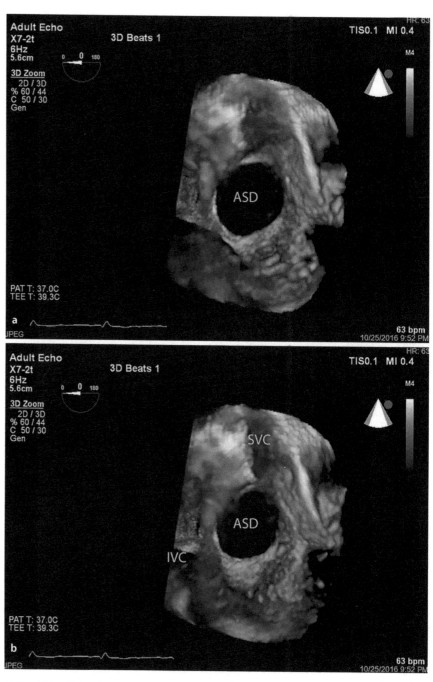

Fig. 12.7 ASD with 3D zoom from right atrial **a**, in this view, superior vena cava (SVC) and inferior vena cava (IVC) can be visualized in 11 and 5 o'clock, respectively **b**

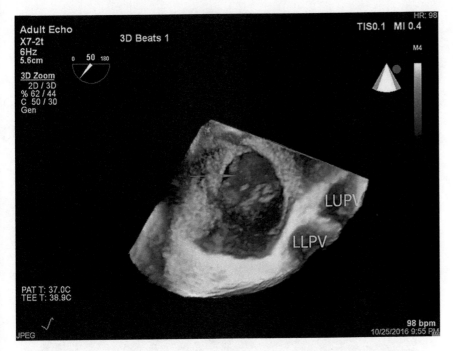

☐ **Fig. 12.8** ASD in 50° from left atrial side by 3D zoom (*arrow*), left upper and lower pulmonary veins are visualized in this view. *LUPV* left upper pulmonary vein, *LLPV* left lower pulmonary vein

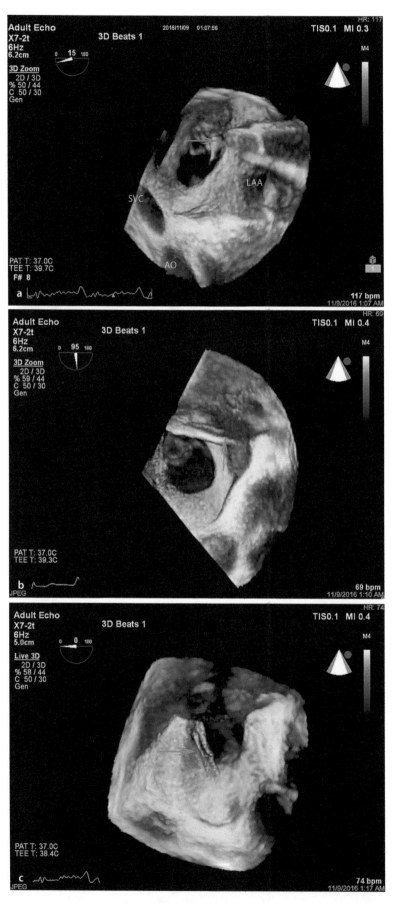

◘ Fig. 12.9 Guide wire in left upper pulmonary vein (LUPV) (*arrows*) for ASD closure by 3D zoom in 15° **a**, 90° **b** and 0° **c** views, superior vena cava (SVC) and aorta (AO) are visualized in this view

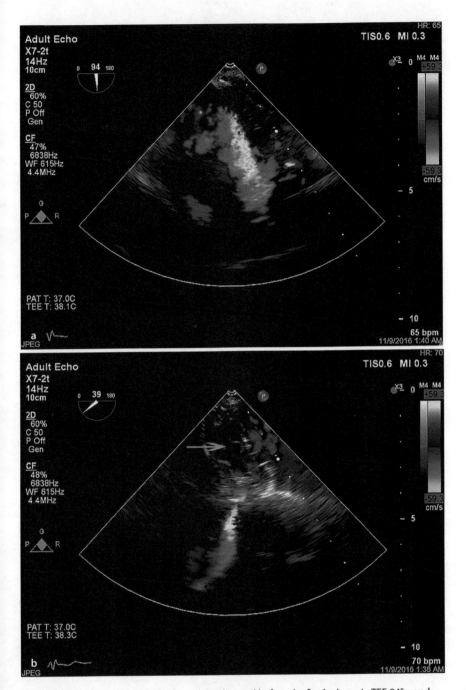

■ **Fig. 12.10** ASD device after opening the disc and before the final release in TEE 94° **a** and short-axis **b** views (*arrows*), no flow passes across interatrial septum

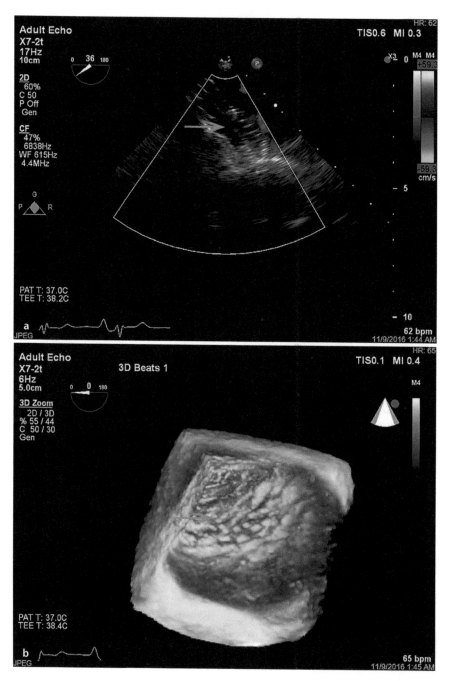

◻ Fig. 12.11   After the final releasing of discs of ASD device closure, no flow passes through interatrial septum and the device is seen in good position by TEE short-axis view **a**, the device is seen by 3D zoom 0° from left atrial side (*arrow*) **b**

Result   Large ASD ostium secundum type, maximum size by TEE 2D = 25 mm and maximum size by TEE 3D 27 mm, the final device used was 30 mm.

It is of notice that the mean difference between TEE 3D and balloon occlusive diameter is about 2 mm.

12.2   Case 2: ASD Device Closure with Loose Inferoposterior Rim

A 39-year-old man referred for ASD closure, he was totally asymptomatic. Transthoracic echocardiography revealed moderate RA and RV enlargement, Qp/Qs = 2 and mild TR with PAPs = 45 mmHg.

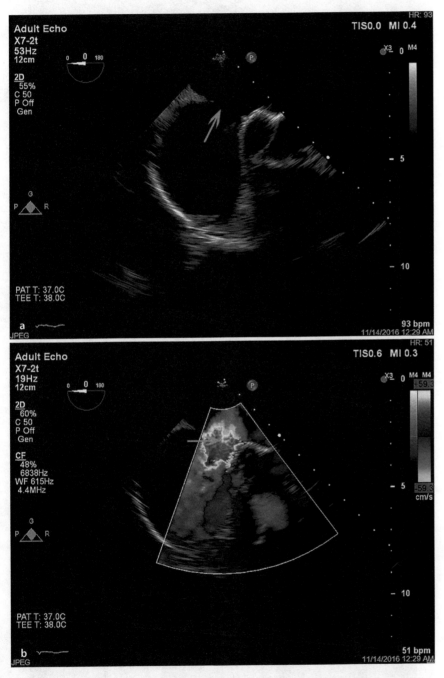

◻ Fig. 12.12 ASD ostium secundum is evident by TEE 0° view with two-dimensional echocardiography **a** and color Doppler study **b** (*arrows*)

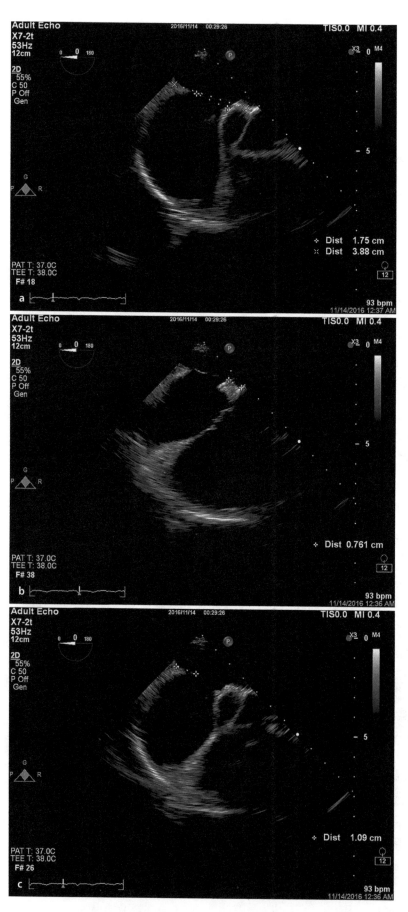

□ **Fig. 12.13**   The ratio of ASD/IAS measures 18/39 mm in TEE 0° view **a**, rim to mitral valve measures 8 mm and posterior rim measures 11 mm in this view **b, c**

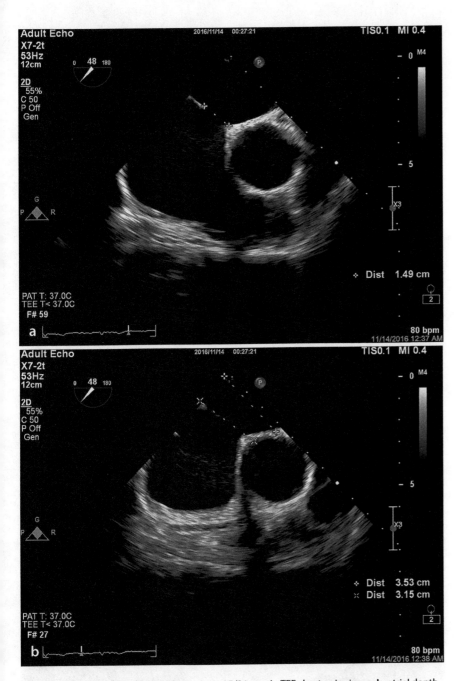

Fig. 12.14 The ratio of ASD/IAS measures 15/31 mm in TEE short-axis view **a**, **b**, atrial depth measures 35 mm in this view **b**

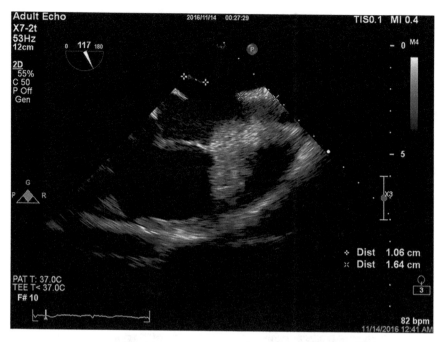

Fig. 12.15 The rim to SVC measures 16 mm and rim to IVC measures 11 mm in TEE bicaval view

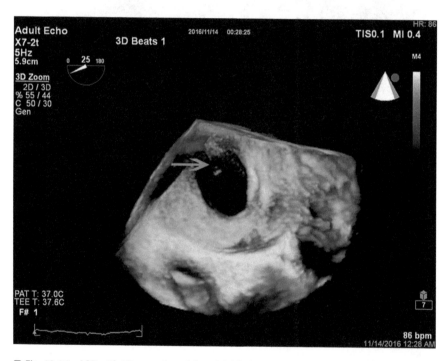

Fig. 12.16 ASD with 3D zoom from left atrial side, loose tissue around ASD is evident (*arrow*)

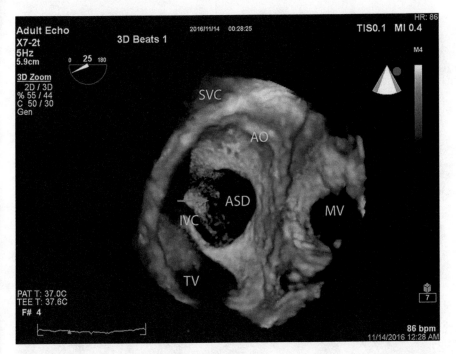

■ **Fig. 12.17** ASD with 3D zoom from right atrial side, loose tissue of interatrial septum near inferior vena cava is seen in this view (*arrow*). *MV* mitral valve, *TV* tricuspid valve, *SVC* superior vena cava, *IVC* inferior vena cava, *AO* aorta

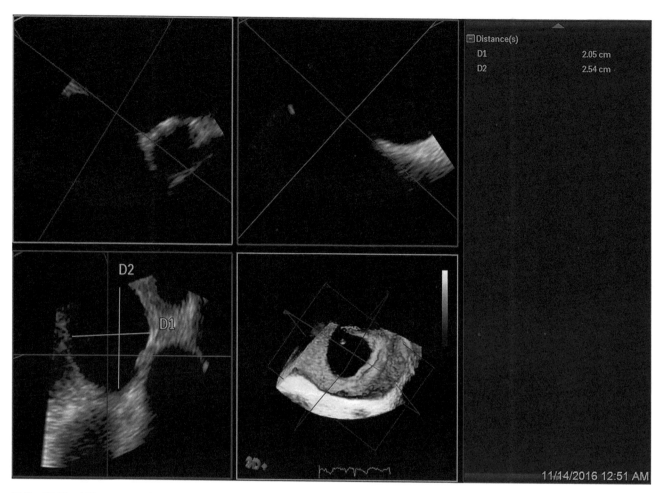

Fig. 12.18 ASD measures 25*21 mm by 3DQ method

Diagnosis Large ASD ostium secundum, maximum size by 2D echocardiography = 19 mm and maximum size by 3D echocardiography = 25 mm and good rims, ASD.

Comment ASD devise closure.
    Successful ASD device closure was done by device 27 mm.

Lesson The presence of loose tissue in the interatrial septum makes measurement of exact size of ASD somehow difficult.

12.3 Case 3: ASD Device Closure Complication

A 28-year-old man with a history of ASD device closure with 3-year duration, he presented with dyspnea on exertion suddenly with 1 week duration. In physical examination fix splitting S2 was heard.

Transthoracic echocardiography shows normal left ventricular size and function and right ventricular dilation.

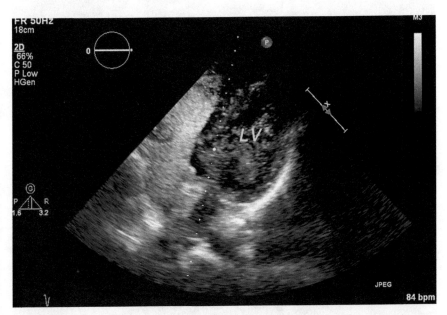

◘ **Fig. 12.19** Apical four-chamber view depicts significant bubble passage through interatrial septum, with force full valsalva maneuver during contrast injection in favor of residual shunt. *LA* left atrium, *RA* right atrium

Transesophageal echocardiography was performed for full evaluation of interatrial septum.

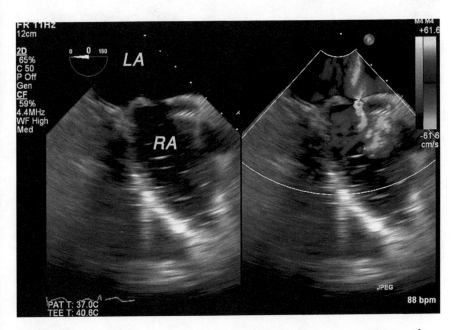

◘ **Fig. 12.20** Mid esophageal 0° view shows residual left to right shunt in posterior area of interatrial septum

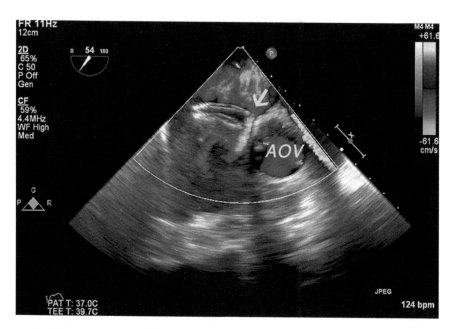

Fig. 12.21   Mid esophageal short-axis view depicts a turbulent shunt flow at the rim to aorta (*arrow*). *AOV* aortic valve

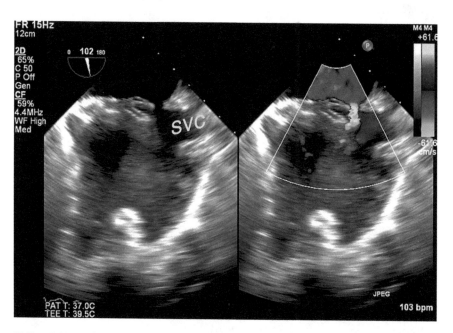

Fig. 12.22   Mid esophageal bicaval view shows residual shunt in the SVC area. *SVC* superior vena cava

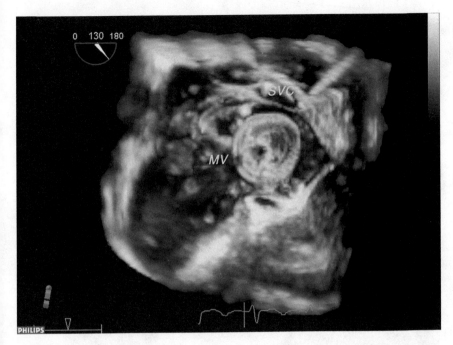

◨ **Fig. 12.23** Live 3D view is taken in 130°, it shows a large crescent shape defect around ASD device. *SVC* superior vena cava, *MV* mitral valve

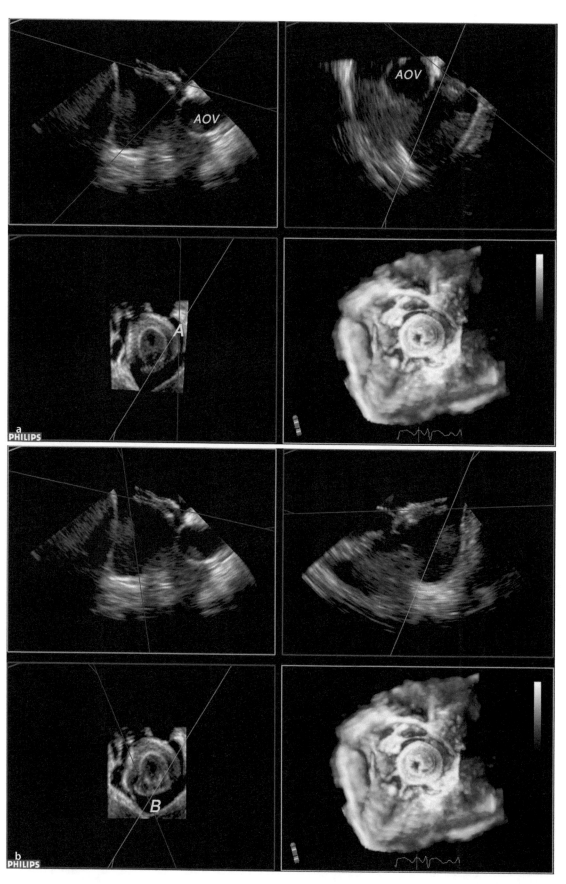

☐ **Fig. 12.24** 3D data set is useful in determination of exact site of defect, A point shows rim to aorta, red and green plane show aortic rim defect and *blue* plane shows enface view of aortic rim defect **a**, B point shows posterior rim **b**, *red* and *green* plane show posterior defect and *blue* plane shows enface view of posterior defect. *AOV* aortic valve

Diagnosis   ASD device impending to dislodgment and a large hole around device is developed most probably due to large device size relative to ASD size.

With respect to pervious echocardiography assessment that it reveals normal right ventricular size and function so interatrial septum necrosis around device is a recent event and complication.

Recommendation   Patient was sent for surgical removal of device and surgical ASD closure.

What are the complications of ASD device closure?

1. The early complications are device emboli, infection.
2. Intermediate complications include the erosion of aorta and hemopericardium after erosion of aorta.
3. Late complication is not reported accurately but necrosis can be a late complication.

Cardiac erosion is reported by deficiency of any rims especially aorta, larger device size, and device size more than 5 mm greater than ASD size [1].

12.4   Case 4: Paravalvular Leak Closure of Prosthetic Mitral Valve

A 31-year-old man with history of factor eight deficiency, he has history of AVR and MVR 3 years ago and at this time he suffered from dyspnea on exertion. In physical examination metallic sound in aortic and mitral area, a pan systolic murmur grade III/VI in mitral area and also a systolic murmur in LSB was heard.

Transthoracic echocardiography showed normal LV size and systolic function and good function of AV prosthetic valve.

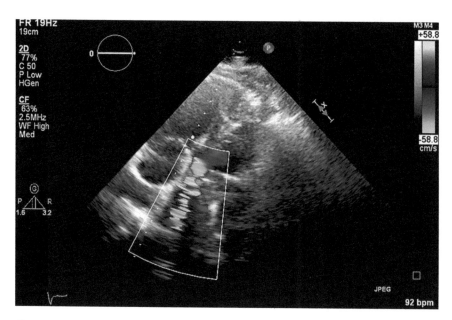

Fig. 12.25   Apical four-chamber view shows a turbulent systolic flow in LA area between AV and MV prosthetic valve suggestive for paravalvular leakage from medial side of MV prosthetic valve

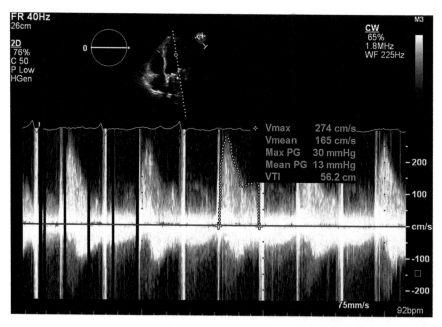

Fig. 12.26   CW Doppler flow study of mitral valve showed MV peak and mean gradients increased significantly (30 and 19 mmHg, respectively) and MV VTI/LVOT VTI was more than 2.2 in favor of MV overflow

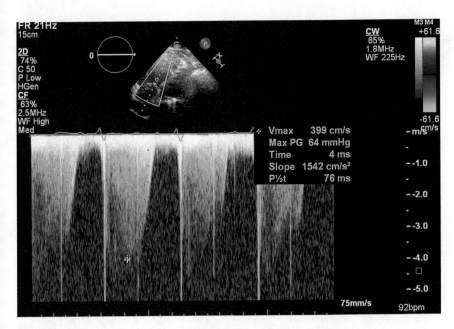

◘ **Fig. 12.27** TV seems normal with mild TR and estimated SPAP was 80 mmHg

Transesophageal echocardiography was performed for better evaluation of MV prosthetic valve.

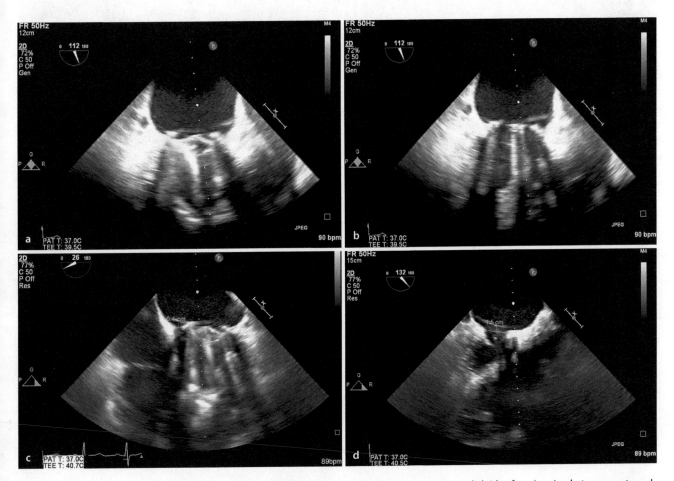

◘ **Fig. 12.28** TEE long-axis view shows good mobility of leaflets **a, b** and a site of defect is seen in medial side of sewing ring between aorta and MV about 4 mm in size in 2D ME 0° **c** and 15 mm in deep LAX view **d** indicative for crescent shape of paravalvular leak

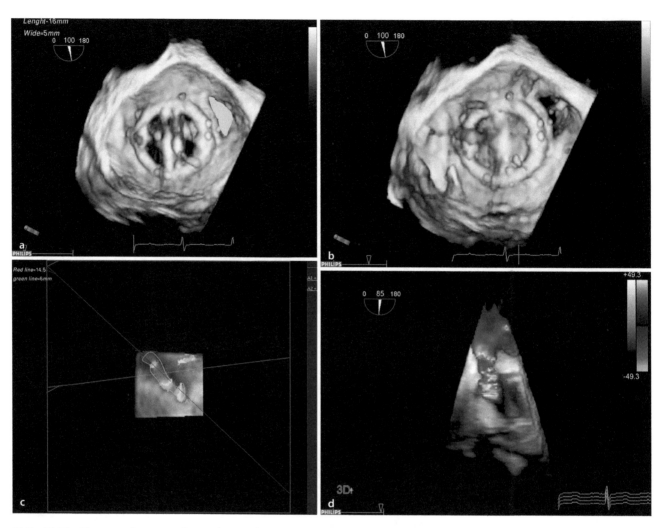

◘ Fig. 12.29   3D zoom enface surgical view of MV confirmed good mobility of MV leaflets **a**, **b** and site of paravalvular defect was in 3 o'clock of this view (aorta in the *top* and LAA in *medial* side in 9 o'clock) and size of defect measured 6 × 14.5 mm **c** and color full volume 3D shows flow across defect **d**

12.4 · Case 4: Paravalvular Leak Closure of Prosthetic Mitral Valve

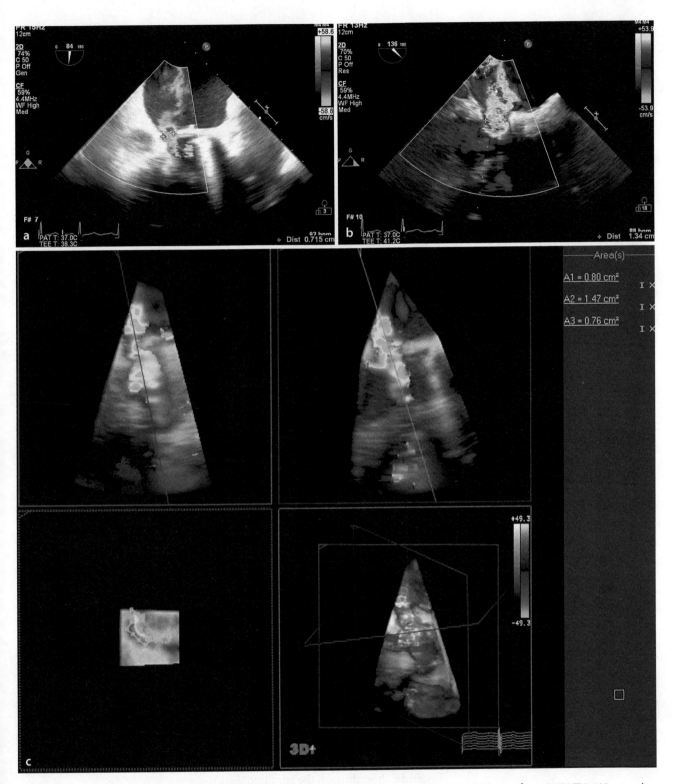

◨ Fig. 12.30 MR VC diameter in 2D measured 7 and 14 mm in SAX and LAX view **a**, **b** and 3D VC area was 0.76 cm² **c** and MR VTI is 100 cm and so estimated paravalvular MR volume by 3D PISA is calculated as follows: 0.76*100 = 76 cm³

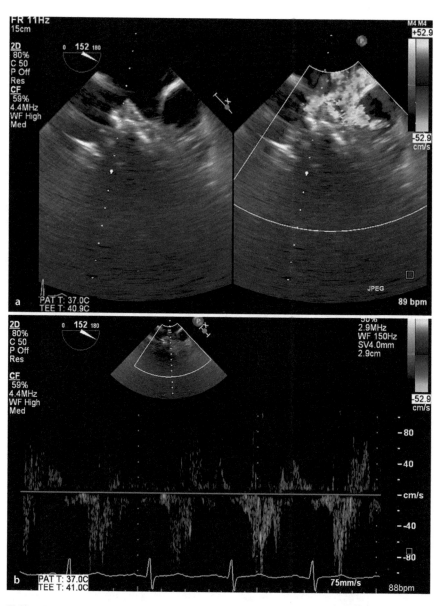

Fig. 12.31 Mid esophageal long-axis TEE view with about 30° clockwise rotation and pulled back of probe visualized left pulmonary veins **a**, CDF and PW study showed systolic flow reversal in left pulmonary veins **b** which confirms severe paravalvular MR

With respect to factor eight deficiency of patient, he was high risk for operation so patient was candidate for trance apical paravalvular device closure.

A work team including surgeon, interventionist, anesthesiologist, and echocardiographist was done this procedure and a paravalve device 6.5 × 14 mm selected.

The patient was anesthetized and after a minimal thoracotomy, the surgeon inserted a sheet through the apex into the LV.

Paravalvular leak closure can be performed with a success rate about 90%, in most cases severity of MR decreased to 1+ [2].

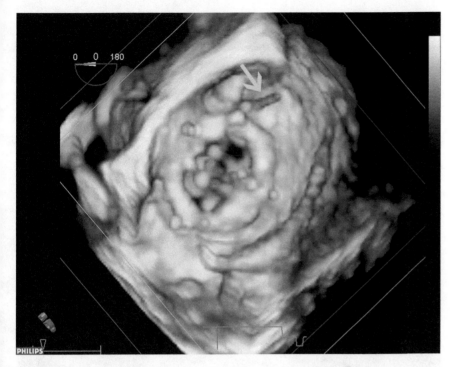

Fig. 12.32 A wire is passed from apex of LV through paravalvular site of leak to LA by interventionist (*arrow*)

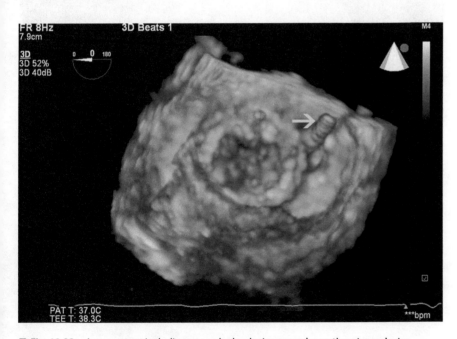

Fig. 12.33 A cover stent including paravalvular device passed over the wire and wire removed (*arrow*)

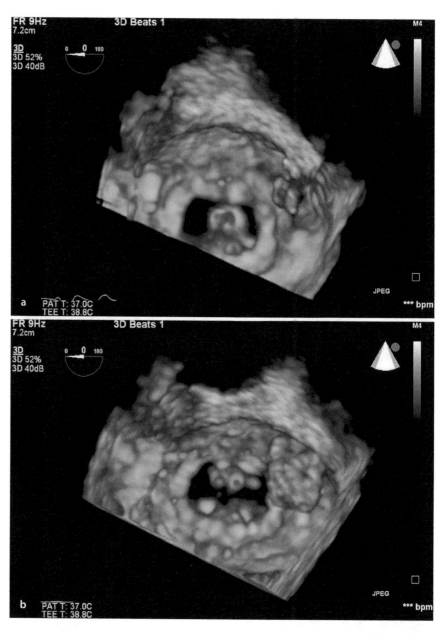

Fig. 12.34 The cover stent was pulled back (*arrow*) **a** and LA side of paravalve device was deployed (*arrow*) **b**

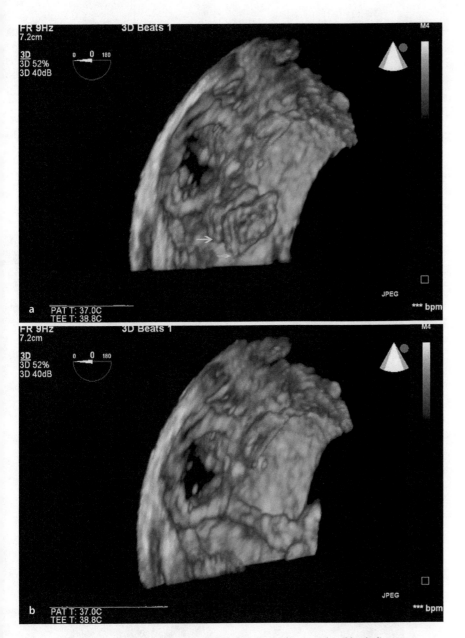

Fig. 12.35 Cover stent was pulled backed slightly more than usual and both discs were deployed (*arrows*) **a** but with echo guide distal disc was covered again and so only one disc remained in LA (*arrow*) **b**

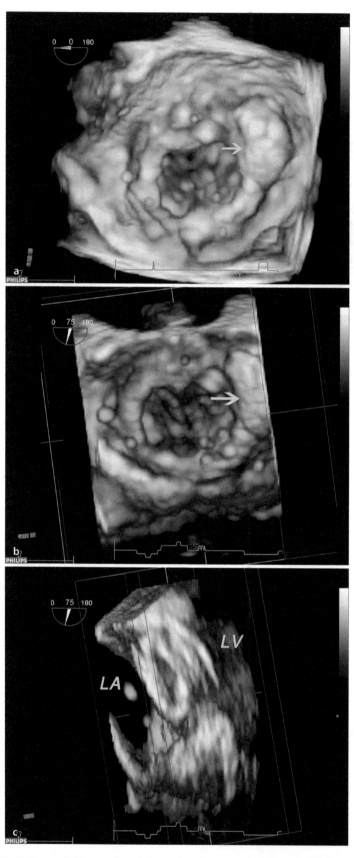

Fig. 12.36 Proximal disc pulled backed and was placed on paravalvular leakage site (*arrow*) **a** and then distal disc was released (*arrow*) (**b**, from ventricular side), *red* crop **c** shows appropriate position of paravalve device, one disc placed in LA side and other disc placed in LV side **b**, **c** (with respect to this device was rectangular, the most important role of echocardiologist was in this stage because echocardiologist must guide interventionist for rotation of device and prevention of MV leaflet motion interaction with device)

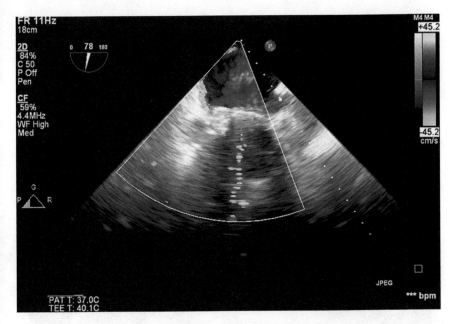

Fig. 12.37 Severe paravalvular change to mild paravalvular leakage with a small VC after 3 day TTE was performed for evaluation of site of device and severity of paravalvular leakage

12

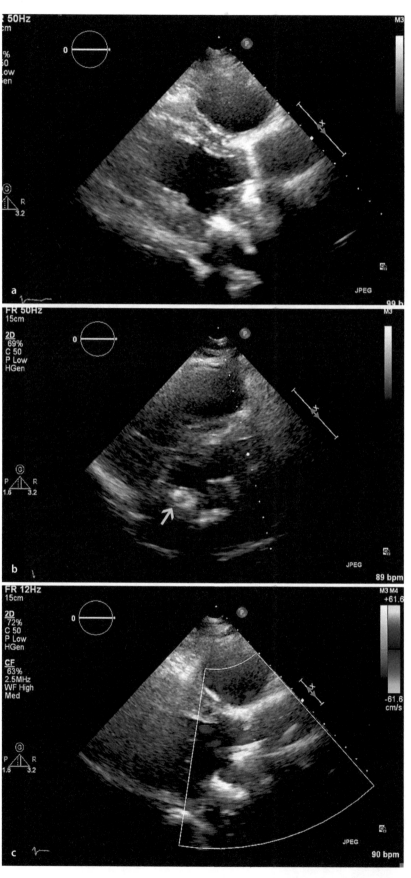

■ **Fig. 12.38** Device was visible in LAX and SAX view **a**, **b** with trivial paravalvular leakage

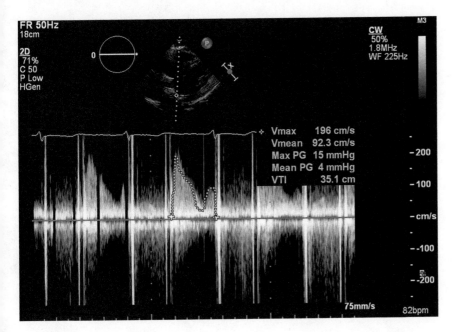

Fig. 12.39 Peak and mean gradients of MV decreased to 14 and 5 mmHg, respectively, indicative for no evidence of overflow

References

1. McElhinney DB, Quartermain MD, Kenny D, Alboliras E, Amin Z. Relative risk factors for cardiac erosion following transcatheter closure of atrial Septal defects: a case-control study. Circulation. 2016;133(18):1738–46.
2. Sorajja P, Cabalka AK, Hagler DJ, Rihal CS. Percutaneous repair of paravalvular prosthetic regurgitation: acute and 30-day outcomes in 115 patients. Circ Cardiovasc Interv. 2011;4(4):314–21.